CW01208765

Bariatric Surgery

BARIATRIC SURGERY

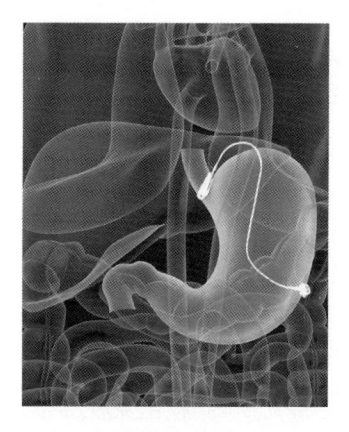

Editors
Nadey S Hakim
Imperial College Healthcare NHS Trust London, UK
Franco Favretti
Vicenza Regional Hospital, Italy
Gianni Segato
Vicenza Regional Hospital, Italy
Bruno Dillemans
St. Jan Hospital, Bruges, Belgium

Imperial College Press

Published by

Imperial College Press
57 Shelton Street
Covent Garden
London WC2H 9HE

Distributed by

World Scientific Publishing Co. Pte. Ltd.
5 Toh Tuck Link, Singapore 596224
USA office: 27 Warren Street, Suite 401-402, Hackensack, NJ 07601
UK office: 57 Shelton Street, Covent Garden, London WC2H 9HE

British Library Cataloguing-in-Publication Data
A catalogue record for this book is available from the British Library.

BARIATRIC SURGERY

Copyright © 2011 by Imperial College Press

All rights reserved. This book, or parts thereof, may not be reproduced in any form or by any means, electronic or mechanical, including photocopying, recording or any information storage and retrieval system now known or to be invented, without written permission from the Publisher.

For photocopying of material in this volume, please pay a copying fee through the Copyright Clearance Center, Inc., 222 Rosewood Drive, Danvers, MA 01923, USA. In this case permission to photocopy is not required from the publisher.

ISBN-13 978-1-84816-588-5
ISBN-10 1-84816-588-9

Typeset by Stallion Press
Email: enquiries@stallionpress.com

Printed in Singapore by Mainland Press Pte Ltd.

Contents

Contributors   xi

Foreword   xvii
(by Michael G. Sarr, Mayo Clinic, USA)

Chapter 1	**Indications for Bariatric Surgery and Selecting the Appropriate Procedure** *John B. Dixon*	1
	Indications for Bariatric Surgery	1
	References	10
Chapter 2	**Anaesthesia in Bariatric Surgery** *Ernesto Pizzirani and Giuseppe Calcarella*	15
	Definitions	15
	Epidemiology	16
	Pathophysiologic Aspects Connected to Obesity	19
	Pharmacologic Considerations	31
	Evaluating the Patient Before Anaesthesia	37
	General Anaesthesia	47
	Loco-Regional Anaesthesia	50
	Post-Operative Treatment	51
	Conclusions	53
	References	53

Chapter 3	**Intragastric Balloon (BIB®) in the Management of Morbid Obesity Disease** *Alfredo Genco, Roberta Maselli and Nicola Basso*	**61**
	Introduction	61
	Results	71
	Discussion and Conclusion	84
	References	86
Chapter 4	**Laparoscopic Adjustable Gastric Banding** *Gianni Segato, Nadey Hakim, Maurizio De Luca and Franco Favretti*	**91**
	Introduction	91
	Indications and Contraindications	91
	Preparation for Surgery	93
	Surgical Instruments	93
	Patient and Surgical Team Positioning	94
	Procedural Steps	94
	References	102
	Suggested Reading	103
Chapter 5	**Long-Term Results in Laparoscopic Adjustable Gastric Banding (LAP-BAND®) for Obese Patients** *Maurizio De Luca, Luca Busetto, Gianni Segato, Nadey S. Hakim and Franco Favretti*	**105**
	Introduction	105
	Laparoscopic Technique	106
	Role of the Balloon	109
	Lap-Band® Series at Vicenza Regional Hospital, Padua	110
	Discussion	118
	Life Expectancy Study	120
	Conclusion	121
	References	122

Chapter 6	**Laparoscopic Adjustable Gastric Banding (LAP-BAND®): Diagnosis, Prevention and Treatment of Complications** *Maurizio De Luca, Luca Busetto, Gianni Segato, Nadey S. Hakim and Franco Favretti*	**125**
	Introduction	125
	Lap-Band® Series at Vicenza Regional Hospital, Padua	126
	Complications	127
	Conclusions	151
	References	152
Chapter 7	**Roux-en-Y Gastric Bypass** *Bruno Dillemans and Sebastiaan Van Cauwenberge*	**155**
	Introduction	155
	Physiology of the Roux-en-Y Gastric Bypass	156
	Preoperative Evaluation	159
	Medical Evaluation	160
	Psychological Evaluation	160
	Technical Aspects of the Laparoscopic RYGB Procedure	161
	Operative Technique of the Fully Stapled Laparoscopic Roux-en-Y Gastric Bypass	164
	Complications of Roux-en-Y Gastric Bypass	171
	Side Effects of Roux-en-Y Gastric Bypass	179
	Weight Evolution After RYGB	183
	Conclusion	188
	Acknowledgements	188
	References	188
Chapter 8	**New Technologies in Bariatric Surgery** *Matthias Lannoo and Andre D'Hoore*	**199**
	Introduction	199

	Sleeve Gastrectomy	199
	New Minimally Invasive Techniques in Bariatric Surgery	214
	References	217
Chapter 9	**Imaging of Complications After Bariatric Surgery**	**223**
	Jose C. Varghese and Shuvro H. Roy-Choudhury	
	Introduction	223
	Laparoscopic Adjustable Gastric Banding	224
	Roux-en-Y Gastric Bypass (RYGB)	245
	Summary	273
	References	275
Chapter 10	**Sequential Treatment of Obesity**	**285**
	Maurizio De Luca, Luca Busetto, Gianni Segato and Franco Favretti	
	Introduction	285
	Classification of Bariatric Operation	286
	Effectiveness/Invasiveness of Various Operations	286
	Undertreatment and Overtreatment	287
	Surgical Treatment of Obesity	290
	Conclusions	291
	References	292
Chapter 11	**Bariatric Surgery: When the Miracle is Not Enough**	**293**
	Melodie K. Moorehead	
	Introduction	293
	Bariatric Surgery is a Behavioural Surgery Too	296
	A Holistic Approach to Bariatric Surgery: Recovery Managed by Healthcare Specialists	302
	Establishing a Three-Stage Psychoeducational Recovery Programme	305
	The Initial Psychoeducational Interview	311
	What is the Value of Speaking the Same Language in Outcomes?	317

	Discussion	320
	Acknowledgements	322
	References	323
	Suggested Reading	324

Chapter 12 Effects of Bariatric Surgery on Co-Morbidities 327
Sebastiaan Van Cauwenberge and Bruno Dillemans

	Introduction	327
	Hypertension	327
	Obstructive Sleep Apnoea	331
	Dyslipidemia	334
	Type 2 Diabetes	337
	Other Co-Morbidities	343
	Quality of Life After Bariatric Surgery	346
	References	348

Chapter 13 Impact on Life Expectancy After Bariatric Surgery 359
Luca Busetto, Elisa Calo', Marco Mazza and Giuliano Enzi

	Introduction	359
	Impact of Morbid Obesity on Morbidity and Mortality	360
	Effects of Bariatric Surgery on Metabolic Co-Morbidities	361
	Effects of Bariatric Surgery on Respiratory Disturbances	371
	Impact of Bariatric Surgery on Health Related Quality of Life	377
	Impact of Bariatric Surgery on Life Expectancy	378
	Conclusion	383
	References	383

Index 389

Contributors

Nicola Basso
Department of Surgery
La Sapienza University
Policlinico Umberto I
Viale Regina Elena 324
00185 Rome, Italy

Luca Busetto
Department of Medical and Surgical Sciences
University of Padova
Via Giustiniani, 2
32128 Padova, Italy
E-mail: luca.busetto@unipd.it

Giuseppe Calcarella
Anaesthesiology Department
Camposampiero Hospital
Via P. Cosma, 1
35012 Camposampiero, Padova, Italy
E-mail: gcalcarella@ulss15.pd.it

Elisa Calo'
Department of Medical and Surgical Sciences
University of Pad
Via Giustiniani, 2
32128 Padova, Italy
E-mail: elisa1002@libero.it

Maurizio De Luca
Department of Surgery
Vicenza Hospital
Via F. Rodolfi, 37
36100 Vicenza, Italy
E-mail: nnwdel@tin.it

Andre D'Hoore
Department of Abdominal Surgery
Hospital UZ Leuven
Gasthuisberg Campus
Herestraat 49, Leuven, Belgium
E-mail: andre.dhoore@uzleuven.be

Bruno Dillemans
Department of General Surgery
Hospital AZ St.-Jan AV
Ruddershove, 10
B-8000 Brugge, Belgium
E-mail: bruno.dillemans@azbrugge.be

John B. Dixon
Head of Obesity Research Unit
Department of Surgery
Monash University
Victoria 3800, Australia
E-mail: john.dixon@med.monash.edu.au

Guiliano Enzi
Department of Medical and Surgical Sciences
University of Padova
Via Giustiniani, 2
32128 Padova, Italy
E-mail: giuliano.enzi@unipd.it

Franco Favretti
Director
Department of Surgery
Vicenza Hospital
Via F. Rodolfi, 37
36100 Vicenza, Italy
E-mail: ffavret@tin.it

Michael G. Sarr
Department of Surgery
Mayo Clinically
200 First Street S.W.
US-Rochester, MN 55905, USA
E-mail: sarr.michael@mayo.edu

Alfredo Genco
Department of Surgery
La Sapienza University
Policlinico Umberto I
Viale Regina Elena 324
00185 Rome, Italy
E-mail: alfredo.genco@uniroma1.it

Nadey S. Hakim
Max Thorek Professor of Surgery
Fellow of the American Society of Bariatric and Metabolic Surgery
Lead Bariatric Surgeon Highgate Hospital London
Surgical Director, West London Transplant Unit
Imperial College Healthcare NHS Trust
Du Cane Road
London W12 0HS, UK
E-mail: nadey@globalnet.co.uk

Matthias Lannoo
Department of Abdominal Surgery
Hospital UZ Leuven
Gasthuisberg Campus
Herestraat 49, Leuven, Belgium
E-mail: matthias.lannoo@uzleuven.be

Roberta Maselli
Department of Surgery
La Sapienza University
Policlinico Umberto I
Viale Regina Elena 324
00185 Rome, Italy

Marco Mazza
Department of Medical and Surgical Sciences
University of Padova
Via Giustiniani, 2
32128 Padova, Italy
E-mail: marco_mazza78@yahoo.it

Melodie K. Moorehead, Ph.D., ABPP
Honorary Member Psychologist
Board Certified by the American Board of Professional
   Psychology in Clinical Health Psychology
1201 Broward Blvd.
Ft. Lauderdale, FL 33301, USA
E-mail: psydrmm@aol.com

Ernesto Pizzirani
Director of Anaesthesiology
Anaesthesiology Department
Camposampiero Hospital
Via P. Cosma, 1
35012 Camposampiero, Padova, Italy
E-mail: epizzirani@ulss15.pd.it

Shuvro H. Roy-Choudhury
Consultant Radiologist
Heart of England NHS Trust
Department of Radiology
Spire Parkway Hospital
1 Damson Parkway
Solihull B91 2PP, UK
E-mail: shuvro.roy-choudhury@heartofengland.nhs.uk

Gianni Segato
Department of Surgery
Vicenza Hospital
Via F. Rodolfi, 37
36100 Vicenza, Italy
E-mail: gsegat@tin.it

Sebastiaan Van Cauwenberge
Department of General Surgery
Hospital AZ St.-Jan AV
Ruddershove, 10
B-8000 Brugge, Belgium
E-mail: sebastiaan.vancauwenberge@azbrugge.be

Jose C. Varghese
Department of Radiology
Boston University Medical Center
88 East Newton Street, 2nd Floor
Boston, MA 02118, USA
E-mail: jose.varghese@bmc.org

Foreword

With the worldwide epidemic of obesity seemingly just around the corner, bariatric surgery has exploded onto the surgery scene, having now become a truly household word. This book, edited by Professor Nadey S. Hakim and colleagues, should serve as a very readable, practical text for a wide range of staff, right from the huge number of medical support staff within a bariatric centre, to the bariatric surgeon, the anaesthesiologist, the bariatrician, and, most importantly, *for the general surgeon* who is NOT a bariatric surgeon! This latter focus on the non-bariatric general surgeon is becoming a topic of both extreme interest and deep concern to many general surgeons, as well as Emergency Room physicians.

Currently, bariatric surgery represents the most common gastric operation in the Western world, since the operative treatment for Peptic Ulcer Disease has all but disappeared. And, with our increasingly mobile population, the ever-increasing number of a spectrum of operations (which are so well reviewed in this book!), and the growth of medical tourism due to first-world costs of bariatric surgery, all physicians, as well as non-bariatric general surgeons, will be exposed on an increasing basis to patients who have undergone surgery. Thus, the education of all physicians who do not have a bariatric practice is vital. This book will do just that — the readability, focus, emphasis, and clinically-oriented approach have been consciously designed to address this topic in a way appealing to both the bariatric and non-bariatric healthcare provider.

This book addresses most of the practical issues in bariatric surgery. Separate chapters address patient selection, different bariatric procedures, including intragastric balloons (this topic is being revisited currently after its dismal failure 15–20 years ago), the "lap band" or the laparoscopic adjustable gastric banding (and its complications/success), Roux-en-Y gastric bypass, and the forms of biliopancreatic diversion. Each procedure obligates a different set of medical concerns, leads to different mechanical and/or functional complications, and requires a unique type of follow-up.

The chapter on anaesthetic issues provides a fabulous focus for the book. These considerations are important, not only for the surgical staff, but also for the entire team in the operating theatre — and not just for just bariatric operations but also for other operations performed on the morbidly obese patient.

Finally, the book finishes with the evidence supporting the efficacy of bariatric surgery from several different aspects — resolution of direct, weight-related medical co-morbidities, improvements in quality of life, and even the concept of impact on life expectancy.

As a general and gastrointestinal surgeon for the last 30 years, I have witnessed (and participated in) the growth, improvements, and finally general acceptance of bariatric surgery by both the lay public but, also importantly, by the medical community. In summary, this book accomplishes its goals — readability, clinical relevance, and the important topic of a global view of bariatric surgery. You will enjoy reading every chapter.

Michael G. Sarr, M.D.
James C. Masson Professor of Surgery
Mayo Clinic, USA

Chapter 1

Indications for Bariatric Surgery and Selecting the Appropriate Procedure

John B. Dixon

Indications for Bariatric Surgery

When is surgery an option for a patient? When should it be recommended as best care?

In 1991, the National Institutes of Health (NIH) criteria for patient selection for gastrointestinal surgery for severe obesity were developed at a consensus conference involving expert surgeons, gastroenterologists, endocrinologists, psychiatrists, nutritionists and other health care professionals as well as the public. After weighing the evidence the panel recommended that:

1. patients seeking therapy for severe obesity for the first time should be considered for treatment in a non-surgical programme with integrated components of a dietary regimen, appropriate exercise and behavioural modification and support;
2. gastric restrictive or bypass procedures could be considered for well-informed and motivated patients with acceptable operative risks;
3. patients who are candidates for surgical procedures should be selected carefully after evaluation by a multidisciplinary team with medical, surgical, psychiatric and nutritional expertise;
4. the operation should be performed by a surgeon substantially experienced with the appropriate procedures and working in a clinical

setting with adequate support for all aspects of management and assessment;
5. lifelong medical surveillance after surgical therapy is a necessity to monitor for complications and lifestyle adjustments.[1]

The patient selection criteria recommendations were that surgery is an option for well-informed and motivated patients who have 'clinically severe obesity' Body Mass Index (BMI) 40, or a BMI 35 and serious co-morbid conditions.

There were many weaknesses with the NIH approach at the time. Recommendations came from an expert panel and were not necessarily evidence-based at the time. The cut-off values of BMI 35 and 40 were arbitrarily chosen although 'patient risk' is clearly a continuous concept which is based on much more than weight corrected for height and the presence of a co-morbid condition. Patient selection involves a clinical assessment of risk versus benefit for the individual patient and while BMI is one consideration, others include age, ethnicity, weight distribution, a wide range of obesity related medical and psychological co-morbidities, and risk factors for future obesity-related morbidity and mortality

An additional concern is the concept of option. The NIH describes a group of patient characteristics and conditions that are required before surgery can be considered. This is a far cry from the description of a recommendation. A recommendation would imply that a caring physician, after identifying a patient's specific conditions, recommends that the patient seek a surgical opinion regarding surgical treatment as best therapy or standard of care. A male aged 25 with BMI 55, severe obstructive sleep apnoea, type-2 diabetes and steatohepatitis may provide an example where recommendation for a surgical opinion is appropriate. To withhold such a recommendation may now be seen as negligent. While it may have been inappropriate in 1991, current evidence regarding the outcomes of surgical versus non-surgical therapy indicates a category of patient where recommendation is now appropriate.

Since 1991 there have also been major advances in our understanding of the benefits of substantial sustained weight loss which include resolution or improvement in obesity related co-morbidity,[2] improved quality of life[3] and psychological conditions, reductions in disease risk factors, and evidence that therapy is cost effective[4] and saves lives.[5,6] We now have considerably more information to use when making a risk–benefit assessment of a patient.

Thus the NIH term 'clinically severe obesity' needs to have plasticity with an ability to mould to a range of important considerations. It also needs to be graded to indicate subjects where surgery should be considered an option and those where a surgical referral and assessment is recommended as best care.

Why have I focused on the NIH criteria? This is simply because they are the most quoted and used. Many surgical societies, health service providers and third party payers around the world have adopted very similar, or at times more restrictive, eligibility criteria for bariatric surgery.

Let us consider some of the factors associated with a patient that should be considered when selecting a patient for a surgical option or consideration.

Age

Age is an important factor in the risk–benefit analysis. Obesity-related excess mortality declines with age at all levels of obesity.[7,8] In a German cohort, older men and women aged 50–74 with a BMI range of 25 to less than 32 had no excess mortality.[7] A US analysis of life table and large health surveys also estimated that years of life lost are significantly greater in younger subjects.[8] The Seven Countries Study found a BMI of up to 30 kg/m^2 was not associated with increased mortality when middle aged men became older.[9] The American Cancer Society's Cancer Prevention Study I also found that the relative risk associated with greater body weight is higher among younger subjects.[10] However, obesity at the age of 40 years is a predictor of a significantly shortened life and has an effect similar to smoking.[11] A Finnish study demonstrated that years of disability and poor health related to obesity were likely to be greater in younger subjects.[12] Elderly patients presenting for bariatric surgery may therefore have limited benefit in both years of life and in years of healthy life gained. Improving shorter term quality of life may be the primary benefit in operating on elderly subjects, but on the other hand older patients have a higher mortality associated with bariatric surgery.[13,14] These findings have important implications when assessing benefit versus risk in older obese subjects presenting for treatment, and emphasizes the importance of treating clinically severe obesity in younger adults. One may use the information concerning age when considering bariatric surgery for adolescents where arguably we may achieve greatest benefit from treating the clinically severely obese. It is in this age group that static BMI cut-off levels have limited value as there is a moving target. Normally with growth and development, BMI rises throughout adolescence in both boys and girls.[15,16] Using age adjusted BMI z-scores and obesity related co-morbidity we may, with further careful evaluation, be able to set guidelines for bariatric surgery in adolescents. Several attempts have been made to define criteria for the use of bariatric surgery in adolescents,[17] but these are flawed by the same lack of sufficient evidence that confronted the NIH in 1991. Fortunately many carefully designed studies are currently in progress and in the near future we should have a better understanding of the relative benefits and risks of intervening early in adolescents. In the meantime adolescent bariatric surgery should only be performed by experienced multidisciplinary teams with experience in managing the issues and nuances of severely obese adolescents, with data collected to evaluate long term clinical outcomes.[17]

Ethnicity

Body Mass Index is used as a surrogate for adiposity and as a marker for risk associated with increasing body weight. However there are major ethnic differences in both the degree of adiposity and risk of obesity related diseases at any given body mass index. The World Health Organization (WHO) consultation has recommended that for those with Asian ethnicity public health BMI action points may be reduced by 2.0–2.5 kg/m^2 to 23.0, 27.5, 32.5 and 37.5 kg/m^2. Recognizing the increased adiposity and co-morbidity risk, the WHO and International Obesity Task Force have also recognized an increased risk of type-2 diabetes at lower BMI levels in Asian populations[18] and the International Diabetes Federation has used ethnic specific waist circumferences for men and women when defining the metabolic syndrome.[19,20] Ethnic differences in adiposity and disease risk should be considered in determining indications for bariatric surgery. It is not acceptable to use cut-off values based on the white population for those of higher risk ethnicity.

Co-morbidity

As already stated there should be graded levels of indications for bariatric surgery: a level where a patient is eligible for surgery and another where it is recommended as best care for the patient's condition (Fig. 1).

On what basis can we assess co-morbidity as an indication or a recommendation for surgery? It would seem logical that a number of criteria could be examined for any particular co-morbidity:

- What is the strength of the relationship between the co-morbidity and obesity?
- How serious is the co-morbidity?
- What is the effectiveness of weight loss for this co-morbidity?
- How effective is current therapy for the patient's condition?

Co-morbidities cluster, and patients often present with a range which all relate to the inflammatory and metabolic consequences of central obesity such as type-2 diabetes, hypertension, obstructive sleep apnoea, non-alcoholic steatohepatitis (NASH) and polycystic ovary syndrome. We

Surgery may be indicated — Eligible for surgery

Surgery is indicated — Should be advised as best care for a patient's condition

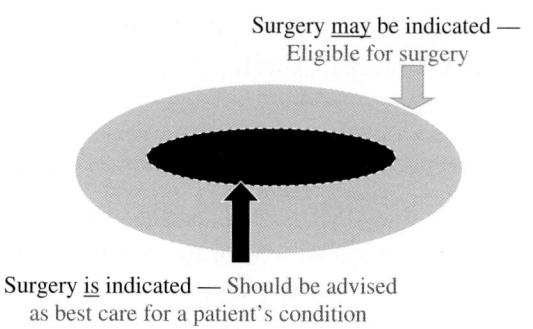

Figure 1. Indications for surgery.

Table 1. Some conditions associated with obesity.

Relative risk > 5	Relative risk 2–5	Relative risk 1–2
Type-2 diabetes	All-cause mortality	Cancer mortality
Dyslipidemia	Hypertension	Breast cancer
Obstructive sleep apnoea	Myocardial infarction and stroke	Prostate and colon cancer in men
Breathlessness	Endometrial carcinoma in women and hepatoma in men	Impaired fertility
Excessive daytime sleepiness	Gallstones and complications, including cancer	Obstetric complications, including fetal abnormalities
Obesity hypoventilation syndrome	Polycystic ovary syndrome	Asthma
Idiopathic intracranial hypertension	Osteoarthritis (knees)	Gastro-oesophageal reflux
Nonalcoholic steatohepatitis	Gout	Anaesthetic risk

need to recognize that we have far less knowledge about the importance and severity of psychological co-morbidities and these are rarely seen as important and pressing indications for bariatric surgery.

Some of the conditions associated with obesity are demonstrated in Table 1. Those with a relative risk greater than 5 are all strongly related to obesity. Of these, type-2 diabetes, obstructive sleep apnoea, obesity hypoventilation syndrome, idiopathic intracranial hypertension and more advanced forms of NASH may be seen as serious. In the context of obesity, these have been shown to respond well to substantial sustained weight loss, but do not respond as well to other therapy.

Bariatric surgery recommended or indicated as 'best care'

Using the NIH notion that BMI is an important marker of adiposity we could argue that those with a BMI > 50 or those with a BMI > 40 with one or more of the serious but responsive co-morbidities should, as best care, be referred for a bariatric surgical assessment (Table 2). Currently we have no indications or guidelines that physicians could use for the obligatory

Table 2. The author's proposed criteria for the two categories.

Surgery an option for therapy*	Surgery is indicated
BMI > 40	BMI > 50
BMI > 35 with a broad range of problems related to obesity	BMI > 40 with serious weight loss — responsive co-morbidity**
BMI > 30 with serious weight loss — responsive co-morbidity	

*For 'at risk' ethnicity the criteria should be dropped by a BMI of 2–3.
**Serious weight loss responsive co-morbidity could include: type-2 diabetes, obesity hypoventilation syndrome, severe obstructive sleep apnoea, obesity related raised intracranial pressure and non-alcoholic steatohepatitis with substantial fibrosis.

referral for bariatric surgical assessment as best practice, and health care providers can use their discretion in providing bariatric surgical services. Further carefully conducted longitudinal studies of long term outcomes of patients in these categories are recommended. There would be ethical concerns about randomized controlled trials for patients with these conditions because it could be seen as negligent not to provide appropriate or 'best care'. There must be equipoise, a balance of risk and benefit, when designing and conducting randomized controlled trials.[21]

Bariatric surgery as an option for therapy

As knowledge about the safety and efficacy of bariatric surgery increases, there has been a growing interest in its utilization in those with a BMI < 35. Our Melbourne group has recently reported two randomized controlled trials including subjects in the BMI 30–35 range.[22,23] The first showed better weight loss, health and quality of life outcomes in participants in the BMI 30–35 range for those randomized to laparoscopic adjustable gastric banding (LAGB) surgery when compared to those randomized to an intensive medical weight loss programme. The second study included participants with type-2 diabetes in the BMI range 30–40. Subjects were randomized to LAGB surgery with conventional diabetes therapy or to a best care lifestyle programme with conventional diabetes therapy. Those randomized to surgery achieved 73 per cent remission of type-2 diabetes compared to only 13 per cent for those on the conventional lifestyle programme when using an intention to treat analysis. The likelihood of remission was directly related to the extent of weight loss. Clearly, evidence such as this provides strong evidence that bariatric surgery is beneficial and may be indicated in those with a BMI < 35. Further randomized controlled trials are needed to strengthen this evidence base. Table 2 shows the hypothetical two-tiered approach to bariatric surgical indications.

Selection of the procedure

Bariatric surgery has evolved as an inexact science. It has advanced through many dedicated surgeons communicating with one another to progress an art, and there have been some wonderful achievements.[24] Experimental designs have almost all been small series on human subjects, with surgeons modifying and changing their procedures to provide greater efficacy and safety, an approach perhaps not unlike the development of many other surgical therapies.

This must change! Bariatric surgery is now considered a 'standard of care'. There are now good data on the efficacy, safety and durability of specific surgical procedures. Deviation from standard techniques should be tested, after appropriate ethical approval, in properly designed clinical trials. If the proposed surgery or technique is a major departure from a standard of care, animal models should be used.

The current most commonly used procedures are shown below in Table 3. The proportion of each procedure used varies enormously from region to region so I have estimated current use based on the 33 international societies and countries surveyed in 2002–3.[25] Since that survey there will have been a marked increase in the number of laparoscopic procedures, a reduction in the proportion of vertical banded and other gastroplasties, and an increase in the proportion of laparoscopic adjustable gastric banding (LAGB) procedures.

While these figures above are hypothetical estimates there is no doubt the RYGB (Roux-en-Y gastric banding) and LAGB dominate the current world scene and there are sufficient data regarding safety, efficacy and durability to justify this trend.

While there are quality data regarding BPD and BPD-DS, the weight loss efficacy and durability have not been a concern, but safety

Table 3. Commonly used surgical procedures.

Procedure	Global estimate
Roux-en-Y gastric bypass (RYGB) — laparoscopic and open (including variants of long limb gastric bypass and banded bypass)	40–55%
Laparoscopic adjustable gastric banding (LAGB)	30–45%
Vertical banded gastroplasty (VBG)	< 5% and falling
Bilio-pancreatic diversion (BPD). (including the duodenal switch variant (BPD-DS)	< 5% and steady
Sleeve gastrectomy (SG)	Unknown, but gaining popularity

is problematic as short and long term nutritional concerns abound.[26,27] Few surgeons have followed the path of performing these procedures as primary bariatric surgical procedures. For sleeve gastrectomy (SG) the efficacy, safety and durability of weight loss remain untested against the RYGB and LAGB standards as a primary bariatric procedure. It was initially utilized as a first stage procedure for those at high risk having BPB-DS, or more recently RYGB, as the definitive procedure.[28,29] This procedure needs further ethical study of a wide range of outcome measures. The American Society for Metabolic and Bariatric Surgery issued a statement of caution regarding the use of SG in 2007. The standard of care provided by RYGB and LAGB means they are the logical choice for primary bariatric procedures today. I will not address failed or revisional surgery. The choice of a primary procedure today is between RYGB and LAGB. There have been a large number of attempts to match the right patient to the right procedure to ensure great results, but to date these attempts have largely failed and lack of hard data means they are not credible.[30] The preoperative unpredictability and variability of weight loss following surgery is problematic. Preoperative BMI, age, co-morbidity, food choices, eating behaviours, personality testing, quality of life testing, motivation and many other variables have been tested, and found to predict a small proportion of weight loss variance.[31–33] These preoperative variables have largely had a common effect on the two candidate procedures and have not really separated them. Perhaps more relevant is that postoperative follow-up and adopted behaviours following surgery are highly predictive of outcome variance.[34,35] Our difficulties with preoperative predictability are perhaps largely driven by our lack of knowledge regarding the actual mechanism of action of bariatric surgery. Just how does surgery have such a profound effect on energy balance and why is any other current therapy so poor in comparison?

One caveat to the comparison of RYGB and LAGB is the very different pattern of weight loss. There is rapid weight loss following RYGB and usually a much steadier loss following LAGB. The difference in mean weight loss between the procedures is quite substantial with better weight loss in those treated with RYGB, but at three years and beyond the percentage of excess weight loss outcomes are comparable.[36] One can argue that more rapid weight loss increases the risk of cholelithiasis, loss of lean body mass and nutritional deficiencies.

The decision as to which procedure a patient should have comes down to a range of issues. Clearly the local experience of the surgeon(s) and multidisciplinary team and their knowledge of the procedures involved are crucial. Most critical is the availability of excellent long term follow-up care.

In addition to this peri-operative mortality, the severity of morbidity and nutritional risk associated with the procedures are important, and clearly LAGB carries a significant advantage in all of these categories.[37] The LAGB procedure is also adjustable and easily reversible providing a more logical choice of adolescents and those considering a pregnancy in the future.[38,39] It also provides a logical choice for patients at high risk of mortality with RYGB.[14,40] On the other hand while weight loss achieved with LAGB surgery has a profound effect on the improvement or resolution of type-2 diabetes, there is growing evidence that in subjects with diabetes, the diversionary aspects of RYGB have benefit in addition to that of weight loss.[23,41] It may be that this benefit is important to those with type-2 diabetes who already have significant beta cell dysfunction. However, the nature and durability of the beta cell stimulatory effects are yet to be fully determined.

References

1. Hubbard, V.S., Hall, W.H. (1991). Gastrointestinal surgery for severe obesity. *Obes Surg* 1(3): 257–265.

2. Buchwald, H., Avidor, Y., Braunwald, E. *et al.* (2004). Bariatric surgery: a systematic review and meta-analysis. *JAMA* 292(14): 1724–1737.
3. Dixon, J.B., Dixon, M.E., O'Brien, P.E. (2001). Quality of life after Lap-Band placement: influence of time, weight loss, and comorbidities. *Obes Res* 9(11): 713–721.
4. Clegg, A., Colquitt, J., Sidhu, M. *et al.* (2003). Clinical and cost effectiveness of surgery for morbid obesity: a systematic review and economic evaluation. *Int J Obes Relat Metab Disord* 27(10): 1167–1177.
5. Adams, T.D., Gress, R.E., Smith, S.C. *et al.* (2007). Long-term mortality after gastric bypass surgery. *N Engl J Med* 357(8): 753–761.
6. Sjostrom, L., Narbro, K., Sjostrom, C.D. *et al.* (2007). Effects of bariatric surgery on mortality in Swedish obese subjects. *N Engl J Med* 357(8): 741–752.
7. Bender, R., Jockel, K.H., Trautner, C. *et al.* (1999). Effect of age on excess mortality in obesity. *JAMA* 281(16): 1498–1504.
8. Fontaine, K.R., Redden, D.T., Wang, C. *et al.* (2003). Years of life lost due to obesity. *JAMA* 289(2): 187–193.
9. Visscher, T.L., Seidell, J.C., Menotti, A. *et al.* (2000). Underweight and overweight in relation to mortality among men aged 40–59 and 50–69 years: the Seven Countries Study. *Am J Epidemiol* 151(7): 660–666.
10. Stevens, J., Cai, J., Pamuk, E.R. *et al.* (1998). The effect of age on the association between body-mass index and mortality. *N Engl J Med* 338(1): 1–7.
11. Peeters, A., Barendregt, J.J., Willekens, F. *et al.* (2003). Obesity in adulthood and its consequences for life expectancy: a life-table analysis. *Ann Intern Med* 138(1): 24–32.
12. Visscher, T.L., Rissanen, A., Seidell, J.C. *et al.* (2004). Obesity and unhealthy life-years in adult Finns: an empirical approach. *Arch Intern Med* 164(13): 1413–1420.
13. Murr, M.M., Martin, T., Haines, K. *et al.* (2007). A state-wide review of contemporary outcomes of gastric bypass in Florida: does provider volume impact outcomes? *Ann Surg* 245(5): 699–706.
14. DeMaria, E.J., Murr, M., Byrne, T.K. *et al.* (2007). Validation of the obesity surgery mortality risk score in a multicenter study proves it stratifies mortality risk in patients undergoing gastric bypass for morbid obesity. *Ann Surg* 246(4): 578–582; discussion 583–574.
15. Cole, T.J., Bellizzi, M.C., Flegal, K.M. *et al.* (2000). Establishing a standard definition for child overweight and obesity worldwide: international survey. *BMJ* 20(7244): 1240–1243.

16. Flegal, K.M., Ogden, C.L., Wei, R. et al. (2001). Prevalence of overweight in US children: comparison of US growth charts from the Centers for Disease Control and Prevention with other reference values for body mass index. *Am J Clin Nutr* 73(6): 1086–1093.
17. Inge, T.H., Krebs, N.F., Garcia, V.F. et al. (2004). Bariatric surgery for severely overweight adolescents: concerns and recommendations. *Pediatrics* 114(1): 217–223.
18. Misra, A., Wasir, J.S., Vikram, N.K. (2005). Waist circumference criteria for the diagnosis of abdominal obesity are not applicable uniformly to all populations and ethnic groups. *Nutrition* 21(9): 969–976.
19. Ford, E.S. (2005). Prevalence of the metabolic syndrome defined by the International Diabetes Federation among adults in the U.S. *Diabetes Care* 28(11): 2745–2749.
20. WHO Expert Consultation (2004). Appropriate body-mass index for Asian populations and its implications for policy and intervention strategies. *Lancet* 363(9403): 157–163.
21. Lilford, R.J. (2003). Ethics of clinical trials from a bayesian and decision analytic perspective: whose equipoise is it anyway? *BMJ* 326(7396): 980–981.
22. O'Brien, P.E., Dixon, J.B., Laurie, C. et al. (2006). Treatment of mild to moderate obesity with laparoscopic adjustable gastric banding or an intensive medical program: a randomized trial. *Ann Intern Med* 144(9): 625–633.
23. Dixon, J.B., O'Brien, P.E., Playfair, J. et al. (2008). Adjustable gastric banding and conventional therapy for type 2 diabetes: a randomized controlled trial. *JAMA* 299(3): 316–323.
24. Buchwald, H., Buchwald, J.N. (2002). Evolution of operative procedures for the management of morbid obesity 1950–2000. *Obes Surg* 12(5): 705–717.
25. Buchwald, H., Williams, S.E. (2004). Bariatric surgery worldwide 2003. *Obes Surg* 14(9): 1157–1164.
26. Newbury, L., Dolan, K., Hatzifotis, M. et al. (2003). Calcium and vitamin D depletion and elevated parathyroid hormone following biliopancreatic diversion. *Obes Surg* 13(6): 893–895.
27. Papadia, F.S., Adami, G.F., Marinari, G.M. et al. (2007). Bariatric surgery in adolescents: a long-term follow-up study. *Surg Obes Relat Dis* 3(4): 465–468.
28. Ren, C.J., Patterson, E., Gagner, M. (2000). Early results of laparoscopic biliopancreatic diversion with duodenal switch: a case series of 40 consecutive patients. *Obes Surg* 10(6): 514–523.

29. Regan, J.P., Inabnet, W.B., Gagner, M. et al. (2003). Early experience with two-stage laparoscopic Roux-en-Y gastric bypass as an alternative in the super-super obese patient. *Obes Surg* 13(6): 861–864.
30. Buchwald, H. (2002) A bariatric surgery algorithm. *Obes Surg* 12(6): 733–746; discussion 747–750.
31. Dixon, J.B., Dixon, M.E., O'Brien, P.E. (2001). Pre-operative predictors of weight loss at 1-year after Lap-Band surgery. *Obes Surg* 11(2): 200–207.
32. Lanyon, R.I., Maxwell, B.M. (2007). Predictors of outcome after gastric bypass surgery. *Obes Surg* 17(3): 321–328.
33. van Hout, G.C., Verschure, S.K., van Heck, G.L. (2005). Psychosocial predictors of success following bariatric surgery. *Obes Surg* 15(4): 552–560.
34. Colles, S.L., Dixon, J.B., O'Brien, P.E. (2008). Grazing and loss of control related to eating: two high-risk factors following bariatric surgery. *Obesity (Silver Spring)* 16(3): 615–622.
35. Colles, S.L., Dixon, J.B., O'Brien, P.E. (2008). Hunger control and regular physical activity facilitate weight loss after laparoscopic adjustable gastric banding. *Obes Surg* 18(7): 833–840.
36. O'Brien, P.E., McPhail, T., Chaston, T.B. et al. (2006). Systematic review of medium-term weight loss after bariatric operations. *Obes Surg* 16(8): 1032–1040.
37. Chapman, A., Kiroff, G., Game, P. et al. (2004). Laparoscopic adjustable gastric banding in the treatment of obesity: a systematic review. *Surgery* 135: 326–351.
38. Dixon, J.B., Dixon, M.E., O'Brien, PE. (2005). Birth outcomes in obese women after laparoscopic adjustable gastric banding. *Obstet Gynecol* 106(5): 965–972.
39. Fielding, G.A., Duncombe, J.E. (2005). Laparoscopic adjustable gastric banding in severely obese adolescents. *Surg Obes Relat Dis* 1(4): 399–405; discussion 405–397.
40. DeMaria, E.J., Portenier, D., Wolfe, L. (2007). Obesity surgery mortality risk score: proposal for a clinically useful score to predict mortality risk in patients undergoing gastric bypass. *Surg Obes Relat Dis* 3(2): 134–140.
41. Rubino, F., Gagner, M. Gentileschi, P. et al. (2004). The early effect of the Roux-en-Y gastric bypass on hormones involved in body weight regulation and glucose metabolism. *Ann Surg* 240(2): 236–242.

Chapter 2

Anaesthesia in Bariatric Surgery

Ernesto Pizzirani and Giuseppe Calcarella

Definitions

On accessing the Medline data-bank, you find the following definition for 'morbid obesity': 'the condition of weighing two, three, or more times the ideal weight, so called because it is associated with many serious and life-threatening disorders'.

This very concise sentence emphasises some aspects which concern the anaesthetist:

- the enormous (pathological) increase in the body mass, to which we attribute the difficulty in performing manoeuvres which are generally simple if related to patients whose weight is close to the ideal;
- the danger due to serious pathophysiologic alterations associated with obesity, that affect the anaesthesiological and intensive care treatment of the obese person; and
- the reference to the ideal weight that compels us to pay attention to the use of drugs in anaesthesia.

Obesity concerns a state of diversity referred to individuals in which, the accumulation of adipose tissue has so increased that both mental and physical health are compromised. The subject's life expectancy is reduced, and it is convenient to divide these individuals into grades or classes according to the severity of the state.

It is useful to underline that in the literature we constantly quote the ideal weight, known by the acronym IBW (Ideal Body Weight), a term coined in 1835 by the Belgian statistician Quetelet. Its value is calculated on the basis of tables worded by insurance companies (for instance the Metropolitan Life Insurance Company) that consider parameters such as height, physical constitution, sex and age. They specify the ideal weight in connection with an estimate of the lower mortality risk relative to the above mentioned parameters.

Others, more simply, are referred to the so-called Broca Index, which allows us to calculate the ideal weight (kg) by subtracting from height (in cm) an x value equal to 100 for adult males and 105 for adult females.

On the other hand, should we calculate the excess of weight, we could refer to the relative weight, which is the connection between real weight and actual weight, or to the most common and widespread system, Body Mass Index (BMI), which represents the numerical ratio between the weight (expressed in kg) and the height squared (expressed in metres).

The BMI is surely the most used measuring parameter for clinical and epidemiologic studies and it has been validated by the World Health Organization and by other acknowledged international institutes. On the basis of its estimate, we can define an individual as underweight if they have a BMI < 18.5 and normal if their BMI is between 18.5 and 25. Overweight is between 25 and 29.9 and covers three obesity classes:

Class I: BMI 30–34.9
Class II: BMI = 35–39.9
Class III: BMI > 40

Subsequently, some specialists in bariatric surgery coined the term 'super obese' for patients whose BMI exceeded 50 and to these patients, according to some specialists, we should reserve the so-called Class IV.[1]

Epidemiology

Once the classification of obesity has been agreed upon, it is easier to study the relative risks of co-morbidity within a specific population. As a matter of fact, the risk is estimated as low, moderate, high and very high according to the passage from the simple overweight to the three obesity

Table 1. Relationship between obesity classes and risks of co-morbidity.

Class	BMI (kg/m^2)	Risks of co-morbidity	Number of fat cells
I	30–35	Low	Normal
II	35–40	Moderate	Normal
III	> 40	High	Normal or increased
IV	> 50	Very high	Increased

Table 2. Obesity classes and treatment.

Class	BMI	Physical activity	Drug treatment	Surgery
I	30–35	1st choice	3rd choice	Not applicable
II	35–40	2nd choice	3rd choice	Not applicable
III	> 40	3rd choice	2nd choice	3rd choice
IV	> 50	3rd choice	1st choice	1st choice

classes, reserving the highest class of risk (IV) for the small subpopulation of the so-called super obese (Table 1).[2]

The proposed classification is considered more efficacious than other general indexes. It allows us to avoid approximate terms such as 'severe', 'morbid' and 'extreme' obesity, and it can be used as a rational approach to the choice of the most appropriate treatment (Table 2).

From the epidemiologic point of view, it is recognized that there is a rising rate of obesity in the world, and in particular in Europe, with an increase of 10–20 per cent, and higher peaks in some regions, resulting in economic fallout. It has been estimated, for example, that in the Netherlands in 1994 the direct and indirect annual sanitary costs associated with overweight and obesity corresponded to 4 per cent of the total sanitary costs.[3] The situation is even worse in the United States. In the first half of the 1990s obesity reached 15 per cent and, according to a later survey, the figure reached 26 per cent (BMI > 30 kg/m^2).[4] Together with these studies highlighting a worrying increase of obesity, a series of other researches came out confirming that subpopulations with very high BMIs

Table 3. Incidence of co-morbidity in obese patients.

Co-morbidity	Incidence (%)
Osteoarthritis	50–65
Hypertension	25–60
Gastro-oesophageal reflux	30–50
Urinary stress incontinence	30–40
Gall-bladder disease	25–45
Depression	20–40
Alteration of lipid metabolism	20–35
↓ HDL-cholesterol	20
↑ blood cholesterol	35
Diabetes	10–20
Hyperisulinemia/increased insulin resistance	10–20
Asthma	10–20
OSA/OSH	5–40
Heart failure	7–12

Table 4. Relative risk of co-morbidity in the obese.

Co-morbidity	Female (%)	Male (%)
Vascular Disease		
Claudicatio	25–100	5
Coronary disease	7–35	15
Myocardial infarction	0.7	5
Stroke	0.7	—
Hypertension		
≥155/ 95 mmHg	1.5–5.3	1.8
≥ 175/ 105 mmHg	1.2–4.2	2.3
Diabetes (glycaemia > 7.1 mmol/L)	8–20	5
Dyspnoea	5.5	4
Low back pain	1.5–2	2
Biliary calculosis	2.5	1

were more susceptible to health risks, with high rates of work absenteeism and higher social costs.[5]

Obesity in general, and high class obesity in particular, are associated with a certain number of alterations in organs and systems, reflecting considerable increases in the mortality rate (Tables 3 and 4).

As underlined by Adams and Murphy,[6] the contemporaneous involvement of cardiovascular, respiratory, endocrine and gastroenteric systems has a substantial impact on mortality and morbidity rates, and in particular is much more likely to expose obese patients to the possibility of a sudden death compared with normal subjects. It is also useful to underline the point that risks are proportional to the duration of obesity, to the level of obesity, and that they are higher for males than for females.[7]

A study published in *JAMA* in 1999 estimates a figure of about 280,000 adult deaths per year due to obesity in the United States, whereas in 2002 the European figure was 279,000 (equal to 7.7 per cent of all deaths), with regional variations ranging from 5.8 per cent (France) to 8.7 per cent (United Kingdom). Of these European deaths, 175,000 occurred in obese subjects and 104,000 in overweight ones. Broken down it was shown that about 70 per cent of the deaths (195,000) were due to diseases in the cardiovascular group and 20 per cent (53,000) due to cancer. In conclusion, at least one death in 13 in the EU is attributed to being overweight.[8]

Today we believe that both the distribution and quantity of fat significantly contribute to the classification of the obese into two groups characterized by specific factors of co-morbidity: those mainly associated with weight (mass), and those associated with an altered metabolism (Tables 5 and 6).[9]

Pathophysiologic Aspects Connected to Obesity

Overweight due to a positive caloric balance in consequence of excessive intake and/or reduced physical activity involves a series of both metabolic and functional alterations at the level of different systems (respiratory, cardiovascular, gastroenteric and endocrine).[10]

Metabolic alterations

The obese patient presents alterations with respect to the metabolism of carbohydrates, proteins and amino acids and other metabolic alterations caused by the thyroid and the sympathetic nervous system.

Table 5. Co-morbidity of the obese associated with weight.

1. Arthropathies
2. Hyperdynamic state with increased intravascular blood volume
   Heart failure
   Fluid imbalance (oedema)
   Prolonged QT tract
   Sudden death
3. Increase of renal blood flow (RBF)
4. Respiratory disease
   Increase of intrathoracic pressure
   Increase of O_2 consumption
   Hypoventilation
   OSA
   Sudden death
5. Skin lesions
   Intertrigo
   Ulceration
6. Increase of intra-abdominal pressure
   Pseudotumor cerebri
   Hernias
   Oesophageal reflux
   Eclampsia
   Urinary incontinence
   Venous stasis
7. Obstetric diseases
   Poor fertility or infertility
   Increased incidence of Caesarian section
   Pre-eclampsia

The increase in fat within the portal system causes the activation of hepatic gluconeogenesis and the secretion of lipoproteins at very low density (VLDL) as well as the reduced clearance of the hepatic insulin.

The hyperinsulinaemia and increased resistance to insulin, increased gluconeogenesis and the reduction in the peripheral uptake of glucose are the cause of the reduced tolerance to glucose and therefore of the development of non insulin dependent diabetes. Furthermore, the hyperinsulinaemia

Table 6. Co-morbidity of the obese associated with an alteration of metabolism.

Sistemic Co-morbidity
1. Neurormonal/behaviour alterations

    Dysfunction of hypothalamo-pituitary axis
    Stress intolerance
    Hypercortisolism
    Gonadic trouble
    Bulimic behaviour, smoke, alcohol, no physical activity, drugs

2. Due to a positive caloric balance

    Glucose intolerance, hyperinsulism, insulin resistance
    Diabetes type II
    Alterations of lipidis metabolism, ↓ HDL-cholesterol, ↑ blood cholesterol
    Inflammatory markers: free radical, oxidative radical, protein C reactive

3. Atherogenic

    Stroke
    Myocardial infarction

4. Carcinogenic

    Breast, endometrial, prostate
    Oesophagus, colon
    Bladder, kidney

5. Trombogenic

    Increase of viscosity
    Increase of fibrinogen
    Decrease of ATIII
    Increase of plasminogen activator inhibitor (PAI-1)

6. Immunologic

    Hypercortisolism
    Disfunction of leucocytes
    Alterations of cytokine

Organ Correlate Co-morbidity
1. Adipose tissue

    Hypertension
    Alteration of gonadic steroids

2. Liver

    Post-hepatic increase of blood glucose
    Steatosis, fibrosis

3. Kidney

    Increase of glomerular filtration volume
    Microalbuminuria
    Sodium reabsorption

4. Pancreas

    Beta-cells hypertrophy

```
                        ┌─────────────────────┐
                        │  ↑ Body Fat Mass    │
                        └─────────────────────┘
                              │
                        ┌─────────────────┐
                        │ Ipercoagulability│
                        └─────────────────┘
```

↑ Abdominal Pressure

↓ Physical Activity

↑ FFA
↑ Fibronectin

Diabetes/ ↑ Blood Glucose
↑ Viscosity
↑ Fibrinogen
↓ ATIII

↑ Lipids

↑ PAI-1*

↓ Plasminogen

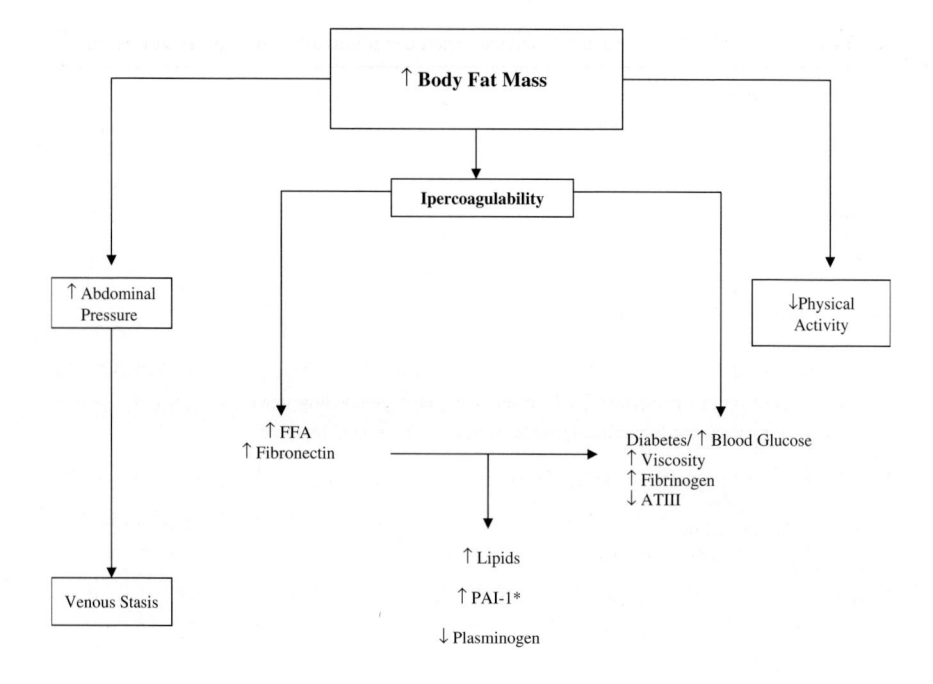

Venous Stasis

* PAI-1 = Plasminogen Activator Inhibitor

Figure 1. Contribution of increased body fat mass to thrombogenesis.

which helps the reabsorption of sodium and stimulates the sympathetic tone, favours the appearance of arterial hypertension.[11]

The factor inhibiting the activation of the plasminogen, which is liberated by the adipose tissue in large quantities, associated with the increase in the concentration of the fibrinogen, would explain the tendency to hypercoagulate that is present in the severely obese patient (Fig. 1).[12]

Respiratory disorders

The most common dysventilatory syndrome associated with obesity is Obstructive Sleep Apnoea (OSA) which includes Obstructive Sleep Hypopnoea (OSH) (Table 7).

Table 7. Definitions of obstructive sleep apnoea and obstructive sleep hypopnoea.

	↓ Airway flow >10 sec	Frequency of apnoea (n°/h)	↓ SaO$_2$	Fragmentation of sleep	Day-time somnolence
OSA	100 per cent	> 5	≥ 4	Yes	Yes
OSH	> 50 per cent	> 15	≥ 4	Yes	Yes

This syndrome is characterized by:

- frequent episodes of apnoea during sleep with the total interruption of flux into the airways for more than ten seconds due to an interrupted inspiratory effort;
- snoring due to the loss of tone in the three pharyngeal segments (veil- or naso-pharynx, oropharynx, laryngo- or hypo-pharynx) during the diaphragmatic contraction in inspiration;
- alteration of the sleep/wake rhythm, fragmentation of nocturnal sleep and day-time somnolence that causes disorders of both concentration and memory;
- pathophysiological alterations resulting from prolonged periods of apnoea involving hypoxia, hypercapnea and systemic pulmonary vasoconstriction.

Description of the obesity is complicated by OSA and OSH which are characterized by an abnormal accumulation of the adipose tissue in the pharyngeal tissues and involve the uvula, tonsils, palatine arches, aryepiglottic plicae and the pharynx side walls.

The increase of fat causes a reduction in the patency of the pharyngeal cavity, which increases the possibility for collapse of the oropharynx due to the muscular relaxation of the upper airways that could occur during sleep. Also, in the obese patient suffering from OSA, the pharyngeal extraluminal pressure (external to airways) is raised due to the deposit of the adipose mass in the neck compressing the upper airways from the outside.[13]

During apnoea, there is a decrease in PaO$_2$, an increase in PaCO$_2$ and a progressive increase in ventilatory effort which corresponds to the duration of the apnoea; finally the pressure in the airways becomes negative. All these phenomena stimulate the ascending reticular system and this causes the subject to regain consciousness. Regained consciousness results in the reinstatement of the muscular tone of the upper airways and reopening of the same. Everything comes together as ventilation restarts, hypoxia is corrected and hypercapnea, which was caused by apnoea, occurs. This sequence of events can occur repeatedly and, if it happens many times, can cause serious pathophysiologic sequences: hypoxia, hypercapnea and systemic vasoconstriction. The first, in particular, can cause secondary polycythaemia involving an increasing risk of ischaemic cardiopathy and cerebrovascular accidents.

It is very important for the anaesthetist to know the impact of both the anaesthetic drugs and sedatives on the patency of airways of the obese suffering from OSA. It is essential to highlight the effect of these drugs on the tone of the pharyngeal muscles that lead to a pharyngeal collapse in a situation already altered by the adipose pharyngeal deposits. Among the most common drugs causing these deleterious effects are thiopental, benzodiazepine, propofol and nitrous oxide. Drugs containing opium, in particular, are characterized by the fact that they lead to a decreased ventilatory response which in turn leads to the occurrence of hypoxia and hypercapnea.

It is useful to complete the general picture of the effects of obesity on the ventilatory parameters. They particularly occur when this kind of patient is under anaesthesia, aside from the presence of OSA. The most important datum, observed in studying the functionality respiratory tests, is the constant reduction in the functional residual capacity (FRC) of the expiratory volume reserve (EVR) and of the total pulmonary capacity (TPC).[14]

The reduction in FRC in the obese patient is explained by the contemporaneous EVR reduction with the conservation of the residual volume (RV) within normal limits, whereas the forced expiratory volume in one second (FEV1) and the forced vital capacity (FVC) can both be kept within normal limits.[15]

All of the changes to both dynamic and static volumes are attributable to the charge effect of the adipose mass on the thorax and abdomen, together with the increased abdominal pressure and the dislocation of the diaphragm in a higher position. These alterations can contribute to reduce FRC over the limit of the alveolar closing capacity (CC), affecting the closure of the small airways, alteration of ventilation/perfusion ratio (V/Q), shunt right–left (up to 20–25 per cent) and arterial hypoxia.[16]

Furthermore, a reduced pulmonary (< 50 per cent) and thoracic (< 30 per cent) compliance and an increase in the elastic pulmonary resistance (>15 per cent) have been observed. The reduced thoracic compliance is the consequence of increased intercostal, peri-diaphragmatic and abdominal adipose tissue. These factors are also associated with both a dorsal kyphosis and a lumbar hyperlordosis (due to the accumulation of abdominal fat).[17]

More recent studies have suggested that the reduction in the total compliance is above all due to the pulmonary compliance reduction due to the increased haematic pulmonary volume.[18]

The combined action of these elements is responsible for the increase in the work of breathing (WOB) and in the reduced efficiency of the respiratory function. In normocapnic obese patients about 30 per cent of WOB is often due to the pulmonary inflation. In hypercapnic obese patients this increases some 100 per cent owing to pulmonary inflation and some 200 per cent owing to the mobilization of the thoracic wall. The explanation for this is that accelerated ventilation, increasing the energetic expenditure and O_2 consumption, might cause alveolar hypoventilation.

Association with the increased mechanic pressure (intra- and extra-abdominal), reduction in the pulmonary compliance and increase in metabolic demands of the respiratory muscles all determine a certain degree of respiratory muscular inefficiency and finally an increase in the WOB. Clinically, all this is characterized by rapid and superficial breathing, together with a limitation of the maximum ventilatory capacity and a very high energetic cost. All this is accentuated when the patient is in a supine position.

The alterations in the ventilatory mechanics in the obese patient bring about important consequences during anaesthesia. The supine position, anaesthetic induction and the use of relaxant drugs causes a reduction in FRC in the healthy patient of normal weight that, in the dependent areas of the lungs, can exceed the closing capacity (CC) of the small airways without any cartilaginous support. This leads to the formation of atelectasis, V/Q mismatch and shunt right–left, with the possibility of reduction in the arterial oxygenation (PaO_2).[19] This mechanism of formation of atelectasic areas is far more accentuated in the obese patient due to the above mentioned alterations of the ventilatory mechanics, so that the occurrence of intra-operative arterial hypoxias is frequent, above all during videolaparoscopic surgeries.

This has led to a study of the ventilation strategies available to alleviate the occurrence of these phenomena. The first measure was to use particularly high current volumes (up to 10–15 ml/kg) and this determined only modest increases in PaO_2.[20] Later, positive end-expiratory pressure (PEEP) was used in anaesthaetized and paralyzed obese patients and a significant increase in O_2 was found in the partial arterial pressure in the group treated with 10 cm H_2O of PEEP.[18]

In 1999 Pelosi et al. measured pulmonary volumes by using the helium technique and recorded the elastance of the respiratory system, lungs and thoracic wall, pressure-volume curves and the endo-abdominal pressure at PEEP 0 and 10 cm H_2O. They reached the following conclusions: during anaesthesia and paralysis, PEEP ameliorates the respiratory function in obese patients, but not in normal subjects.[21] It is important to notice that application of PEEP has unpleasant side-effects, in particular on the cardiac output (CO), as underlined by Santesson in 1976.[22]

More recently it has been suggested that one should carry out the recruitment manoeuvres followed by the high level PEEP in order to open the atelectasic pulmonary areas and keep them open.[23] In particular, Whalen et al.[24] proposed high level PEEP for at least three respiratory acts from 4–20 cm H_2O as a recruitment manoeuvre, making sure the peak pressures of 50 cm H_2O, followed by a 12 cm H_2O PEEP, are not exceeded. This ventilatory strategy has been applied to two groups of obese patients subject to laparoscopic surgeries. The results in terms of an increase in PaO_2 have been significant, as have those concerning the improvement in dynamic compliance, and no substantial difference has been registered in the occurrence of post-operative respiratory complications. Therefore, these manoeuvres are effective in the prevention of intra-operative atelectasis but their effect is to be considered as transitory. Further and wider studies are necessary so that the utility of these strategies in the prevention of post-operative complications can be assessed; however we should not exclude the possibility that post-operative, non invasive ventilatory techniques of positive pressure such as continuous positive airway pressure (CPAP) with helmet or facial-nasal mask could also be used.

Cardiovascular disorders

Cardiovascular disorders are a consequence not only of the adaptation of the cardiovascular system to obesity and to increased metabolic request but also to the anatomic changes to the cardiac structure caused by obesity. They are also a consequence of the accumulation of adipose tissue in the myocardium which provokes severe consequences on mechanic and electric performance. It has been observed that cardiovascular diseases play a major role in the clinical situation of the obese. Cardiovascular disease affects both morbidity and mortality and all the studies underline that an increase in BMI corresponds to an increase in cardiovascular diseases.[25]

It is however useful to note that the highly reduced mobility of obese patients is able to utterly conceal the presence of cardiovascular diseases, even serious ones. Consequently the clinical occurrence of the disease appears only when the subject makes a physical effort, even if moderate, or if he is under stress, such as undergoing surgery. In these cases the onset of certain symptoms such as polypnoea, dyspnoea, and anginous crises are very common. This compels the anaesthesiologist to request very detailed cardiovascular tests in order to look for the symptoms of possible cardiorespiratory deficiency (increase of venous pressures, symptoms of pulmonary stasis, hepatomegaly, etc.). The clinical examination must be completed with a series of instrumental tests in order to quantify the severity of the dysfunction. An ECG, echocardiography and a chest X-ray can give us all the information necessary in drawing up a therapeutic pre-operative plan and to quantify the risk associated with planned surgery (Fig. 2).

The genesis of obese myocardiopathy is due to the strict relationship between hypertension, ischemic cardiopathy and pneumopathy. The latter, affected by ventricular dilatation and increase in stroke volume, stresses the wall of the left ventricle leading to hypertrophy.[26] This left eccentric ventricular hypertrophy, accompanied by a reduction in the efficiency of the left ventricle, compromises the ventricular filling up and results in increasing left ventricular tele-diastolic pressure (LVEDP) and also of pulmonary oedema.[27] It is clear that the possibility of a dilated ventricle being hypertrophized is rather unlikely, so that when the parietal thickness cannot increase due to the excessive dilatation, one immediately observes the occurrence of a systolic dysfunction.[28]

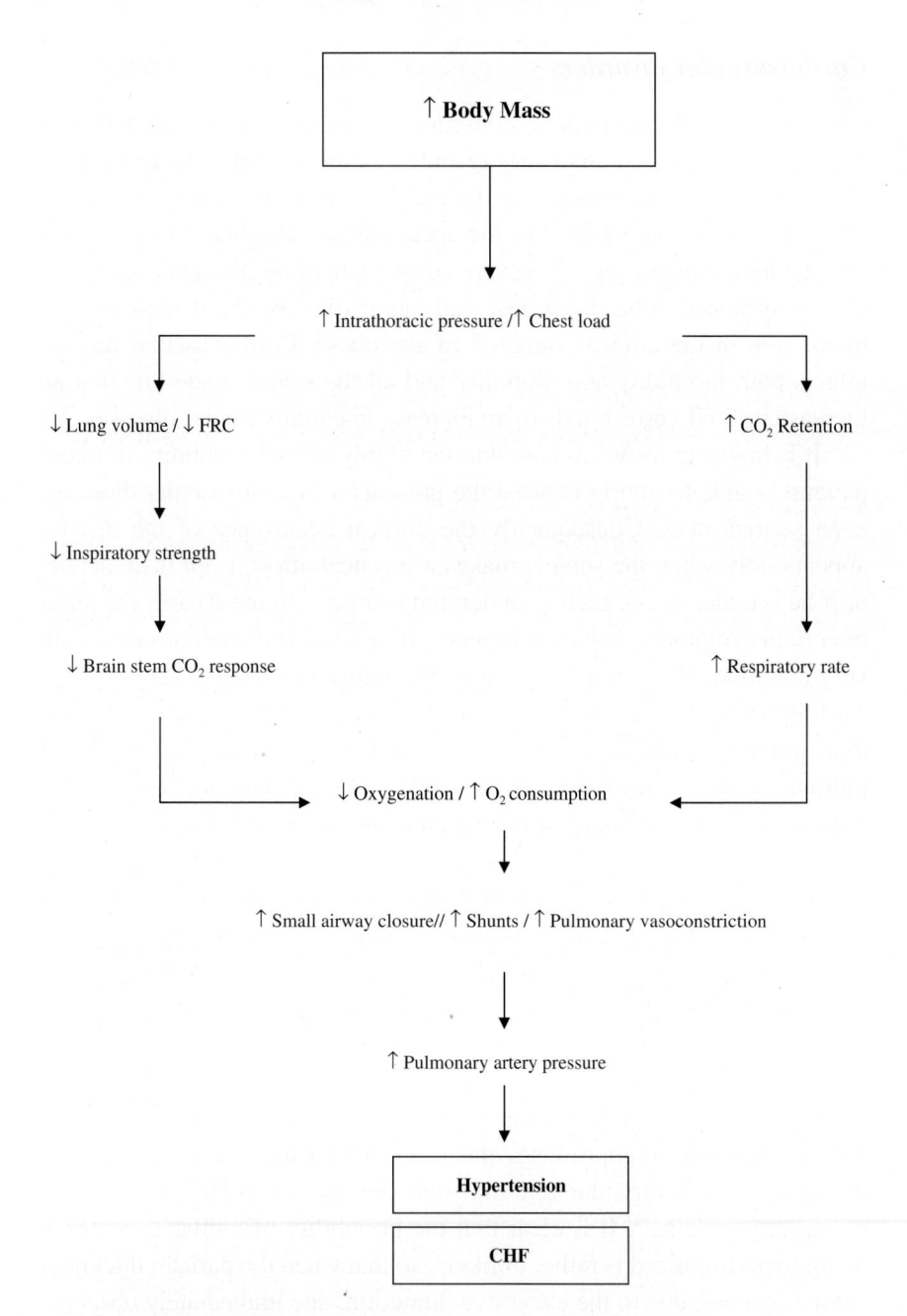

```
                    ┌─────────────────┐
                    │  ↑ Body Mass    │
                    └────────┬────────┘
                             │
                             ▼
              ↑ Intrathoracic pressure / ↑ Chest load

   ↓ Lung volume / ↓ FRC                    ↑ CO₂ Retention

   ↓ Inspiratory strength

   ↓ Brain stem CO₂ response                ↑ Respiratory rate

                  ↓ Oxygenation / ↑ O₂ consumption

          ↑ Small airway closure// ↑ Shunts / ↑ Pulmonary vasoconstriction

                      ↑ Pulmonary artery pressure

                      ┌─────────────────┐
                      │  Hypertension   │
                      ├─────────────────┤
                      │      CHF        │
                      └─────────────────┘
```

Figure 2. The role of increased body mass in the pathophisiology of hypertension and cardiac heart failure (CHF).

A review of the factors involved in cardiovascular disorders of the obese includes:

- *An increase in both the circulating blood volume and the cardiac output* necessary to satisfy the needs of an abnormal body mass. The increase in volume is not proportional to the increase in body mass (haematic volume/body weight ratio of the obese patient = 45 ml/kg instead of the corresponding value 75 ml/kg in the non obese patient) and the majority of the haematic volume is distributed in the adipose tissue.[29] In the meantime, we observe a splanchnic haematic flux increased by 20 per cent whereas the cerebral and renal fluxes are normal.
- *Reduced vascular systemic resistance* due to the increase in the cardiac output together with a constant arterial pressure. It is not clear whether this situation is caused by alterations of the sympathetic tone since there have been cases of some patients with increased, normal or reduced sympathetic activity.
- *Cardiac frequency* is generally normal, although some studies establish a positive relation between obesity and increased cardiac output.[30]
- *Increase in cardiac output*, essentially due to the increase in the systolic volume and/or the cardiac work (increases up to 40 per cent) even if the indexed parameters are normal, which indicates that the increase is proportional to obesity. As a result of dilatation and eccentric hypertrophy of the left ventricle, the reduction in compliance and the increase in the filling up pressures, there is a predisposition to the occurrence of cardiac insufficiency. Studies have also described reductions in the left ventricular function,[31] which exceed 50 per cent in the obese patients (without symptoms), whereas the hypertrophic dilatative pathology of the left ventricle is more often observed in patients suffering from Pickwickian syndrome.
- *Systemic arterial hypertension (IPT)* due to different factors including the increased activity of the renin–angiotensin–aldosterone system, the increase in the haematic volume, sympathetic tone and hyperinsulinism. It has also been observed that 50–60 per cent of obese patients suffer from light or moderate IPT, whereas only 5–10 per cent have the severe form,[32] but the exact mechanism causing IPT in the

obese patient is not perfectly known even if many researchers attribute it to a mix of haemodynamic, genetic and hormonal factors. It is important to stress that weight loss reduces hypertension.[33]

- *Arterial pulmonary hypertension* due to the increase in the cardiac output, hypoxic pulmonary vasoconstriction and increase in left ventricle diastolic and pulmonary pressure (Fig. 2).
- *Cardiac arrhythmias* due to the combined action of different factors: myocardial hypertrophia, hypoxia, hypokalaemia due to diuretic therapy, coronary disease, increase in circulating catecolamine and infiltration of the adipose tissue into the conductive tissue of the myocardium. We should notice that in serious obesity associated with OSA, episodes of sinusal bradycardia occur during apnoea and sinusal tachycardia when the patient starts to breathe again.
- *The coronary pathology* present in a high percentage of the obese[34] results in an increase in myocardial infarction, coronary insufficiency and sudden death. Most of the epidemiologic studies have shown a strong connection between the amount of adipose tissue with a central distribution and ischemic cardiac disease, so that nowadays it is accepted that obesity represents an independent risk factor for ischemic cardiopathy (Fig. 2).[35]

Gastroenteric disorders

These consist of an increased prevalence of gastro-oesophageal reflux and hiatal hernia, and are strictly correlated with an increase in intra-abdominal pressure. According to certain studies, 75 per cent of obese patients had a gastric stagnation greater than 25 ml with pH < 2.5. This condition is associated with increased abdominal pressure and was correlated to the risk of inhalation of the gastric content and the development of pneumonia *ab ingestis*. Later studies attributed these possible complications more to the pathology of the gastro-oesophageal junction than to the increase in the gastric stagnation, which in the obese has not been observed as increased if compared to the normal subject.[36]

At the hepatic level, we find processes of steatosis, fibrosis, cirrhosis and biliary calculosis more frequently than in normal patients. Tests of hepatic functionality often do not indicate the real gravity of the pathology even if the determination of a decrease in blood albumin concentration, an increase in the duration of prothrombin time and an increase in serum transaminases, indicate a serious hepatopathy.

Endocrine disorders

Obese patients show an increased production of triiodothyronine (T3) and also a consequential increase in metabolism with which an increased sympathetic tone is associated.

In females a state of hyper-androgenesis has been observed and in males the opposite condition[3] and this could explain the different distribution of the adipose tissue in both males and females.

Pharmacologic Considerations

In the obese patient the distribution of drugs is altered. This is due to various factors:

- lower corporal water content;
- increased content of adipose tissue;
- reduced lean mass;
- changes in the linking capacity of the tissue proteins;
- increased haematic volume and cardiac output;
- increased haematic concentration of free fatty acids, cholesterol and alpha-glycoproteins.

Liposoluble drugs

Liposoluble drugs such as thiopental, xilocaine and most benzodiazepines have an increased distribution volume, a more selective accumulation in the adipose tissue and a longer elimination half life, even though clearance values are normal or increased.[37]

Hydrosoluble drugs

Drugs in this category react in the same way both in the obese patient and in those of normal weight. The increased haematic concentration of alpha 1 glycoproteins and hyperlipidemia modify the proteic bond of drugs, reducing the quantity of free drugs in circulation.

Renal clearance is increased due to the greater renal haematic flow, glomerular filtration and tubular secretion, and consequently there is an increase in the elimination of all those substances which are not biotransformed before renal excretion and which are filtered by glomerula.

Anaesthetic drugs

A summary of some anaesthetic drugs is shown in Table 8.

Thiopental

This highly lipophilic drug has an increased distribution volume, a more selective accumulation in the adipose tissue and a longer elimination

Table 8. Pharmacokinetic alterations of anaesthetics drugs in obese patients.

	Induction drugs		
Drugs	Thiopental	Propofol	Midazolam, Diazepam
Pharmacokinetic alterations	1. ↑ Vd.*		1. ↑ Vd associated with weight
	2. ↑ Elimination half-life	1. Vd normal	2. ↑ Elimination half-life
Clinical evidence	1. ↑ Total dose	1. ↑ Total dose	1. ↑ Total dose
	2. ↓ Dose/Kg	2. Dose/kg correlated to the corrected body weight**	2. ↓ Dose/kg
	3. ↑ Recovery time		3. ↑ Recovery time
	Neuromuscolar blockers		
Drugs	SCH	Atracurium	Vecuronium	Pancuronium
Pharmacokinetic alterations	↑ Pseudo-cholinesterase activity	None	1. ↑ Vd 2. ↓ Hepatic Clearence 3. ↑ Recovery Time	Liposolubility
Clinical evidence	1. ↑ Total Dose 2. ↓ Dose/kg	None	Dose/kg sec LBW***	= Dose/kg

(Continued)

	Opiates		
Drugs	Fentanyl	Alfentanyl	Morfina
Pharmacokinetic alterations	None	Increase of elimination half time	No information available
Clinical evidence	None	Dose/kg sec. LBW	None

	Local anaesthetics	
Drugs	Xilocain	Bupivacain
Pharmacokinetic alterations	1. ↑ Vd 2. = Vd/kg	No information available
Clinical evidence	1. = Dose/kg e.v. 2. ↓ Dose/kg (25%)	Unpredictable extension of subaracnoidal block

	Volatile agents		
Drugs	N$_2$O	Enflurane	Sevoflurane
Pharmacokinetic alterations	No information available	1. ↓ Partition coefficient 2. High levels of fluoride catabolites	None
Clinical evidence	Impossibility to use high percentages of FiO$_2$	1. ↓ MAC**** 2. ↑ risk by fluoride metabolites	None

Vd = Distribution volume; ** = correct weight = ideal weight + (0.4 × excess of weight) *** LBW = Lean body weight MAC = ****Minimum alveolar concentration.

half life, even though the clearance values are normal. Doses between 4 and 7 mg/kg of the ideal body weight are suggested.[38]

Benzodiazepines

Benzodiazepines behave in almost the same way as thiopental and there are no precise recommendations about the dosage. Diazepam has a volume of systemic distribution which is almost the same in obese and normal weight patients, so increased doses should be used. An increased half life has been demonstrated for midazolam: 2.7 hours in non obese patients, and 8.4 hours in obese subjects.[39]

Propofol

This drug shows normal distribution at steady state and an accelerated clearance so that after 24 hours of infusion there is no accumulation present.[40]

An empirical formula has been used for the drug dosage, correlated to the correct body weight (correct weight = ideal weight + [0.4 × excess of weight]), which has highlighted how the pharmacokinetics of propofol are similar to those observed in non-obese patients.[41]

Synthetic opiates

This group behaves differently. There are no variations in the kinetics as far as fentanil is concerned, but there is an increase in the elimination half life for alfentanil and sulfentanil.[37] Among the new opiates, remifentanil is worthy of particular attention for its pharmacokinetic characteristics which can be summarized as follows:

- short action onset (1 minute);
- rapid distribution;
- half life singularly short and independent of the duration of infusion (3.7 minutes after an infusion of 240 minutes);
- ultra-short action duration (5–10 minutes);
- organ-independent metabolism: the drug is hydrolyzed by plasmatic and tissue esterase with the formation of substantially inactive derivatives.

These characteristics make remifentanil extremely adaptable with regards to dosage levels, suitable for administration for a short or long period of time without protracting the recovery time. Furthermore, the steady state is reached in 5–10 minutes. A precise titration of the analgesia is possible, so a rapid recovery, predictable and independent of the dose and the duration of infusion is therefore possible.

Due to the high percentage of adipose tissue and therefore an increased accumulation of lipophilic drugs in the obese patient, a prolonged elimination half life is observed. In fact, the majority of authors have highlighted a reduction in the clearance and in the distribution volume of such drugs.[42]

A study by Egan[43] has revealed that in the obese patient, the dosage of remifentanil, correlated to the IBW rather than to the total body weight (TBW), has the same tendency as that found in the normal population. The absolute distribution volume and clearance (not correlated to the body weight) are similar in both groups, but if correlated to the total body weight are reduced in the first group. Instead, these same parameters show a strict correlation to lean body mass (LBM). It is very complicated to extrapolate this value in everyday practice, therefore, the authors advise us to refer to IBW, which is representative of LBM, when we calculate the optimal dosage of the opiate.

Finally, it is correct to highlight that the short ECS of remifentanil should be used in laparoscopic surgery in obese patients, resulting in an early recovery from surgery and an early discharge from hospital.[9]

Depolarizing muscle relaxants

Succinylcholine (SCH)

This is used in different dosages. The obese patient generally has increased pseudo-cholinesterase activity and it is advisable to use doses of 1.2–1.5 mg/kg on the basis of the ideal body weight. Moreover, studies show different behaviours, since some have revealed that dosages of 120–140 mg were satisfactory as far as the tracheal intubation is concerned (in patients whose weight is over 140 kg), whereas others have successfully used dosages of 75–100 mg (in patients whose weight is between 130 and 135 kg).

More recently in a study by Lemmens et al.[44] the administration of a dose of 1 mg/kg of SCH has been studied on the basis of the ideal body weight, lean body weight and total body weight. The study reveals that complete paralysis suitable for an optimal laryngoscopy can be obtained with the dose of 1 mg correlated to the total weight.

Pancuronium bromide

Pancuronium bromide is a drug with low liposolubility. Some authors maintain dosages that do not need to be altered from those used in non-obese patients,[45] but according to other authors, higher dosages would be needed.[46]

Vecuronium

This drug should be administered according to ideal body weight.[17] In fact the use of doses proportional to actual body weight leads to a prolonged recovery time, which, according to some authors, correlates only with overdosage, but according to others, with the modification of hepatic and renal clearance and with a higher haematic distribution volume.[47]

Atracurium

Atracurium is used in doses per kilogram of body weight, and has the same recovery time for both obese and non-obese patients when used as such.[48] There are no variations in the distribution volume, clearance or elimination half life. This is probably because this last molecule is independent of the function of the organ, even if major haematic concentrations have been found, when compared with those found in non-obese patients. The meaning of this is not clear; the hypothesis is that alterations have taken place in the proteic link or in the acetylcholine receptors.[49]

Nitrous oxide

A gaseous, inhaling agent with low liposolubility and which is difficult to metabolize, this represents a rational choice in the obese patient. The only limitation is the impossibility of using high percentages of O_2 in the inspiratory mixture in order to always provide adequate oxygenation.

Volatile agents

It was suggested in the past that these resulted in a prolonged recovery time as a result of the accumulation in the adipose tissue.[50,51] This has not been confirmed by further studies, which suggests that reduced tissue perfusion could inhibit the formation of deposits of these substances.

Halothane and enfluorane are metabolized producing high levels of urinary catabolites,[50,52] whereas isofluorane and desfluorane, which are less metabolized, are considered the drugs of choice. With regards to sevofluorane, the first studies on its biotransformation and plasmatic fluoride levels gave similar results in both obese patients and those of normal weight. In particular Frink et al.[53] demonstrated that, with a Minimal Alveolar Concentration (MAC) = 2.05 (1.4 MAC/h) the concentrations of fluoride ions during and after anaesthesia did not differ in either group.

In contrast, Higuchi et al.,[54] with a MAC of a much higher dosage of sevofluorane (MAC 4.5/h), found haematic peaks of fluorides higher than 50 nmo/l for about two hours and an increased urinary secretion of the same in the first 24 hours without the occurrence of alterations in the renal functionality in the first 48 hours after surgery.

In the same study, the authors compared isofluorane and sevofluorane, showing that there are no differences in the MAC-awake of the two agents (0.14 per cent for isofluorane; 0.17 per cent for sevofluorane), even when varying their concentration, the duration of the inhalation and the class of obesity.[54]

Local anaesthetics and opiates

Intrathecally administered, the kinetics and dynamics of these drugs have only been partially explained. It is understood that as a result of the higher content of extradural fat, a greater initial dose of the drug is required, and this factor together with the venous blockage, which reduces the dimensions of the extradural space, would increase the segmental distribution of the anaesthetic, with anaesthetic levels larger than those we would have expected.

For these reasons doses of the drug required for surgery analgesia, calculated on the basis of the total body weight, must be reduced by 20–25 per cent,[55–57] whereas for the post-operative analgesia variations are unnecessary for non-obese patients.[58]

Evaluating the Patient Before Anaesthesia

Obese patients with positive anamnesis regarding pneumopathy and/or cardiopathy who are subject to abdominal or thoracic surgery present an increased morbidity due to the higher incidence of post-operative complications.[59] For hysterectomies via the abdomen and in major abdominal surgery[60] the mortality is increased. Emergency surgery involves an additional risk, even if the data at our disposal do not always agree on this subject.

Different anaesthesiological approaches have been recommended, but no technique has demonstrated advantages when compared to others.

Pre-operative visit

A scrupulous evaluation is necessary during the pre-operative visit in order to assess the cardiovascular, pulmonary and metabolic situation. A meticulous anatomic inspection is needed in order to find predictable parameters for difficult intubations. As usual, it is in this phase that all necessary information must be obtained, including the chosen anaesthesiological technique and its related problems. It also covers any need for post-operative analgesic treatments such as epidural analgesia and possible admission to ITU. The usefulness of early post-operative mobilization should be emphasized and the opportunity taken to highlight the advantages of both passive and active physiotherapy. It is useful to stress that the overweight person has often been taking antidepressants and/or sedatives for years and is therefore subject to a psychological weakness which strongly affects his behaviour both in the pre- and post-operative phases. Furthermore it is vital that a trusting relationship is formed between the anaesthetist and the patient. This should be based on an exhaustive exchange of information, which is fundamental in achieving a calm induction phase and it is also an aid to achieving a post-operative regaining of consciousness without uncontrolled reactions.

Cardiovascular evaluation

This is based on the study of:

- ECG (12 derivations) in order to look for ventricular (left or right) ischemia and hypertrophy signs;
- the measurement of non invasive blood pressure (NIBP) with a cuff as large as the patient's arm (since the standard one easily overestimates the real values of the blood pressure);
- a chest X-ray, used to check for myocardial hypertrophia and/or signs of pulmonary congestion and atelectasic areas.

The presence of increased cardiac diameters together with a hypertrophic left ventricular wall is frequently associated with a hypertensive status. This condition results in a normal ventricular reaction to exercise, which does not occur in the obese when there is no increase in the augmentation of the left ventricle, if body weight is more than 100 pounds in excess of the norm. Instead, in patients whose weight exceeds 170 per cent of the ideal, a decrease in the ventricular reaction to the effort occurs with the progressive increase in the thickness of the left ventricle.[61] This is particularly significant as the cardiovascular stress suffered by patients in the peri-operative period is similar to that observed during physical effort.[62]

Respiratory apparatus evaluation

This is still based on the study of the chest X-ray, pulmonary function tests and arterial blood–gas analysis in both sitting and supine positions. In anamnesis we have to look for episodes of obstructive apnoea occurring during sleep, secondary to obstructions and/or closing of the upper airways.[63]

Haematochemical evaluation

Evaluation includes:

- determining the haemoglobin level for evidence of polycythaemia which must suggest the presence of chronic hypoxia;
- serum chemistry studies;
- renal and hepatic functionality tests;
- a study of coagulation parameters.

Finally, in the case of positive anamnesis a precise definition of thyroid function is recommended considering the serious haemodynamic disorders due to thyroid disease which may occur in both the intra- and post-operative phases.

The pre-operative visit finishes with the search for possible pharmacological therapies which could interfere with anaesthesia, for example amphetamine,[64] anti-hypertensive drugs, antidepressants, oral anti-diabetic drugs and treatments with insulin. All of these are frequently found in the treatment of different organ pathologies affecting the obese patient, even though they could create problems that are difficult to resolve in both the intra- and post-operative phases. It is not recommended that treatment be varied from that which would be given to a person of normal weight, with the exception of post-operative glycaemia for which one should remain particularly alert.

Pre-medication

Opinions vary on the use of sedative and opiate drugs in pre-medication due to the concrete risk of causing prolonged respiratory depression that would be hard to treat.[65] Opiates should certainly be avoided, whereas short and ultra short action duration benzodiazepines (midazolam) seem not to cause problems of this kind.[66,67] These drugs should be administrated by intravenous injections or sublingual pills, since subcutaneous and intramuscular administration involves a certain level of unpredictable absorption. In cases where a patient needs to be intubated whilst conscious and at discretion in other cases, it is good practice to administrate a vagolytic agent to reduce possible sialorrhoea. Anti-H_2 drugs, such as Ranitidine (100 mg e.v.), are better than Cimetidine for their more prolonged action and lack of side effects on the hepatic metabolism, and Metoclopramide, a prokinetic drug, which has a constrictor effect on the oesophageal sphincter.[65] This pre-treatment in the obese patient is always necessary because unexpected and difficult orotracheal intubation (OTI) is frequent. This can lead to repeated attempts to intubate the patient by laryngoscopy with the possibility that regurgitated gastric juice might end up being accidentally inhaled.

Intubation

Particular attention should be paid to all the parameters that can predict a difficult intubation. Morbidly obese patients represent a difficult test even for a skilled anaesthetist since they are the extreme expression of unfavourable anatomic conditions.[68]

In synthesis, these patients present all or part of the following 'negative' characteristics:

- large tongue;
- poor cervical spine mobility;

- limited atlanto-occipital articulation;
- accumulation of fat in the oropharyngeal spaces;
- short or 'absent' neck.

Poor cervical spine mobility is present at different levels and it is at times worsened by the presence of a conspicuous adipose gibbus which does not allow the extension of the head over the neck. Furthermore, the obese have conspicuous accumulations of tissue in the para-tonsilar and para-glottic areas that can mask both the visibility and the accessibility of the glottis during the laryngoscopy.[56]

A large tongue is highlighted by the characteristic print of the teeth on the lateral edges of the tongue and by the disproportion between the latter and the oral cavity.

Together with these evident anatomic limitations we have to consider pathophysiologic alterations which do not allow exploration of the airways by laryngoscopy during sedation. This depends on the fact that these patients are very often affected by Obstructive Sleep Apnoea Syndrome (OSAS) and by other ventilation disorders due to the obstruction of the pharynx–larynx area that make spontaneous breathing difficult. Sometimes a modest degree of sedation can unbalance an already precarious situation and cause a sudden fall of coronary flow rate (CFR) resulting in acute respiratory insufficiency.[55,69] It is important to correlate the problematic OTI in the obese patient with 'difficult airways' and evaluate according to external parameters such as:

- Mallampati classification (to evaluate the relative dimensions of the tongue with respect to the oral and pharyngeal capacity);
- thyromental distance (to evaluate the mandibular space);
- mobility of atlanto-occipital and temporo-mandibulary articulations;
- view of head and neck seen opposite and in profile (to evaluate the morphologic characteristics such as dimensions, shape, congenital anomalies).

If we refer to the decisional algorithms for difficult intubation, the obese must be placed in the patient category in which a certain difficulty could be predictable. This difficulty, often evaluated as severe, is associated with a further disadvantage related to the kind of patient who is difficult or impossible to ventilate by mask. Therefore, it might be prudent to proceed with OTI, with a colleague and equipment for difficult ventilation and intubation, in order to apply all the alternative techniques appropriate to difficult airways which are illustrated in decisional algorithms approved by scientific societies.[70]

If the patient agrees, the possibility should be considered of intubating him whilst still conscious, using a local anaesthetic without sedation and through the use of the flexible fibreoptic bronchoscope (FOB).

It has been useful, in many cases, for the anaesthetist to delicately perform a laryngoscopic manoeuvre in order to create a working area enough large to allow a good articulation of the distal tip of the FOB. This procedure has been chosen in order to help those who use the endoscope when adopting an orotracheal approach. Furthermore, it is important to remember that if we adopt a rhino-tracheal approach, one must first go beyond the nasal duct with the FOB and then, when the instrument is well placed in the trachea, to move past the choanae with the tracheal tube, and to delicately move it through the FOB in the trachea. This sequence of manoeuvres is necessary to avoid a nasal haemorrhage caused by an attempt to move the tube too early. The nasal haemorrhage would mask the laryngeal entrance making it difficult to see both the glottis and the trachea with the scope and it may cause the conditions for blood inhalation.

In connection with these problems, we recommend the use of a scope expressly developed for this kind of manoeuvre and equipped with a large aspiration canal. Such an instrument can quickly eliminate possible secretions and, having thick distal end, is suitably resistant to the considerable pressures to which it is often subject during these manoeuvres.

Other procedures using retrograde OTI must be avoided, as they conflict with the unfavourable anatomy of the obese patient. This anatomy is characterized by abundant pre-tracheal panniculus adipose tissue in a generally short or absent neck. This makes exploratory injections, in order to safely introduce metallic mandrels, difficult if not impossible.

Therefore, in the case of anticipated difficult intubation, the decision–action procedure is very linear if the patient is collaborative. On the other hand, everything is much more difficult when the patient does not collaborate or when they absolutely oppose the above mentioned manoeuvres. In that case, the specialist has to continue, as the eventual operation could present urgent characteristics and it might not be possible to delay. As it is impossible to operate using loco-regional anaesthesia, the specialist must adopt a rapid induction followed by neuromuscular block with depolarizing drug, carefully pre-oxygenating the patient and positioning them on the operating table in the best way.[71]

Correct pre-oxygenation, a precaution which is not always respected, is fundamental to execute one or more attempts with OTI whilst maintaining good levels of arterial O_2 saturation. It is well known that the necessary time to execute laryngoscopy and subsequent intubation is directly proportional to the extent of difficulty in exposing the larynx and inversely proportional to the ability of the performer of the manoeuvre.

A pre-oxygenation with high percentage of O_2 in the mask is always recommended since even an experienced anaesthetist needs 30–60 seconds to complete laryngoscopy, intubation and control over the success of the manoeuvre. Pre-oxygenation can be obtained by asking the patient to inhale deeply and very frequently for one minute, or with low current volumes and low frequencies for 3–4 minutes. The comparison between the two techniques (ventilation with current volume with O_2 100 per cent with a flux of 4 litres per minute for 5 minutes and ventilation with four respiratory acts at high volumes with O_2 100 per cent) has revealed that both have been equally successful in raising the PaO_2 up to values such as 300 mmHg. Furthermore, the time for desaturation ($SaO_2 < 90$ per cent) in the obese patient (with a weight not exceeding 45 kg compared to the ideal weight) was 247 seconds, and 163 seconds in the super-obese by oxygenation for 5 minutes.[71]

Before proceeding with laryngoscopy, it is necessary to correctly position the head. A direct laryngoscopy, ending up with an intubation, involves the alignment of the oral, pharyngeal and laryngeal axes so that the passage from the incisors to the glottis is rectilinear.

If the head is simply placed on a horizontal plane (without any support underneath), the oral, pharyngeal and laryngeal axes form a C-shaped figure.

To obtain the alignment of the laryngeal axis with the pharyngeal axis, the neck must be flexed on the thorax to an angle of about 30° raising the head about 10 cm with supports placed under the occiput (shoulders remaining on the operating table). To align the oral axis with both the pharyngeal and the laryngeal ones, we have to extend the head over the neck (extension at the level of the atlanto-occipital articulation) so that the angle between the occipital-nasal axis would be 80–85 per cent with the long axis of the neck and the facial plane at a 15° angle to the horizontal plane. This position of head over neck is commonly called sniffing position and it is a light flexion of neck on thorax and marked extension of head on neck at the level of the atlanto-occipital articulation.[72]

To obtain a correct sniffing position in the obese, it is always useful to raise the scapular area, shoulders and the base of neck with some supports, such as rolled sheets, elastic materials, etc., in order to allow an appropriate flexion of neck on thorax and extension of head on neck. The aim of the supports placed under scapula, shoulders and neck is to allow the head to extend on the neck. The correct position must be evaluated when viewed laterally because only this perspective gives us precise information about the thoracic, neck, face and head axes. The complete extension of head without the elevation of the occiput is contraindicated, because this position increases the distance of the lips from the glottis, makes the larynx turn to the front, places the oral axis on different levels with both the pharyngeal and laryngeal ones and the teeth can cause lever movements with the blade of laryngoscope.

It has also been observed in practice that it is necessary to search for the optimal position of both head and neck before adopting anaesthesiologic induction and the subsequent laryngoscopy, since it is very difficult to adopt them later after different unsuccessful attempts of OTI.

As to the pharmacological choices, in complex cases, when intubation is difficult and the optimal sniffing position is not reached, it seems logical to adopt drugs which induce both anaesthesia and a neuromuscular blocking agent with a short lasting action (propofol, succinylcholine or mivacurium) in order to allow a quick recovery of consciousness and muscular strength suitable for spontaneous respiration, in case of OTI failure.

In conclusion, what is the right approach towards a morbidly obese patient who needs OTI?

Firstly it is always necessary to consider them a 'difficult' patient and, therefore, to mentally and physically prepare oneself for possible problems. Therefore, a trolley is necessary, equipped with all the instruments suitable for a patient who could undergo a difficult intubation.

The trolley should be equipped with the following instruments:

- flexible fibreoptic bronchoscope and ventilation mask with nozzle for the insertion of instruments;
- faryngoscopic blades in different sizes;
- introducers;
- mandrils;
- laryngeal mask;
- combitube;
- set for cricothyroidotomy;
- system for Jet ventilation;
- Bullard laryngoscope (optional).

It is important that each anaesthetist uses the FOB correctly and that every effort is made to acquire the instruments and knowledge (theoretical and practical courses) required to become a specialist.[73,74]

Positioning in the operating theatre

Positioning on a standard operating table can be difficult, so some operating theatres are equipped with two operating tables side by side which are jointly able to support weights of up to 300 kg.[48]

The anaesthesiologic induction must be performed on the operating table where the patient has been positioned when he was awake. In this way the patient, before undergoing anaesthesia, can signal any discomfort and avoid complications due to nervous compression in limbs and caused by prolonged uncomfortable positions.

As we have already explained, to obtain an optimal position for the intubation, the patient has to be in the sniffing position (light flexion of neck on head and extension of head on neck).

As to intra-operative positions for particular surgical demands, it is well-known that some of them, such as the Trendelenburg and lithotomic positions are not well tolerated since they modify endo-abdominal pressures, and movements alter the mechanical ventilatory parameters.

Prone positioning, instead, have to be considered. In a study performed on obese (BMI > 30 kg/m^2) patients[75] undergoing surgery on a herniated disc, it has been verified that the application of thoracic and pelvic supports, used to keep abdominal mobility and to avoid the pressure of the viscera on the diaphragm, improved the respiratory parameters. An increase in CFR may be observed due to both the reduced rising of the diaphragm and/or to the re-opening of atelectasic areas. Furthermore, pulmonary compliance, which decreases when in the supine position, improves due to a mechanism of alveolar recruitment of areas previously hypo-ventilated. On the other hand, the compliance of the thoracic wall was reduced, probably due to the action of the positioning supports, whereas total resistance and its components were not modified. Finally, the improvement of both CFR and static compliance (STC) turned out to be consistent with an increase in oxygenation.[75]

The lateral position, allowing a greater diaphragmatic range, turns out to be well tolerated as has been demonstrated by Brodsky *et al.* in the mono-pulmonary anaesthesia with FiO$_2$ corresponding to 1 in obese patients.[76]

Monitoring

The general criteria used to determine what kind of monitoring should be adopted depend on the type of surgical operation and the conditions from which the patients are suffering. In the obese these criteria are not wholly effective, because the general condition of these patients compels the specialist to scrupulously survey a wide range of parameters in order to have the best opportunity of overcoming all the possible complications linked to anaesthesia carried out on those with multiple organ and system deficiencies. The standards of monitoring proposed by the scientific societies can certainly fit the obese, but it is opportune to introduce a correction, that is recommending the extensive application of monitoring standards and the elimination of the habitual distinction between minor and major interventions. Furthermore, the need to monitor the degree of neuromuscular block with Peripheral Nerve Stimulator (PNS) must be highlighted, since the consequences of an over-dosage of neuromuscular blocking agent could, during emergence from anaesthesia, be much worse than those seen in normal subjects. For the same reason we should not disregard the monitoring of body temperature in the intra- and post-operative phases, due to the well-known side effects on the patient's haematosis.

General Anaesthesia

The induction of anaesthesia is a particularly delicate procedure, so that some authors recommend the contemporaneous presence of more than one anaesthetist in order to avoid possible difficulties represented by mask ventilation and difficult OTI. Furthermore, as mentioned above, it is necessary to have a trolley close at hand with all the necessary instruments for solving problems of any sort.

In our personal case histories, which include about 2,000 patients with as average BMI of 47 (range 37–72) we have observed a 3 per cent rate of difficult intubation (defined as an OTI which needed more than three laryngoscopies and non conventional procedures) while other studies even record a prevalence of 13 per cent.

Pre-oxygenation is necessary, as in the obese patient an inverse correlation between the degree of obesity and desaturation time has been demonstrated. Pre-oxygenation allows us to make further improvements to laryngoscopic manoeuvres without running the risk of early desaturation.[77]

Drugs used for induction can be both thiopental and propofol, whereas muscular relaxation is obtained with succinylcholine (1.2–1.5 mg/kg of IBW). We must always remember that the obese can have a pseudocholinesterase activity which is higher than normal[41] and which can determine a rapid metabolization of the drug.

Should the laryngoscopic vision be reduced (2nd degree: arytenoid cartilages; 3rd degree: epiglottis; 4th degree: soft palate) it would be useful to manipulate the larynx by pushing it backwards, upwards, right and in a posterior position (BURP: Back–Up–Right–Posterior). This manoeuvre generally improves laryngoscopic vision by at least one degree.

With respect to maintenance of anaesthesia, the superiority of one determined anaesthesiologic technique over another has not been demonstrated, but it seems that a balanced anaesthesia, whenever possible, is preferable. This is because it allows a better dosage of single drugs, a greater concentration of O_2, all the while reducing the concentration of volatile anaesthetics. It also results in an earlier extubation, reduces post-operative complications and gives a more satisfactory post-operative analgesia.[78]

Among opiates remifentanil is widely used for its pharmacokinetic characteristics, which make it the first drug of choice whenever a rapid post-operative recovery is needed.

As to neuromuscular blocking agents, one tends towards vecuronium and cisatracurium, favouring the latter due to its elimination (not organ dependent), and which even in the case of prolonged operations is not particularly affected by the numerous organ pathologies which can afflict the obese.

Mechanical ventilation is practised using an initial current volume of about 7–8 ml/kg of IBW which, associated with the reduced compliance of the thoracic wall and the rising of the diaphragm due to an increase in the intra-abdominal pressure, can cause the development of high peak pressures.

Premature hypoxia, observable in the first phases of anaesthesia, is linked to the reduced CFR, as a reduction in this parameter of about 50 per cent already occurs in the phase of anaesthesiologic induction (from 2.2 l to 1 l). It has been demonstrated that both manual hyper-inflation[58] and application of PEEP < 10–15 cm H_2O increase the CFR and improve oxygenation.[22]

Should decreases in SaO_2 occur, ventilation techniques which involve manoeuvres of increasing recruitment and the subsequent application of high PEEP, can also be useful. Pulmonary recruitment can be particularly valuable during laparoscopic operations where, due to a further increase in the intra-abdominal pressure, the rising of the diaphragm can be more marked. These manoeuvres must not result in exceeding determined values of peak pressure (not over 50 cm H_2O) and they must be conducted under strict haemodynamic monitoring.

The risk of intra-operative hypoxia can involve the use of elevated FiO_2 especially in patients with serious pulmonary and/or cardiovascular pathologies, and this can affect the choice of the inhaled gaseous mixture. Therefore it would be preferable to use a mix of air and O_2 with hypnosis maintained by anaesthetic vapours or intravenous drugs.[40]

During surgery it is possible, thanks to the aid of end tidal CO_2 (ETCO$_2$), analysis of arterial O_2 saturation and blood–gas analysis, to adjust the current volume and the extrinsic PEEP to avoid the hypocapnic conditions (PaCO$_2$ < 30 mmHg) responsible for an increase in shunt (as a result of the vasodilatation induced) and a reduction of the venous return. Moreover mere ETCO$_2$ is not a sufficient parameter for good ventilation because in the obese the difference between PaCO$_2$ and PetCO$_2$ is very marked due to the increase in the alveolar dead space.

We have little information on the haemodynamic alterations which occur during general anaesthesia in the obese. In a prospective study on patients subject to major abdominal surgery, a reduced correlation between LVSW and PAWP has been highlighted. This is an index of reduced left ventricular contractility, both during intubation and in the post-operative period, with consequent reduction in the cardiac index of 20–30 per cent.[31]

A recent study by El-Dawlatly[79] shows a significant reduction in the cardiac index of obese patients compared with patients of normal body weight subject to laparoscopic surgery. However the meaning of this alteration is not clear.

Extubation must be performed to achieve a complete resolution of the muscular blockage. It should be measured with a neuro-stimulator, and the presence of an adequate cough reflex could be considered appropriate. It may be prudent to suggest the use of a tube exchanger, in case it is necessary to facilitate a rapid reintubation, and to prevent the inhalation of the gastric contents.

Patients with positive anamnesis linked to respiratory and/or cardiovascular disease, serious endocrinopathy and uncontrollable hypertension are expected to be admitted to intensive care. This is also expected for patients subject to major abdominal or thoracic operations. It is possible that an incomplete resolution of neuromuscular block, a state of maintained post-anaesthetic sedation or a particularly intense post-operative shivering can all compromise post-operative recovery, even after simple operations. In these cases therefore it is advisable to be very cautious and to monitor the patients in intensive care units until post-operative recovery is complete.

Loco-Regional Anaesthesia

Loco-regional anaesthesia, when possible, is recommended by the majority of authors. The difficulties in its execution are essentially linked to the loss of the traditional anatomic landmarks. Epidural or subarachnoidal anaesthesia can be less difficult than expected since the median dorsal line presents a minor layer of fat compared to the lateral zones. With both techniques, epidural or subarachnoidal needles longer than 10 cm make procedures particularly difficult. To carry out the procedure it is preferable to have the patient sit down, the epidural space then being more easily identifiable through the loss of resistance technique.

A subarachnoidal block is technically less difficult than an epidural block, but its extension is often unpredictable, the onset is slower and latency time is longer, even over 30 minutes for its completion.[58]

The major cephalic diffusion of the anaesthetic occurring after the block is linked to the increase in the adipose tissue, with consequent reduced dimensions of the subarachnoid space. It has been observed that blocks extending to levels higher than T5 can cause serious respiratory repercussions in obese patients with pre-existing pulmonary diseases and also severe vascular collapses due to sympathetic block. This can be partially compensated for by preventive infusion of liquids. With the epidural technique, doses of local anaesthetic necessary for surgical anaesthesia are generally reduced by 20–25 per cent. This is due to the reduced volume in the epidural space in consequence of the conspicuous presence of adipose tissue and the increase in the haematic venous content shifted by the vena cava due to the increase in abdominal pressure. The difficulties in executing peripheral regional blocks can be limited by using isolated needles of the appropriate length and a neuro-stimulator[80] which naturally amplifies the sensibility of the operator and limits the consumption of drug. Intra-venous anaesthesia (Bier block) is contra-indicated by the frequent diffusion of the anaesthetic which, even if used in doses related to IBW, can cause serious episodes of cardiac and neurological toxicity.[81]

When these loco-regional techniques are adopted, it is desirable that the patient has adequate monitoring, oxygen therapy and a very mild sedation in order not to alter a very labile equilibrium. In these cases all the necessary instruments must be available to deal with probable respiratory and/or cardiovascular complications, as well as all that is necessary to convert this technique into a general anaesthesia.

Morbid obesity during pregnancy is frequently associated with diabetes, hypertension, pre-eclampsia, high incidence of caesarean section and premature births affected by macrosomia. In these patients, in addition to the technical problems linked to obesity and its related pathologies, there are the difficulties related to the need to operate in a state of emergency.[82] Such operations often include respiratory complications resulting from a difficult intubation and more frequently than in other situations, it is necessary to follow a decisional algorithm.

Post-Operative Treatment

This focuses on:

- prevention and treatment of the probable cardiocirculatory, respiratory and thromboembolic complications;
- endocrine disorders or imbalances;
- inadequate control of post-operative pain.

In the post-operative phase, respiratory complications are three times higher in the obese. Body weight, BMI or tests of respiratory preoperative functionality do not seem to correlate to the occurrence of such complications. What is more frequently observed is respiratory insufficiency accompanied by more or less marked degrees of hypoxia. These are natural consequences of a reduction in CFR and a high incidence of basal atelectasis which are produced in the first phases of surgery under general anaesthetic.

Two particularly effective techniques in preventing the development of atelectasic areas have been described: ventilation at two different pressures (BIPAP) and ventilation with continuous positive non-invasive[83] pressure (CPAP). Each technique must be carried out with a scrupulous monitoring of the vital parameters (ECG, FC, SaO_2, PA, FR) and signs such as muscular effort, cough efficiency, level of consciousness of the patient, the appearance of bronchial obstruction and development of infection.

Patients with OSA can be subject to serious obstructions of the upper airways. Some post-operative deaths have in the past been attributed to pulmonary embolism, seemingly caused by acute and severe post-operative hypoxia.

Respiratory insufficiency more frequently appears in the first three days post-operatively and can last for 4–6 days. The need for mechanical ventilatory support is fairly rare and is necessary only for anxious and non-collaborative patients, the over 50s, cardiopathic patients and those who suffer pre-operatively from hypercapnea and who develop fever in the post-operative period when they undergo major surgical operations.

Different measures can be taken to reduce the incidence of these kinds of complications:

- keep the patient in a semi-sitting position (30–45°) for several days;
- early mobilization;
- active respiratory physiokinesitherapy;
- optimization of the post-operative analgesia.[78]

Cardiomyopathy linked to reduced left ventricular contractility, observed in the immediate post-operative phase, contributes to increased post-operative mortality rates. Pulmonary embolic complications, which according to some studies are often fatal, are observed post-operatively in 5–12 per cent of obese patients[84,85] and are promoted by the frequency of deep vein thrombosis resulting from polycythaemia, increased haematic volume, reduced fibrinolytic activity and stasis of vena cava secondary to the increased abdominal pressure and prolonged immobilization.

On this subject, a recent study of the coagulation function in pre-operative morbidly obese patients has revealed the presence of anomalies such as accelerated formation of fibrin, activation of the blood platelet function and of interaction between fibrinogen and blood platelets.

These elements, correlated with the pre-operative presence of an increased concentration of fibrinogen and the factor inhibiting the activation of plasminogen (released by the adipose tissue), confirm the tendency to hyper-coagulation present in these patients.[86]

This condition could also explain the increased frequency of thromboembolic complications connected to the insertion of canula in central veins observed by some authors.[87]

As to the percentage of post-operative mortality, opinions differ, but there is consensus on the evidence of increased morbidity due to respiratory, embolic and infective complications.[88] What is more, with the exception of an improvement in PaO_2 as a result of slimming, no study has demonstrated that pre-operative weight loss reduces the frequency of morbidity and/or post-operative mortality.

Conclusions

Different anaesthesiologic techniques have been recommended for the obese patient, but none of them have demonstrated real advantages over others. In general both the anaesthetist's knowledge and experience in avoiding complications are determining factors in improving the outcome of surgery. What we can conclude from the above-mentioned problems is that these kinds of patients require the greatest level of concentration on the part of the anaesthesiologists, even when the procedure is brief and straightforward. All these procedures are more complex (both from the point of view of human effort and the equipment required) than those required for patients of normal body weight.

References

1. Bray, G.A. (1992). Pathophysiology of obesity. *Am J Clin Nutr* 55: 488s–494s.
2. Shenkman, Z., Shir, Y., Brodsky, J.B. (1993). Perioperative management of the obese patient. *Br J Anaesth* 70: 349–359.
3. Schwartz, A.E., Matteo, R.S. Ornstein, E. *et al.* (1992). Pharmacokinetics and pharmacodynamics of vecuronium in the obese surgical patient. *Anesth Analg* 74: 515–518.
4. Tsueda, K., Warren, J.E., McCafferty, A. *et al.* (1978). Pancuronium bromide requirement during anesthesia for the morbidly obese. *Anesthesiology* 48: 438–439.

5. Burton, W.N., Chen, C.Y., Shultz, A.B. et al. (1998). The economic costs associated with body mass index in a workplace. *J Occup Envir Med* 40 (9): 786–792.
6. Adams, J., Murphy, P.G. (2000). Obesity in anaesthesia and intensive care. *Br J Anaesth* 85: 91–108.
7. Kushner, R.F. (1993). Body weight and mortality. *Nutr Rev* 51: 127–136.
8. Banegas, J.R., Lopez Garcia, E., Gutierrez Fisac, J.L. et al. (2003). A simple estimate of mortality attributable to excess weight in the European Union. *Eur J Clin Nutr* 57(2): 201–208.
9. Sjostrom, L.V. (1992). Morbidity of severely obese subjects. *Am J Clin Nutr* 55: 5085–515S.
10. Bjorntorp, P. (1997). Obesity. *Lancet* 350: 423–426.
11. Braunwald, E., Isselbacher, K., Petersdorf, R.G. et al. (1987). *Harrison's Principles of Internal Medicine*, 11th ed. New York, McGraw-Hill.
12. Pivalizza, E.G., Pivalizza, P.J., Weavind, L.M. (1997). Perioperative thromboelastography and sonoclot analysis in morbidly obese patients. *Can J Anaesth* 44: 942–945.
13. Benumof, J.L. (2000). Obstructive sleep apnea in the adult obese patient: implication for airway management. *J Clin Anesth* 13: 144–156.
14. Alexander, J.K., Burthie, A.E., Sakaguchi, H. et al. (1959). Lung volume changes with extreme obesity. *Clin Res* 7: 171.
15. Ray, C., Sue, D., Bray, G. et al. (1983). Effects of obesity on respiratory function. *Am Rev Respir Dis* 128: 501–506.
16. Vaughan, R.W. (1982). Anesthetic management of the morbidly obese patient. In: Brown, B.R., Blitt C.D. et al. (eds). *Anesthesia and the Obese Patient*, pp. 71–94, New York, Davis Company.
17. Seidell, J.C., Deerenberg, I. (1994). Obesity in Europe: prevalence and consequences for use of medical care. *Pharmacoeconomics* 5(Suppl 1): 38–44.
18. Pelosi, P., Croci M., Ravagnan I. et al. (1996). Total respiratory system, lung and chest wall mechanics in sedated-paralyzed postoperative morbidly obese patients. *Chest* 109: 144–151.
19. Hedenstierna, G., Santesson, J., (1976). Breathing mechanics, dead-space and gas exchange in the extremely obese, breathing spontaneously and during anaesthesia with intermittent positive ventilation. *Acta Anaesthesiol Scand* 20: 248–254.

20. Bardoczky, G.I., Yernault, J.C., Houben, J.J. et al. (1995). Large tidal volume does not improve oxygenation in morbidly obese patients during anesthesia. *Anesth Analg* 81: 385–388.
21. Pelosi, P., Ravagnan, I., Giuriati, G. et al. (1999). Positive end-expiratory pressure improves respiratory function in obese but not in normal subjects during anesthesia and paralysis. *Anesthesiology* 91(5): 1221–1231.
22. Santesson, J. (1976). Oxygen transport and venous admixture in the extremely obese. Influence of anaesthesia and artificial ventilation with and without positive end-expiratory pressure. *Acta Anaesthesiol Scand* 20: 387–394.
23. Lachmann, B. (1992). Open the lung and keep the lung open. *Intensive Care Med* 18: 319–322.
24. Whalen, F.X., Gajic, O., Thompson, G.B. et al. (2006). The effects of the alveolar recruitment maneuver and positive end-expiratory pressure on arterial oxygenation during laparoscopic bariatric surgery. *Anaesth Analg* 102: 298–305.
25. Lean, M.E. (1999). Obesity and cardiovascular disease: the waisted years. *Br J Cardiol* 6: 269–273.
26. Alpert, M.A., Hashimi, M.V. (1993). Obesity and the heart. *Am J Med Sci* 306: 117–123.
27. Berkalp, B., Cesur, V., Corapcioglu, D. et al. (1995). Obesity and left ventricular diastolic function. *Int J Cardiol* 52: 23–26.
28. Wirth, A. (2001). Hypertension and cardiomyopathy in obesity. Treat the heart simultaneously. *MMW Fortschr Med* 143(42): 39–42.
29. Alexander, J.K. (1963). Obesity and the circulation. *Mod Concepts Cardiovasc Dis* 32: 799–803.
30. Buckley, F.P., Robinson, N.B., Simonowitz, D.A. et al. (1983). Anasthesia in the morbidly obese. A comparison of anaesthetic and analgesic regimens for upper abdominal surgery. *Anaesthesia* 38: 840–851.
31. Agarwal, N., Shibutani, K.J., Sanfilippo, J.A. et al. (1982). Haemodynamic and respiratory changes in surgery of the morbidly obese. *Surgery* 92: 226–234.
32. Alexander, J.K. (1964). Obesity and cardiac performance. *Am J Cardiol* 14: 860–865.
33. Benotti, P.N., Bistrain B., Benotti J.R. et al. (1992). Heart disease and hypertension in severe obesity: the benefits of weight reduction. *Am J Clin Nutr* 55: 586–590.

34. Oberg, B., Poulsen, T.D. (1996). Obesity. An anaesthetic challenge. *Acta Anaesthesiol Scand* 40: 191–200.
35. Duflou, J., Birmani, R., Burke A. et al. (1995). Sudden death as a result of heart disease in morbid obesity. *Am Heart J* 130: 306–313.
36. Harter, R.L., Kelly, W.B., Kramer, M.G. et al. (1998). A comparison of the volume and pH of gastric contents of obese and lean surgical patients. *Anesth Analg* 86(1): 147–152.
37. Seidell, J.C., Deerenberg, I. (1994). Obesity in Europe: prevalence and consequences for use of medical care. *Pharmacoeconomics* 5(Suppl 1): 38–44.
38. Jung, D., Mayersohn, M., Perrier, D. et al. (1982). Thiopental disposition in lean and obese patients undergoing surgery. *Anesthesiology* 56: 269–274.
39. Greenblatt, D.J., Abernethy, D.R., Locniskar, A. et al. (1984). Effect of age, gender and obesity on Midazolam kinetics. *Anesthesiology* 61: 27–35.
40. Frederique, J., Farinotti, R., Haberer, J.P. et al. (1993). Propofol infusion for maintenance of anesthesia in morbidly obese patients receiving nitrous oxide. *Anesthesiology* 78: 657–665.
41. Bentley, J.B., Bond, J.D., Vaughan, R.W. et al. (1982). Weight, pseudocholinesterase activity and succinylcholine requirements. *Anesthesiology* 57: 48–49.
42. Cheymol, G. (2000). Effects of obesity on pharmacokinetics implications for drug therapy. *Clin Pharmacokinetic* 39(3): 215–231.
43. Egan, T.D., Huizinga, B., Gupta S.K. et al. (1998). Remiphentanil pharmacokinetics in obese versus lean patients. *Anesthesiology* 89: 562–573.
44. Lemmens, H.J., Brodsky J.B. (2006). The dose of succinylcholine in morbid obesity. *Anesth Analg* 102: 438–442.
45. Matteo, R.S., Schwartz, A.E., Ornstein, E. et al. (1989). Pharmacokinetics and pharmacodynamics of pancuronium in the obese surgical patient. *Abstract J Anesthesiol* 71: A820.
46. Taivainen, T., Tuominen, M., Rosenberg, P.H. (1990). Influence of obesity on the spread of spinal analgesia after injection of plain 0.5 per cent bupivacaine at the Ll3–L4 and L4–L5 interspace. *Br J Anaesth* 64: 542–546.
47. Schimth, V.D., Fielder-Kelly, J., Phillis, L. et al. (1997). Prospective use of population pharmacokinetics/pharmacodynamics in the development of Cisatracurium. *Pharm Res* Jan 14(1): 91–97.
48. Sarr, M.G., Felty, C.L., Hilmer, D.M. et al. (1995). Technical and practical considerations involved in operations on patients weighing more than 270 kg. *Arch Surg* 130: 102–105.

49. Van Itallie, T.B. (1994). Worldwide epidemiology of obesity. *Pharmacoeconomics* 5(Suppl 1): 1–7.
50. Blovin, R.A., Kolpek, J.H., Mann, H.J. (1987). Influence of obesity on drug disposition. *Clin Pharm* 6: 706–714.
51. Fischer, A., Waterhouse, T.D., Adams, A.P. (1975). Obesity: its relation to anaesthesia. *Anaesthesia* 30: 633–647.
52. Miller, M.S., Gandolfi, A.J., Vaughan, R.W. et al. (1980). Disposition of enflurane in obese patients. *J Pharmacol Exp Ther* 215: 292–296.
53. Frink, E.J. Jr, Brown, E.A., Morgan, S. et al. (1993). Plasma inorganic fluoride levels with Sevofluorane anesthesia in morbidly obese and non obese patients. *Anesth Analg* 76: 1333–1337.
54. Higuchi, H., Satoh, A., Kanno, M. (1993). Endoserum inorganic fluoride levels in morbidly obese patients during and after sevofluorane anesthesia. *Anesth Analg* 6: 260–270.
55. Connolly, L.A. (1991). Anesthetic management of obstructive sleep apnea patients. *J Clin Anesth* 3(6): 461–469.
56. Lee, J.J., Larson, R.M., Buckley, J.J. et al. (1982). Airway maintenance in the morbidly obese. *Anesthesiol Rev* 7: 33–36.
57. Shenkman, Z., Shir, Y., Brodsky, J.B. (1993). Perioperative management of the obese patient. *Br J Anaesth* 70: 349–359.
58. Hodgkinson, R., Hussein, F.J. (1980). Obesity and the spread of analgesia following epidural administration of bupivacaine for caesarean section. *Anesth Analg* 59: 89–93.
59. Cooper, J.R., Brodsky, J.B. (1987). Anesthetic management of the morbidly obese patient. *Semin Anesth* 6: 260–270.
60. McCulloch, W.J., Littlewood, D.G. (1986). Influence of obesity on spinal analgesia with isobaric 0.5 per cent Bupivacaine. *Br J Anaesth* 58: 610–614.
61. Alpert, M.A., Singh, A., Terry, B.E. et al. (1989). Effect of exercise on left ventricular systolic function and reserve in morbid obesity. *Am J Cardiol* 63: 1478–1482.
62. Paul, D.R., Hoyt, J.L., Boutros, A.R. (1976). Cardiovascular and respiratory changes in response to change in posture in the obese. *Anesthesiology* 45: 73.
63. Ryan, C.F., Lovel, L. (1996). Mechanical properties of the velopharynx in obese patients with obstructive sleep apnea. *Am J Resp Critic Care Med* 154: 806–812.

64. Jeffers, L.A. (1996). Anesthetic considerations for the new antiobesity medications. *AANA J* 64(6): 541–544.
65. Damia, G., Mascheroni, D., Croci, M. *et al.* (1988). Perioperative changes in functional residual capacity in morbidly obese patients. *Br J Anaesth* 60: 574–578.
66. Brodsky, J.B. (1986). Anesthetic management of the morbidly obese patient. *Int Anesthesiol Clin* 24: 93–103.
67. Robertson, I.K., Eltringam, R.J. (1985). Anaesthetic management of the morbidly obese. *Br J Hosp Med* 42: 224–228.
68. Bond, A. (1993). Obesity and difficult intubation. *Anaesth Intensive Care* 21: 828.
69. Biro, P., Kaplan, V., Block, K.E. (1995). Anesthetic management of a patient with obstructive sleep apnea syndrome and difficult airway access. *J Clin Anesth* 7(5): 417–421.
70. Benumof, J.L. (2004). Obesity, sleep apnea, the airway and anesthesia. *Curr Opin Anaesthesiol* 17(1): 21–30.
71. Berthoud, M.C., Peacock, J.E., Reilly, C.S. (1991). Effectiveness of preoxygenation in morbidly obese patients. *Br J Anaesth* 67: 464–466.
72. Adnet, F., Baillard, C., Borron, S.W. *et al.* (2001). Randomized study comparing the "sniffing position" with simple head extension for laryngoscopic view in elective surgery patients. *Anesthesiology* 95(4): 836–841.
73. Erb, T., Hampl, K.F., Schürch, M. *et al.* (1999). Teaching the use of fiberoptic intubation in anesthetized, spontaneously breathing patients. *Anesth Analg* 89(5): 1292–1295.
74. Rosenblatt, W.H., Wagner, P.J., Ovassapian, A. *et al.* (1998). Practise patterns in managing the difficult airway by anesthesiologists in the United States. *Anesth Analg* 87(1): 153–157.
75. Pelosi, P., Croci, M., Calappi, E. *et al.* (1996). Prone positioning improves pulmonary function in obese patients during general anesthesia. *Anesth Analg* 83: 578–583.
76. Brodsky, J.B., Wyner, J., Ehrenwerth, J. *et al.* (1982). One-lung anesthesia in morbidly obese patients. *Anesthesiology* 57: 132–134.
77. Jense, H.G., Dubin, S.A., Silverstein, P.I. *et al.* (1991). Effect of obesity on safe duration of apnea in anesthetized humans. *Anesth Analg* 72: 89–93.

78. Rawal, N., Sjostrand, U., Christofferson, E. et al. (1984). Comparison of intramuscular and epidural morphine for postoperative analgesia in the grossly obese. Influence on postoperative ambulation and pulmonary function. *Anesth Analg* 63: 583–592.
79. El-Dawlatly, A.A. (2006). Hemodinamic profile during laparoscopic cholecystectomy versus laparoscopic bariatric surgery. The impact of morbid obesity. *Middle East J Anesthesiol* 18: 733–742.
80. Buckley, F.P. (1989). Anesthetizing the morbidly obese patient. *ASA Refresher Courses* 243: 1–6.
81. Holmes, C.M. (1963). Intravenous regional anaesthesia. *Lancet* 1: 245–246.
82. Hood, D.D., Dewan, D.M. (1993). Anaesthetic and obstetric outcome in morbidly obese parturients. *Anesthesiology* 79(6): 1210–1218.
83. Joris, J., Sottiaux, T., Chiche, J.D. et al. (1994). Bi-level CPAP (BIPAP) reduces the postoperative restrictive pulmonary syndrome in obese patients after gastroplasty. *Br J Anaesth* 72(Suppl 1): A111.
84. Fox, G.S., Whalley, D.G., Bevan, O.R. (1981). Anaesthesia for the morbidly obese: experience with 110 patients. *Br J Anaesth* 53: 811–816.
85. Fox, G.S. (1975). Anaesthesia for intestinal short circuiting in the morbidly obese with reference to the pathophysiology of gross obesity. *Can Anesth Soc J* 22: 307–315.
86. Postlethwaite, R.W., Johnson, W.D. (1972). Complications following surgery for duodenal ulcer in obese patients. *Arch Surg* 105: 438–440.
87. Mason, E.E., Renquist, K.E., Jiang, D. (1992). Perioperative risk and safety of surgery for severe obesity. *Am J Clin Nutr* 55: 573S–576S.
88. Song, D., Whitten, W., White, P.F. (2000). Remifentanil infusion facilities early recovery for obese outpatients undergoing laparoscopic cholecystectomy. *Anest Analg* 90: 1111–1113.

Chapter 3

Intragastric Balloon (BIB®) in the Management of Morbid Obesity Disease

Alfredo Genco, Roberta Maselli and Nicola Basso

Introduction

The natural history of patients suffering from pathological obesity is chequered with the repeated failures of dietary, behavioural and pharmaceutical therapies. Nowadays, only 6 per cent of the overweight patients who rely on diet treatment alone find an effective and radical solution to their serious problems.

The indications inherent to surgical treatment are, on the other hand, strictly specific, limited and even today, far from acceptable even to severely overweight patients. Bariatric surgery has, moreover, been shown to lead to a greater incidence of intra- and post-operative complications, directly correlated to the numerous diseases resulting from obesity.[1] It is often difficult to intubate and mechanically ventilate super-obese patients.[2] Studies have demonstrated that the probability of problematic intubation is proportionate to the circumference of the patient's neck, ranging from 5 per cent per 40 cm circumference, to 35 per cent per 60 cm circumference.[1] They have also shown that, because body weight is the chief factor underlying the determination of the arterial oxygenation tension in anaesthetized, overweight patients, there is less than 30 per cent respiratory compliance compared to normal-weight patients.[3] Most bariatric operations are now carried out laparoscopically. Technical-surgical and systemic problems induced by the pneumoperitoneum are far more evident than in other types of patients.[1] The presence of a considerable amount of intestinal fat leads to numerous technical difficulties: the operating area is often badly visualized, increased omental fat frequently obstructs visualization of the stomach, a 'fatty liver' cannot easily be mobilized by the retractors,[4] leading to a high rate of conversion to open surgery.[5]

As early as 1986 Pasulka *et al.* demonstrated how a modest preoperative weight loss (10–20 per cent) reduced surgical complications,[6] whether anaesthesia-based or not, resulting from bariatric surgery.

Consequently, over the last few years, the interest of 'insiders' operating in the sector has turned to remedies able to help patients to maintain restrictive and long-term diet programmes. These programmes aim at making dietary therapy more 'aggressive' and effective, thus leading to greater control of the co-morbidities in view of radical surgical treatment. One of these remedies is the intragastric balloon.

The concept underlying the use of an intragastric balloon in the treatment of obesity first saw the light in 1921 when Davies observed that patients with *bezoars* (partially digested agglomerates of hairs or vegetable fibres called, respectively, hair-balls or food-balls (tricobezioars or phytobezoars), often complained of post-prandial fullness, nausea and vomiting. This led to the idea of contriving a device which would imitate an intragastric bezoar by partially filling the stomach.[7]

The first intragastric balloon to be marketed was the Garren-Edwards Gastric Bubble (GEGB, American-Edwards Laboratories, Irvine, CA, USA), approved in 1985 by the Food and Drug Administration as a device co-adjuvant to diet and behaviour-modification treatments. The GEGB was a cylindrical, polyurethane contrivance, with a self-filling valve at one end through which a removable catheter for air inflation was inserted. It was placed inside the stomach by means of a dedicated introducer, then inflated with 220 ml of air. Removal was carried out endoscopically after puncturing the bubble (Fig. 1).

The device was used in the USA up to 1988, with over 25,000 placements. Between 1987 and 1989 numerous scientific studies devoted to it were published, expressing the unanimous conclusion that the GEGB was no more successful in achieving weight loss than dieting alone or modified alimentary behaviour.[8–14] The complications reported included: gastric

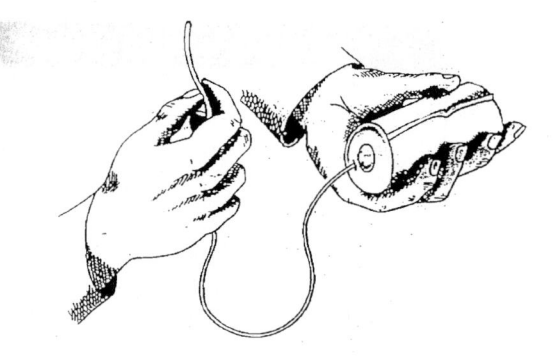

Figure 1. Garren-Edwards balloon.

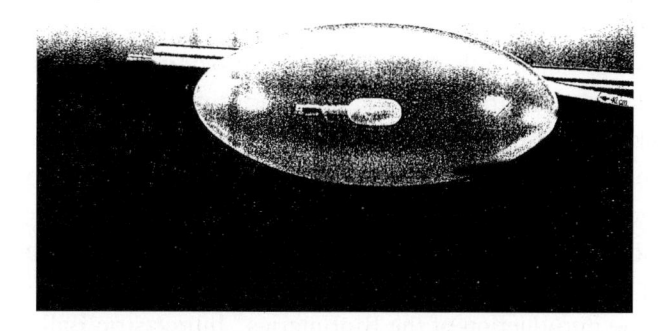

Figure 2. Ballobes intragastric balloon.

erosion (26 per cent), gastric ulcers (14 per cent), intestinal obstruction (2 per cent), Mallory–Weiss syndrome (11 per cent), oesophageal tears (1 per cent).[12] Due to the considerable collateral effects and lack of data supporting its efficacy, GEGB is no longer used and is now unavailable commercially.[15,16]

After the GEGB numerous modified intragastric balloons were introduced and evaluated in minor scientific studies. GEGB's lack of safety and efficacy was attributed, by some critics, to the low air-volume inflated into the balloon and to the material used in its fabrication. Among the various balloons presented, the 'Ballobes intragastric balloon' (DOT ApS, Rodovre, Denmark) deserves some attention (Fig. 2).

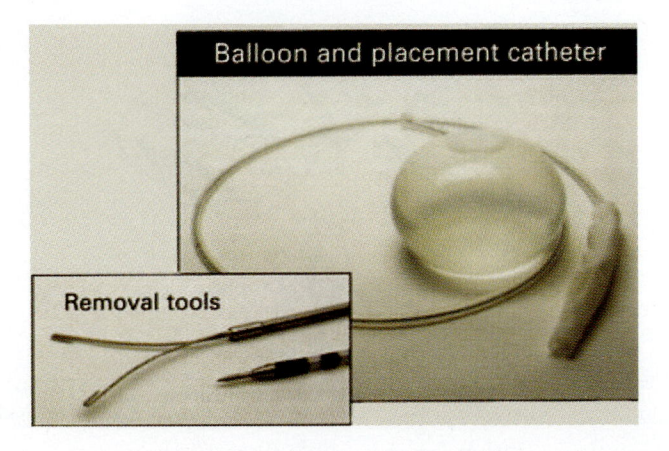

Figure 3. Intragastric Balloon BIB®.

This was inflated with about 475 ml of air but, in this case too, the relevant studies demonstrated no additional advantages of the balloon over dieting, physical exercise and modified eating habits. Despite the variations adopted, with respect to the original concept of a space-occupying, intragastric bubble, none of the devices conceived seemed to be effective and complication-free. For this reason they were, and are, no longer used in clinical practice.

With the introduction of the BioEnterics® Intragastric Balloon (BIB®, Allergan Inc., Irvine, CA, USA), a new chapter in the history of intragastric balloons is being written (Fig. 3).

BIB®: Characteristics and differences compared with the 1980s bubbles

In March 1987 a team of experts at Tarpon Springs (Florida, USA) defined the specifications of the ideal intragastric balloon (Table 1). Subsequently the BIB® intragastric balloon was launched on the market.

The BIB® system is made up of a soft, transparent, silicone balloon connected, by means of a radiopaque valve, to a 'placement' catheter with a 6.5 mm external diameter, also made of soft silicone. This catheter is stiffened by a metal guide-wire, which facilitates the movement of the balloon down the oesophagus during placement and is

Table 1. Ideal intragastric balloon characteristics.

Efficacy
Variable volume
Spherical shape
Soft surface
Filled with liquid
Radiopaque valve

---

connected to the valve, at both ends, by a 'Y-shaped' loop connected, in its turn, to the filling system. The fill volume advised is 500–700 ml of physiological solution and removal after 180 days is recommended. The addition of 10 ml of viable staining (methylene blue) to the physiological solution will colour the urine blue should the intragastric balloon break.[17]

Three fundamental factors clearly distinguish the BIB® intragastric balloon from the 1980s bubbles:

- the liquid content which makes it definitely more effective (greater sense of repletion);
- the 'self-sealing' radiopaque valve which increases safety because it gives the BIB® freedom of movement inside the gastric cavity rendering breakage before 180 days extremely rare;
- the spherical form and silicone structure which render the complication of ulcers extremely rare.

How it works

The efficacy of the BIB® in inducing weight loss is due not to a placebo effect but to the characteristics which make it effective 'in itself'.[18] How it actually works is only partially known and chiefly depends on the characteristics of the device:

- Its weight (the BIB® is filled with 500–700 ml of liquid), which massively stimulates the baroceptors located at the gastric wall level. These, through the brain-gut axis, stimulate the satiety centre located

at hypothalamic level; this mechanism is particularly active in the first two–three months post placement and diminishes during the following months.
- *Delayed gastric emptying:* an ultrasonographic study on gastric emptying pre- and post-placement of the BIB® was carried out at our institution. This highlighted the fact that in patients without the balloon, food could already be visualized by ultrasound in the antrum 32 minutes ± 12 minutes after the consumption of a solid, 800 Kcal meal. Thirty days after BIB® placement in the same patients, this study only visualized food in the antrum after 300 minutes ± 23 minutes. These data are supported in a recent study by Torres-Barrera *et al.* who demonstrated a reduced electric gastric activity deriving from intragastric balloon placement.[19]
- Reduction of unoccupied gastric volume by about 750 cm^3 due to the presence of the device.
- *Discomfort:* this term means the overall disorders (nausea, precocious sense of satiety, vomiting, epigastric pain) suffered during the first 24–30 hours post-placement and which may reappear during the six-month treatment, above all if the patient fails to adhere to the prescribed dietary regime.
- *Hormonal mechanisms:* in our experience during treatment with the BIB® in the first three months a significant increase in the plasmatic ghrelin levels was observed. This was followed by a gradual reduction until the basal levels were reached after removal, despite the persistence of the weight-loss. Other studies show hormonal variations in patients with the BIB®. Mion *et al.*[20] show that during BIB® treatment plasma ghrelin levels were significantly decreased (–3.8 to –20.7 ng/ml), despite concomitant weight loss. Weight reduction was significantly correlated to the ghrelin variations (0.212–0.885 ng/ml). We already know that the ghrelin is correlated to weight loss, but we still do not know exactly how.

Indications

The BIB® system is indicated for temporary use associated with a specific slimming programme using diet treatment under direct medical control, in patients with a history of obesity (at least five years), after numerous failures of dietary treatment only.

Present indications suggest BIB® placement in patients with:

- < 35 BMI if there are concurrent obese-related co-morbidities (e.g. cardiovascular, orthopaedic, metabolic etc.) whose resolution or improvement require mandatory weight loss;
- > 35 BMI, within the framework of anti-obesity treatment where the balloon plays a pre-surgery role in patients with co-morbidities, before any other type of surgery (orthopaedic, cardiac etc.), or in patients who refuse surgery;
- 'BIB® Test' to evaluate capacity to comply with a pre-established diet programme, in patients who are candidates for restrictive-type surgery and whose eating behaviour is difficult to pinpoint.

At the moment there are no specific limitations as regards age. The device can, therefore, also be used for children.

Contraindications

Placement of the BIB® is contraindicated, at present, in:

- voluminous hiatal hernia (>5 cm);
- oesophagitis > Grade II;
- duodenal ulcer;
- potential bleeding conditions of the upper gastrointestinal tract;
- outcomes of prior, major surgical operations on the gastrointestinal tract and/or certified adhesion syndrome;
- neoplasias;
- patients receiving chronic treatment with gastric irritants or anti-coagulants;
- patients with major or non-collaborative psychiatric disorders;
- alcohol or drug dependent patients;
- certified pregnancy;
- all inflammatory pathologies of the gastrointestinal tract (e.g. Crohn's disease, etc.).

Work up

All patients undergo the following clinical procedures:

- complete haemato-chemical tests;
- ECG and cardiologic video;
- diagnostic oesophago–gastro–duodenoscopy with HP analysis;
- endocrinologic/dietologic examination to exclude endocrine-based obesity;
- psychiatric examination to exclude psychiatric illness and to ascertain, if they exist, the type of the eating disorders (e.g. 'sweet eating', 'binge eating' etc.).

A chest X-ray, respiratory function tests and anaesthesiologic examination are required for super-obese patients with breathing difficulties. All the patients, after receiving accurate and exhaustive information, have to give their written consent.

Placement and removal technique

BIB® placement and removal can be performed in conscious sedation with Diazepam or Midazolam (80 per cent), in unconscious sedation with Propofol (15 per cent) or with orotracheal intubation (5 per cent). During placement the patient is in left lateral decubitus and a diagnostic oesophago–gastro–duodenoscopy is performed. The balloon is then positioned with the valve under the cardia and is filled, under endoscopic vision, with 500–700 ml of physiological solution and 10 ml vital staining solution (methylene blue). The connection catheter is removed and the valve checked for possible leaks. The mean duration of the procedure is 12 minutes.

Methylene blue is used for early identification of balloon rupture or valve leaks: should the intragastric balloon break, the solution will be absorbed and will colour the urine blue. For this reason it is important to sensitize the patient to ongoing urine observation before discharge from the hospital.

A diligent anamnesis is essential to exclude the presence of glucose-6-phosphate-dehydrogenase (G-6-PDH) deficit. Patients with this disease, like those afflicted with 'favism' could, in fact, suffer a haemolysis crisis due to the methylene blue. In these cases methylene blue cannot be used and possible balloon rupture or valve leaks can be ascertained ecographically.

BIB® removal is carried out after six months. Due to the delayed gastric emptying achieved with the balloon, the removal procedure should be preceded by a 72 hour, no-'roughage' diet and by a 24 hour semi-liquid diet (yoghurt, mashed potatoes, puréed vegetables). It is very important that the patient respect this diet in order to avoid '*ab ingestis*', chiefly when the procedure is performed in unconscious sedation. In these cases the patient should never lose the cough reflex.

The procedure foresees an oesophago–gastro–duodenoscopy to facilitate identification of the balloon and its subsequent deflation with a specific device. The BIB® is removed with a dedicated 'grasper' when completely deflated. Stomach observation is necessary to exclude possible mucosal lesions.

BIB® placement can be performed on in-patients, out-patients and in day hospitals; in Italy, to be able to claim refunding from the National Health Service, it is usually carried out on in-patients with at least two days' hospitalization. When it is performed on out-patients or in day hospitals, the patient must always be properly informed as to the adverse symptoms which may arise. It is essential, moreover, that close, ongoing follow-up be carried out to facilitate diagnosis and to be able to treat complications such as hydro-electrolitic imbalance or gastric dilation.

Post-placement pharmacological treatment

Due to the secondary effects deriving from the presence of the BIB® (nausea, regurgitation or vomiting, cramp-like epigastric pains) and from the almost total impossibility of eating during the first 24–36 hours, all patients must receive support treatment consisting in the infusion of electrolytic solutions, proton pump inhibitors, antispasmodic and antiemetic drugs.

Post-placement diet

On the first day the patient receives a liquid diet only. From the second and up to the sixth or seventh day a semi-liquid diet (yoghurt, mashed potatoes, puréed vegetables) is followed. The dietetic regime to be associated with the intragastric procedure has not yet been fully standardized but, as of the seventh or eighth day our patients receive a diet programme, prepared by the nutritionists. This foresees a daily intake of about 1000–1200 Kcal (68 g protein, 18 g lipids, 146 g glucids — at least 1 g protein/kg ideal weight), consumed over three main meals and two snacks. For the first three months, moreover, a multi-vitamin supplement is added. This dietetic regime is maintained until removal of the BIB®. Our experience shows that the daily consumption of a high volume of vegetables is inadvisable because they are difficult to digest. They clog up the gastric cavity and cause vomiting. It is therefore advisable to prescribe vegetables in soup form.

Follow-up

All patients are contacted by phone every day for the first seven days. On the eighth day they undergo an in-office clinical-nutritional examination. During the remaining period the patient undergoes every two weeks, alternatively, a clinical-nutritional examination and an evaluation carried out by one of the team of physicians that performed the procedure. The psychological assistance for the entire treatment (six months) is performed only if requested during the first pre-treatment work-up meeting, by the patients or by the psychologists themselves.

When there are signs (e.g. blue urine) or symptoms indicating a possible complication, an immediate clinical evaluation of the patient, and a possible oesophago–gastro–duodenoscopy, is essential. Decubital ulcers or gastrectasia indicate the need to remove the BIB®.

Before discharge the patient is made aware of the importance of optimum hydration and of ongoing urine checks, in order to diagnose in time the premature rupture of the BIB® or a possible valve leak. All the patients are, obviously, informed of the increased chance of balloon rupture if it remains in the gastric cavity for longer than the prescribed six months.

At the end of the sixth month the BIB® will, in any case, be removed. The following alternatives are then evaluated: (a) starting the patient of on a 'maintenance' diet programme; (b) subjecting him/her to the consensual placement of a second BIB® (multiple treatment); (c) performing the previously planned bariatric surgery.

Results

Secondary post-placement effects

In our experience the secondary post-placement effects were: nausea for 24–36 hours in 87 per cent of the patients; vomiting (a mean two episodes) in 51 per cent; slight epigastralgia in 61 per cent, regressed with antispasmodic drugs; increased intestinal meteorism in 36 per cent; diarrhoea (5–6 episodes/day) in 5 per cent; and halitosis in 12 per cent (Table 2).

Weight loss

From March 1998 to November 2006 our case histories recorded 640 placements of BIB® in 583 patients (181 male/402 female). The mean age was 37.5 (19–69); mean BMI 42.7 (30.7–56.5); mean EW percentage 68.3 (43–117.6). The incidence of intra-operation complications during placement and removal was nil. At the end of the treatment the patients presented: BMI 34.8, EWL 34.4 per cent (Table 3). These results

Table 2. BIB® post placement symptom.

Nausea	87%
Vomiting	51%
Epigastralgia	61%
Meteorism	36%
Diarrhoea	5%
Halitosis	12%

Table 3. Results of 583 patients that have undergone BIB placement.

	BMI	EW % — EWL %
BIB placement	42.7	68.3 EW %
BIB removal	34.8	35.4 EWL %

Table 4. GILB results of 2,515 patients.

	BMI	EW % — EWL %
BIB placement	44.4	59.5 EW %
BIB removal	35.4	33.9 EWL %

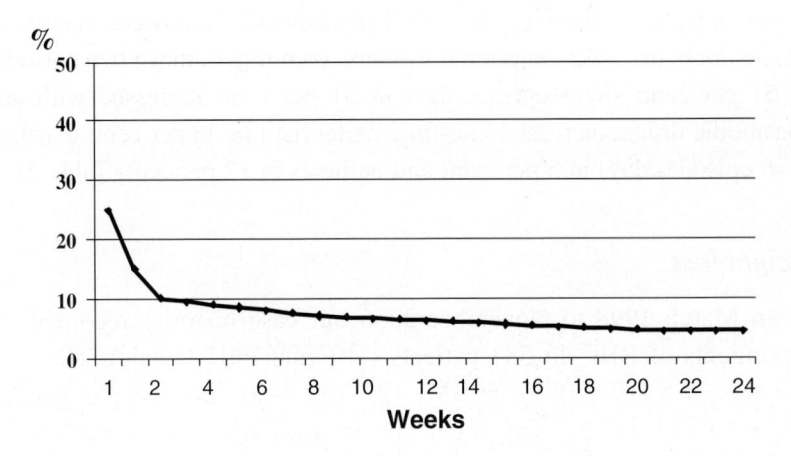

Figure 4. Weight loss/weeks.

can be superimposed on those reported by the Italian LAP-BAND® and BIB® group (GILB) relevant to 2,515 cases with a mean weight-loss of 9.0 BMI and 33.9 per cent EWL[21] (Table 4). As regards the modality of the weight loss, about 60 per cent occurs within the first 6–8 weeks, then evens out over the remaining months (Fig. 4). The best results are obtained in hyperphagic patients without specific modification of alimentary behaviour. Eating disorders influence the quantity and modality of the weight loss. In patients suffering bulimic crises the results are discouraging when evaluated with respect to weight loss; it must be emphasized, however, that as regards to the bulimic patients group, some of them reduced the number of their crises considerably (Fig. 5) from a mean of 8–10 a week to 1–2 a month. This condition is, however, limited to the BIB® treatment period, because after removal there is a gradual renewal of the eating disorder.

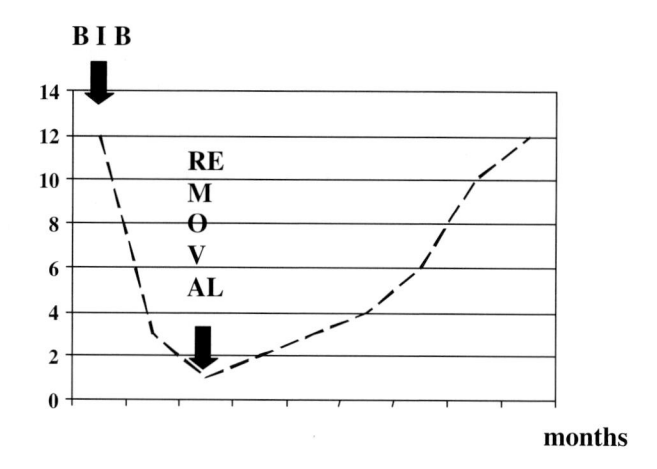

Figure 5. Bulimic crisis pre and post BIB®.

Other important results derive from our study which compares weight loss achieved by BIB® combined with dietary instructions versus a tapered diet therapy at six months, when the balloon was removed, and at eighteen months, twelve months after BIB® removal. The experimental group (BIB® + diet) consisted in 122 obese patients (81 females, 41 males) mean age 37.7 ± 11 years and mean BMI 41.8 ± 6.8; the control group (diet alone) comprised 128 patients (84 females, 44 males) mean age 39 ± 12.3 years and mean BMI 42.0 ± 6.

Weight loss was significantly higher in patients treated with BIB® when compared to a matched group of patients treated by diet alone (weight loss 16.2 versus 6.6 kg, BMI decrease 5.7 versus 2.5 kg/m^2) at six months. The difference persisted to a lesser degree but was still significant at follow-up (twelve months), both groups showing a tendency to regain weight at the follow-up (twelve months) after the treatment. In the patients treated with BIB® the average weight loss from baseline was reduced to 11.2 kg and the BMI loss to 3.5 kg/m^2, while in the control group, treated by diet, weight loss from baseline was 5.5 kg and BMI loss was 2.0 kg/m^2.

These results demonstrate that intragastric balloon combined with dietary instructions induces significantly higher weight loss then simple dietary therapy in the first six months of treatment and persists at twelve months of follow-up.[22]

Long-term results

It is difficult to consider the long-term efficacy of a device such as the intragastric balloon, created for temporary treatment. There are actually no data in the literature concerning long-term BIB® results. The longest follow-up reported (Melissas et al.[23]) is 1.5 years (range 6–30) when:

> 100/140 patients (71.4 per cent) lost ≥ 25 per cent of their EW on balloon extraction and were categorized as *successes*, while 40 patients (28.6 per cent) did not achieve that weight loss and were categorized as *failures* of the method. During the follow-up period, 44 of the originally successful patients (31.4 per cent) regained weight and were categorized as *recurrences*, while the remaining 56 patients (40 per cent) maintained their EWL of ≥ 25 per cent and were considered '*long-term successes*'.

In a prospective study carried out on a 100-patient sample, Herve et al.[24] report that:

> at BIB® removal mean weight loss was 12.0 kg. Mean EWL per cent was 39.8. 12 months after removal of the BIB®, mean weight loss was 8.6 kg and mean EWL was 26.8 per cent for the group as a whole.

The Brazilian experience, performed on a 483 patients between 2000 and 2004, indicates that after a six-month follow-up subjects showed significant reductions in weight (15.2 ± 10.5 kg), EWL percentage (48.3 ± 28.1), and BMI (–5.3 ± 3.4 kg/m^2). The 85 patients who completed one year follow-up after BIB® placement (six months after BIB® removal), (34 per cent of the 250 patients who completed 1 year after BIB® placement), maintained a substantial weight reduction, even if their one-year percentage EWL (50.9 ± 28.8) was significantly lower than their six-month percentage EWL (57.4 ± 26.4 per cent). However, 17 patients who were followed up two years after BIB® placement (11 per cent of the 158 patients who completed two years follow-up after BIB® placement) showed two-year percentage EWL 56.9 ± 36.5, which was not significantly different from their six-month percentage EWL of 66.1 ± 28.0.[25] This experience also shows the results relating to adolescents: 21 adolescents (age < 18 years) changed from a pre-treatment BMI of 36.5 ± 8.4 to a six-month BMI of 31.5 ± 9.1 (BMI reduction –5.0 ± 3.6), with a mean percentage EWL of 57.4 ± 37.0. The five adolescents who completed a one-year follow-up maintained a mean percentage EWL of 46.5 ± 30.4, a result statistically not different from their six-month percentage EWL of 49.2 ± 27.3.

Within the framework of our experience[26] from our database pertinent to obese patients undergoing the BIB® from March 1998 to July 2006 (total number of patients 613), we selected those having at least a 48 months post-removal follow-up (n = 145). We excluded patients who had undergone bariatric surgery after BIB® removal (n = 52) and who had a sequential BIB® placement or other non-surgical weight loss treatment (n = 30). The remaining patients (n = 45) were contacted and submitted to clinical evaluation. Weight fluctuations and any further interventional therapy requested by the patients after balloon removal were recorded. Excess weight loss (EWL) ≥ 25 per cent when the BIB® was removed was considered a success. Thirty patients (69 per cent) lost ≥25 per cent (range 25.0–69.0) of their excess weight on balloon removal and were classified as 'successes', while 15 patients (31 per cent) lost from 0 to 21.0 per cent of their excess weight and were categorized as 'failures'. At 60 months follow-up (60 months ± 21.47; range 48–96) 30 per cent (9/30) of the 'success' group had an EWL percentage of ≥25 and were categorized as 'long term successes'; whereas 70 per cent (21/30) of them had an EWL percentage of <25 and were categorized as 'long term failures'. To individualize possible predictive factors in long-term success, we evaluated the association between follow-up results and three factors: initial BMI (<35, 35–40, 40–50, >50), pre-BIB® age (>35 years, <35 years), and sex (male/female). A statistical analysis was done on the investigated predictive factors that have confirmed the associations: female gender, age <35 years and initial BMI from 35 to 40 are long-term success predictive factors. The results of this study confirm the safety and the short-term efficacy of the BIB®: at six months about the 70 per cent of the treated patients lost at least 25 per cent of their excess weight. At 60 months follow-up 30 per cent of the patients were able to control their weight loss and had at least 25 per cent of their EWL percentage. These results indicate a possible role for BIB® in long-term weight loss control.

As far as the predictive factors are concerned, we have singled out three different factors that bias long-term results; if they could be confirmed by larger studies, BIB® use could be recommended in those younger than 35 years, women and those patients with an initial BMI between 35 and 40.[27] The BIB® has been used only as a short-term treatment, but if prospective studies involving a larger number of patients confirm these results, our study suggests utilizing BIB® as a possible long-term treatment in selected patients.

Effects of the weight loss on associated diseases; BIB® and surgery; pre-operative strategy; sequential treatment

In our series the rapid weight-loss induced by the BIB® drastically affects the progression of obesity-related diseases, thus determining the suspension or reduction of the pharmacological therapy (Table 5). The dyslipidemic values improve in 58 per cent; there is significant hypertension control in 38 per cent. In 61 per cent joint diseases improved, including pain regression and in 80 per cent the rapid weight loss led to the prompt improvement of respiratory function and sleeping difficulties with the disappearance of apnoea (breath-holding) attacks.[28] As can be observed in Fig. 6, after BIB® treatment the apnoea index ranged from 33 to 5 episodes/hour. Furthermore, weight loss induced by the intragastric balloon, as demonstrated by various studies in the literature, led to a significant reduction in intestinal fat and liver volume (Fig. 7): the role and importance of the pre-surgery use of the intragastric balloon is clearly

Table 5. Weight loss effects on co-morbidities.

	Cleared up (stopped drug treatment) (%)	Improved (reduction of drug treatment) (%)	Unchanged (%)
Hypertension	38	52	10
Diabetes	36	45	19
Dislipidemia	58	28	14
Joint diseases	61	—	39
Respiratory function	80	—	20
Hyperinsulinemy	56.6	—	43.4

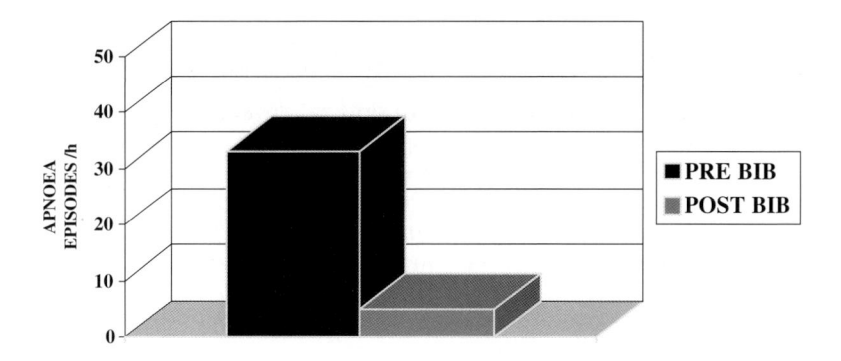

Figure 6. Apnoea episodes pre and post BIB® treatment.

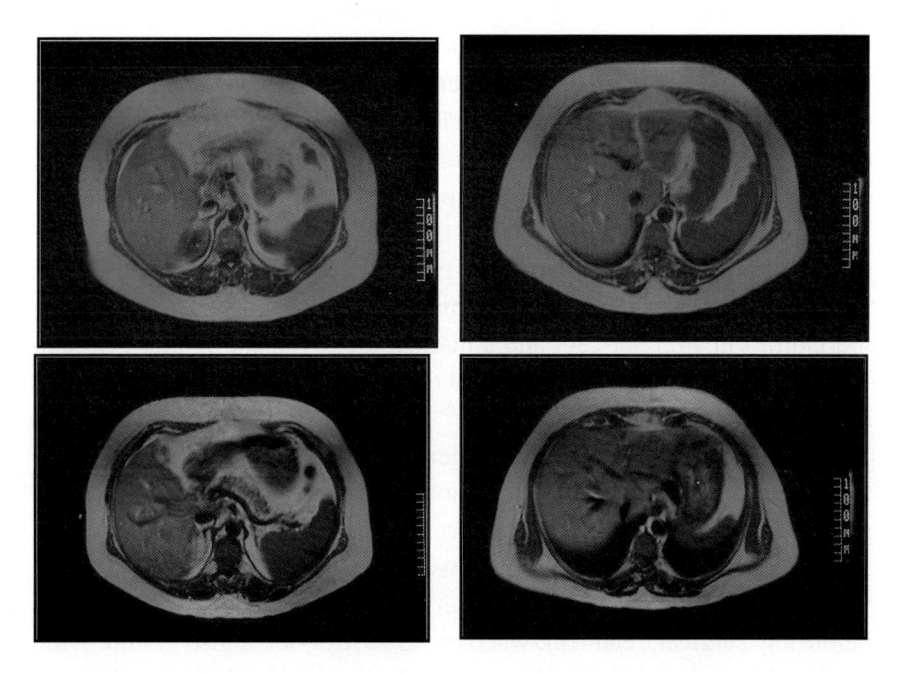

Figure 7. Intestinal fat and liver volume pre and post BIB.

shown also in Busetto's study,[29] where the pre-LAP-BAND® treatment together with BIB® induces a weight loss that shortens operating time and reduces the intraoperative complications, the conversion rate for patients subsequently subjected to gastric banding and hospital stay when compared

Table 6. Busetto's study data on operating time, hospital staying, conversion rate and intra-operative complications.

	BIB-LAPBAND (case pts)	LAPBAND (control pts)
Op time	82.5 ± 20.9	102.6 ± 35.1*
H stay	3.0 ± 0.2	3.3 ± 0.8*
Conversion	0/43 (0%)	7/43 (16.3%)*
IO Compl	0/43 (0%)	3/43 (7.0%)

with patients submitted directly to LAP-BAND® (Table 6). This is a fundamental condition for any patient candidate for surgery, in order to reduce morbidity and intra- and post-operative complications. Moreover, the weight loss induces an improvement in the size of the pharyngeal cross-sectional areas related to the reduction of neck circumference, determining a reduction in the problems relating to orotracheal intubation, often encountered with super-obese patients.[1]

In conclusion, the findings of the Italian LAP-BAND® and BIB® (GILB group), in a study on 2,515 patients, indicate that the use of the intragastric balloon induced an immediate normalization of the co-morbidities in 44.3 per cent and a marked improvement in 44.8 per cent. In only 10.9 per cent of the cases did the co-morbidities show no positive effects whatever from the treatment.[21]

In addition, the Brazilian experience of 483 patients illustrates how the BIB® affects obesity-related pathologies: clinical co-morbidities were regarded as unchanged in 7 (9.2 per cent), improved in 31 (40.8 per cent), and solved in 38 (50 per cent) patients.[25]

The use of the intragastric balloon is defined as 'sequential treatment' before any surgical treatment, whether bariatric or not, aimed at improving co-morbidities in order to reduce surgical and anaesthesiologic complications deriving from such surgery.

When pre-operatively evaluating patients who are candidates for bariatric surgery, careful attention must be paid to cardiologic, respiratory diseases and functionality. Patients with morbid obesity frequently present intubation and mechanical ventilation problems.[1]

In particular, pre-operative weight-loss achieved by means of an intragastric balloon, which induces a significant improvement in obesity-related pathologies, has been proposed, over the last few years, as an effective way of reducing the intra, post and anaesthesiologic risks connected with surgery on super-obese patients.[30]

The weight loss is associated with a reduction in the intestinal fat: prospective studies have shown how, in relation to the weight loss (reduction of about 10 per cent of the initial weight) the volume of abdominal–intestinal fat can vary (from 4.2 to 3.3, and even to 2.7), with a weight loss of about 16 per cent.[29]

Similar modifications can also be seen with regard to hepatic volume. It has been found that a weight reduction of about 10 per cent corresponds to a reduction of 0.24 litres of hepatic volume, corresponding to a relative decrease of 12.3 per cent.[31] These modifications of the intra-abdominal anatomy probably explain the positive impact on laparoscopic surgery of the pre-operative weight loss achieved with the intragastric balloon. It is evident that such changes are related to the weight loss and not to the use of the BIB® *per se*. In any case, it has been demonstrated that the weight loss obtained with the balloon is greater than the reduction achieved by dieting alone.[18,31,32]

Another important role to be played by the intragastric balloon derives from the results achieved by one of our studies which relates the results obtained with BIB® to those achieved with the first step of the bilio-pancreatic diversion.[33] We must, however, bear in mind that laparoscopic biliopancreatic diversion with duodenal switch represents the evolution of the operation described by Scopinaro[34] and one of the most successful surgical procedures for severe obesity.[35,36] Long term studies demonstrate that it is effective in super-obese patients with well known results (EWL 75 per cent at ten-year follow-up).[37] In 1999 Michel Gagner described the first laparoscopic BPD and 'duodenal switch'.[38] In order to decrease operative time and preoperative complications, the procedure has been divided into two stages[39]:

- a restrictive operation[40] with tubulisation of the stomach and preservation of the pylorus (sleeve gastrectomy);
- a malabsorptive stage (BPD-DS)[41,42]

However, this technique demands two operations. For this reason the purpose of this retrospective study was to verify the possibility of using BIB® placement as an alternative approach in the preoperative setting for patients who are candidates for major bariatric surgery.

The main result of the study is represented by the curve showing the weight decrease in super-obese patients: the curves show no difference in the slope between the two treatments: at six months follow-up there is no statistically significant difference between the weight loss in the group of patients treated with endoscopic placement of BIB® and the group of patients operated on with a sleeve gastrectomy (Fig. 8). This result confirms that BIB® placement is an effective option in the bariatric procedures. In fact when the BIB® is removed patients stop losing the same amount of weight or even start gaining weight. At ten months follow-up this trend is clearer and the difference between the two procedures begins to appear significant. However, this fact confirms that in the short period the endoscopic approach still maintains its value and appears particularly useful when a temporary weight-loss is required. The study also showed an influence on co-morbidities. In a recent study Gagner *et al.* have shown similar results in terms of weight loss suggesting a possible role for BIB® placement in a selected group of patients as a first stage of BPD.[43] In particular, BIB® placement appears highly advisable in those patients who are candidates for BPD-DS, when operative and anaesthesiologic risks due to co-morbidities are very high. The endoscopic approach could reduce the entire treatment to a single stage surgical procedure avoiding the operative complications of two operations.

Multiple treatment: What it is, why and when it is appropriate

This consists of placing two intragastric balloons one after the other, respecting an interval of at least 30 days between the removal and the second balloon placement.

The reason underlying the delay of at least one month is the need to allow the patient to 'get the feel' of the balloon again. After about five months' treatment, in fact, the majority of patients feel a diminished sense of satiety when compared with the first months of the treatment. This is

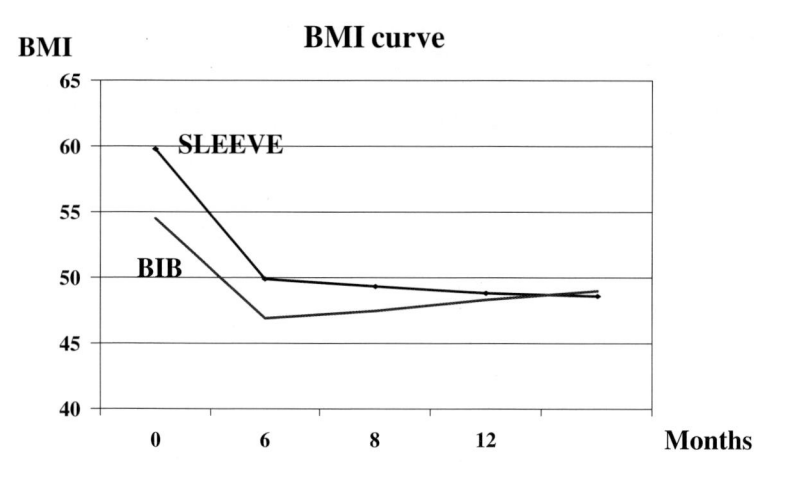

Figure 8. Weight loss achieved with BIB vs Sleeve gastrectomy in super obese patients.

probably due to the saturation of the gastric receptors which 'adapt' to the presence of the intragastric prothesis. We observed that the placement of the second BIB® (equal or higher volume compared to the first), after at least one month's delay, allows the patient to recover part of the sensitivity lost over the last few months of treatment with the first device. In any case weight loss obtained with the second BIB® never exceeds 50 per cent of the weight loss achieved with the first balloon.

The multiple treatment, as mentioned above, is to be taken into consideration only under the following three conditions:

- success of the first treatment (weight loss of at least 15 per cent of the initial weight);
- refusal of surgery;
- as already observed, serious failure to alter eating behaviour (e.g. sweet eating).

In our study 57 patients underwent multiple treatment. The mean weight loss achieved with the second BIB® was 4.0 BMI and the overall weight loss (with first and second BIB®) was 11.1 BMI (Table 7).

Table 7. Results of the multiple treatments on 57 patients (personal series).

	Pre-BIB	First BIB	Second BIB
BMI	47.6	40.4	36.7

Complications

Minor complications

In the Italian BIB® experience of 3,252 patients the incidence of minor complications was 2.1 per cent (71 patients). The intragastric balloon was removed due to intolerance in 13 patients (0.39 per cent). These patients, although they had been suitably informed before placement as to the appearance and modalities of what was likely to occur, decided to have it removed because they found the symptoms intolerable. Breakage of the device occurred in 19 patients (0.58 per cent) and, except in two cases, always after the period advised by the company (6 months). Oesophagitis diagnosed after removal of the BIB® occurred in 39 patients (1.2 per cent), probably due to the discontinuous use of the proton pump inhibitors (Table 8).[44]

The Brazilian study performed by Sallet *et al.* reports, among the minor complications, reflux oesophagitis in 40/683 patients (12.4 per cent) and symptomatic gastric stasis in 28/683 patients (8.7 per cent).[25]

Major complications

The overall major complication was 32/3252 (0.9 per cent)[44] in 19 (0.58 per cent) patients the device became displaced in the cavity causing a typical case of gastric obstruction which totally blocked gastric emptying (Fig. 9).

This condition was resolved with medical treatment in three cases by inserting a naso-gastric tube for 24–48 hours, but in 16 cases this proved to be ineffective and removal of the BIB® was required. Another complication is gastric ulceration, very frequently experienced with the 1980s balloons, but very rare today (due to the spherical shape, the improved characteristics and the use of the proton pump inhibitor). This complication occurred in 0.15 per cent (five patients) (Table 9). As far as we know

Table 8. BIB minor complication in 3,252 patients.

BIB intolerance	0.39%
BIB breakage	0.58%
Oesophagitis	1.2%

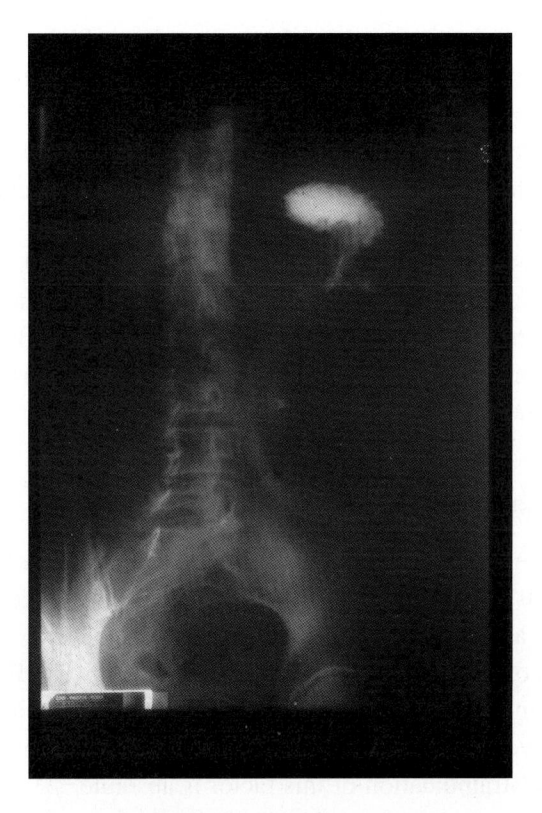

Figure 9. Gastric obstruction.

intestinal obstruction occurred in three of the 7000 patients treated in Italy, each case entailing surgical treatment. Gastric perforation, the most frightening complication, occurred in five patients (0.15 per cent). Four of the latter had already undergone surgery: three at gastric level (fundoplication according to Nissen, a vertical gastroplasty complicated by fistula, gastric banding removed because of intragastric migration) and one due to

Table 9. BIB major complication in 3,252 patients.

Gastric obstruction	0.58%
Gastric ulceration	0.15%
Gastric perforation	0.15%

prior, thoracic–abdominal trauma. In three patients this complication was treated and solved by surgical means. Two other patients died: one during surgery and the other during diagnostic tests.

In the Brazilian experience Sallet et al.[25] also include balloon impaction in the antrum with gastric hyperdistension among the major complications, requiring removal of gastric content under general anaesthesia (two cases, 0.6 per cent). There was one case (0.3 per cent) of spontaneous deflation of the balloon and migration into the small bowel, causing intestinal obstruction after five months of the BIB®, treated conservatively for the first 24 hours without satisfactory results and subsequently removed surgically.

Discussion and Conclusion

Our experience, and the literature illustrated here, indicate that the intragastric BIB® is a totally different prothesis from that used in the 1980s because, over a short term, it is a safe and effective device. Even though the incidence of major complications is <1 per cent (GILB data), its use solely for cosmetic purposes is not at the moment advisable, and because four of the five perforations occurred in patients with previous gastric surgery, the contraindication of this factor is absolute.

The placement and removal procedures are easy, both for gastroenterologists and for surgeons who perform endoscopies. Physicians must, however, take great care to follow-up their patients very closely, particularly in the first seven days after placement. Only an attentive and rigorous follow-up permits the timely diagnosis and appropriate treatment of the dangerous complications which could arise in this first phase: gastric ischemic ulcer, with subsequent perforation (4/5 occurred during the first five days after placement, GILB data) and dehydration.

Despite the adverse symptoms felt by the patient during the first two days after placement, the incidence of 'psychological intolerance' and subsequent early removal is, in the Italian experience, very low (0.39 per cent). This is certainly due to two factors: the first is the lengthy, complete and repeated information given to the patient before treatment and, the second, keeping the patients in hospital, where they feel definitely more 'protected', for two days.

In patients suffering from morbid obesity, incapable of keeping to any diet, and who are candidates for bariatric or other types of surgery, the intragastric balloon is the only non-surgical procedure able to induce a rapid and consistent weight-loss which positively affects all the obesity-related co-morbidities and reduces the risks of surgery and anaesthesia.

The ongoing trend relating to the use of the device points to sequential treatment, i.e. before and in preparation for surgery. In this respect the data relating to super-obese patients (BMI > 50) indicated in the study comparing it with sleeve-gastrectomy[33] is very encouraging. The effective control of co-morbidities induced by the use of the intragastric balloon authorizes the hypothesis of a possible role for the device as the first step in a complex surgical treatment. If further prospective studies, involving a greater number of patients, confirm the data obtained up to now, it is reasonable to hypothesize for the future performance, for example, of the biliopancreatic diversion with sleeve gastrectomy in one sole step, after a six-month treatment with the intragastric balloon.

The unexpected results deriving from the evaluation of our experience in patients with five year follow-up,[26] lead us to think that the BIB® will be able to play a important role in the prevention of super-obesity, so little discussed even by the experts in this field. The fact that one-third of female patients, younger than 35 years and with a BMI lower than 40, are able to maintain, or even optimize their weight loss five years after the treatment, should stimulate the 'precocious' use of the BIB® in the prevention of super-obesity and its correlated diseases.

Use of the intragastric balloon in adolescent and paediatric patients is another possible and important field.

To be truthful, however, there is not enough scientific evidence at the moment to support verified affirmations. The study of 21 adolescents reported by Sallet[25] can be supplemented by that of Dr F. De Peppo's group at the Paediatric Hospital Bambino Gesù in Rome, where 11 children suffering from the Prader–Willi syndrome (mean age 11 years) were given BIB® multiple treatment, with good results.[45]

At the present time there is no medical cure for obesity and, despite the numerous dietary treatments, the natural course of the disease is characterized by an ongoing, sometimes unstoppable, weight gain. There are now one billion overweight or obese persons worldwide. Only some of these patients, however, express the desire or are able to undergo a surgical operation. In this context the intragastric balloon can play a very clear role in interrupting the ongoing and inexorable weight gain in patients with first degree obesity and in achieving positive control or resolution or improving of the relevant co-morbidities.[24,46] In super-obese patients, where there are numerous co-morbidities, the weight loss obtained with the BIB® represents, on the other hand, a chance to reduce the surgical and anaesthesiologic complications deriving from bariatric surgery. Other endoscopic procedures such as Endobarrier and POSE have a real potential and have been added to the armamenterium of bariatric endoscopic procedures.[47]

References

1. Ogunnaike, B.O., Jones, S.B., Jones, D.B. et al. (2002). Anesthetic considerations for bariatric surgery. *Anesth Analg* 95: 1793–1805.
2. Sprung, J., Whalley, D.G., Falcone, T. et al. (2003). The effects of tidal volume and respiratory rate on oxygenation and respiratory mechanics during laparoscopic in morbidly obese patients. *Anesth Analg* 97: 268–274.
3. Bloostom, M., Zervos, E.E., Camps, M.A. et al. (1997). Outcome following bariatric surgery in super versus morbidly obese patients: does weight matter? *Obes Surg* 7: 414–419.
4. Weiner, R., Gutberlet, H., Bockhorn, H. (1999). Preparation of extremely obese patients for laparoscopic gastric banding by gastric balloon therapy. *Obes Surg* 9: 261–264.
5. Angrisani, L., Furbetta, F., Doldi, S.B. et al.. (2002). Results of the Italian multicentre study on 239 super-obese patients treated by adjustable gastric banding. *Obes Surg* 12: 846–850.

6. Pasulka, P.S., Bistrian, B.R., Benotti, P.N. et al. (1986). The risks of surgery in obese patients. *Ann Intern Med* 104: 540–546.
7. Neiben, O.G., Harboe, H. (1982). Intragastric balloon as an artificial bezoar for treatment for obesity. *Lancet* 1: 198–199.
8. Goustout, C., Rajan, E. (2005). Endoscopic treatments for obesity: past, present and future. *Gastrointest Clin N Am* 34: 143–150.
9. Dillon, J.G., Hughes, M.K. (1992). Degradation of five polyurethane gastric bubbles following *in vivo* use: SEC, ATR-ir and DSC studies. *Biomaterials* 13(4): 240–248.
10. Geliebter, A., Melton, P.M., Gage, D. et al. (1990). Gastric balloon to treat obesity: a double-blind study in nondieting subjects. *Am J Clin Nutr* 51(4): 584–588.
11. Hogan, R.B., Johnston, J.H., Long, B.W. et al. (1989). A double-blind, randomized, sham-controlled trial of the gastric bubble for obesity. *Gastrointest Endosc* 35(5): 381–385.
12. Kirby, D.F., Wade, J.B., Mills, P.R. et al. (1990). A prospective assessment of the Garren-Edwards gastric bubble and bariatric surgery in the treatment of morbid obesity. *Am Surg* 56(10): 575–580.
13. Benjamin, S.B., Maher, K.A., Cattau, E.L. Jr et al. (1988). Double-blind controlled trial of the Garren-Edwards gastric bubble: an adjunctive treatment for exogenous obesity. *Gastroenterology* 95(3): 581–588.
14. Lindor, K.D., Hughes, R.W. Jr., Ilstrup, D.M. et al. (1987). Intragastric balloons in comparison with standard therapy for obesity — a randomized, double-blind trial. *Mayo Clin Proc* 62 (11): 992–996.
15. Benjamin, S.B. (1988). Small bowel obstruction and the Garren-Edwards gastric bubble: an iatrogenic bezoar. *Gastrointest Endosc* 34(6): 463–467.
16. Ulicny, K.S., Goldberg, S.J., Harper, W.J. et al. (1988). Surgical complications of the Garren-Edwards gastric bubble. *Surg Gynecol Obstet* 166(6): 535–540.
17. Wahlen, C.H., Bastens B., Herve J. et al. (2001). The Bioenterics Intragastric Balloon (BIB): how to use it. *Obes Surg* 11: 524–527.
18. Genco, A., Cipriano, M., Bacci, V. et al. (2006). BioEnterics Intragastric Balloon (BIB): a short-term, double-blind, randomised, controlled, crossover study on weight reduction in morbidly obese patients. *Int J Obes (Lond)* 30(1): 129–133.

19. Torres-Barrera, G. (2006). Gastrical electrical activity before and after Bioenterics Intragastric Balloon (BIB) placement. *Digest Dis Week* 20–25 May.
20. Mion, F., Napoleon, B., Roman, S. *et al.* (2005). Effect of intragastric balloon on gastric emptying and ghrelin plasma levels in non-morbid obese patients. *Obes Surg* 15(4): 510–516.
21. Genco, A., Bruni, T., Doldi, S.B. *et al.* (2005). Bioenterics Intragastric Balloon: the Italian experience with 2,515 patients. *Obes Surg* 15: 1161–1164.
22. Genco, A., Balducci, S., Bacci, V. *et al.* (2008) Intragastric Balloon or diet alone? A retrospective evaluation. *Obes Surg* 18(8): 989–992.
23. Melissas, J., Mouzas, J., Filis, D. *et al.* (2006). The intragastric balloon — smoothing the path to bariatric surgery. *Obes Surg* 16(7): 897–902.
24. Herve, J., Wahlen, C.H., Schaeken, A. *et al.* (2005). What becomes of patients one year after the intragastric balloon has been removed? *Obes Surg* 15(6): 864–870.
25. Sallet, J.A., Marchesini, J.B., Paiva, D.S. *et al.* (2004). Brazilian multicenter study of the intragastric balloon. *Obes Surg* 14: 991–998.
26. Genco, A. Bioenterics Intragastric Balloon (BIB) in morbid obesity treatment: 5 years results. In press.
27. Busetto, L., Enzi, G., Inelmen, E.M. *et al.* (2005). Obstructive sleep apnea syndrome in morbid obesity: effects of intragastric balloon. *Chest* 128(2): 618–623.
28. Busetto, L., Segato, G., De Luca, M. *et al.* (2004). Preoperative weight loss by intragastric balloon in super-obese patients treated with laparoscopic gastric banding: a case-control study. *Obes Surg* 14(5): 671–676.
29. Weiner, R., Gutberlet, H., Bockhorn, H. (1999). Preparation of extremely obese patients for laparoscopic gastric banding by gastric balloon therapy. *Obes Surg* 9: 261–264.
30. Busetto, L., Tregnaghi, A., De Marchi, F. *et al.* (2002). Liver volume and visceral obesity in women with hepatic steatosis undergoing gastric banding. *Obes Res* 10: 408–411.
31. Doldi, S.B., Micheletto, G., Perrini, M.N. *et al.* (2002). Treatment of morbid obesity with intragastric balloon in association with diet. *Obes Surg* 12: 121–127.
32. Hodson, R., Zacharoulis, D., Goutzamani, E. *et al.* (2001). Management of obesity with the new intragastric balloon. *Obes Surg* 11: 327–329.

33. Genco, A., Cipriano, M., Materia, A. et al. (2010). Laparoscopic sleeve gastrectomy versus intragastric balloon: a case control study. *Surg Endosc* 23(8): 1849–1853.
34. Scopinaro, N., Adami, G.F., Marinari, G.M. et al. (1998). Biliopancreatic diversion. *World J Surg* 22: 936–946.
35. Van Hee Robrecht, H.G.G. (2004). Biliopancreatic diversion in the surgical treatment of morbid obesity. Editorial update. *World J Surg* 28(5): 435–444.
36. Biron, S., Hould, F.S., Lebel, S. et al. (2004). Twenty years of biliopancreatic diversion: what is the goal of the surgery? *Obes Surg* 14(2): 160–164.
37. Scopinaro, N., Gianetta, E., Adami, G.F. et al. (1996). Biliopancreatic diversion for obesity at eighteen years. *Surgery* 119: 261–268.
38. Ren, C.J., Patterson, E., Gagner, M. (2000). Early results of laparoscopic biliopancreatic diversion with duodenal switch: a case series of 40 patients. *Obes Surg* 10: 514–523.
39. Regan, J.P., Inabnet, W.B., Gagner, M. et al. (2002). Early experience with two-stage laparoscopic Roux-en Y Gastric bypass as an alternative in the super-super obese patients. *Obes Surg* 12: 245–248.
40. Rabkin, R.A., Rabkin, J.M., Metcalf, B. et al. (2003). Laparoscopic technique for performing duodenal switch with gastric reduction. *Obes Surg* 13: 263–268.
41. Baltasar, A., Bou, R., Miró, J. et al. (2002). Laparoscopic biliopancreatic diversion with duodenal switch: technique and initial experience. *Obes Surg* 12(2): 245–248.
42. Marceau, P., Hould, F.S., Lebel, S. et al. (2001). Malabsorptive obesity surgery. *Surg Clin North Am* 81(5): 1113–1127.
43. Milone, L., Strong, V., Gagner, M. et al. (2005). Laparoscopic sleeve gastrectomy is superior to endoscopic intragastric balloon as a first stage procedure for super-obese patients (BMI > or =50). *Obes Surg* 15(5): 612–617.
44. Genco, A. (2006). Italian Society for Bariatric Surgery, Italian Congress on Obesity Surgery — SICOB — Florence, September.
45. Crinò, A., Di Giorgio, G., De Peppo, F. et al. (2009). Bioenterics intragastric balloon may represent an alternative and effective treatment for body weight control in Prader–Willi syndrome. *Obes Surg* 19(5): 674–675

46. Mathus-Vliegen, E., Tytgat, G. (2005). Intragastric balloon for treatment-resistant obesity: safety, tolerance, and efficacy of 1-year balloon treatment followed by a 1-year balloon-free follow-up. *Gastrointest Endosc* 61: 19–27.
47. Bonanomi, G., Di Caro, S., Traina, M. *et al.* (2006). Pilot study of Preoperative Weight Loss in Super Morbid Obese Patients: The Additional Effect of Endoscopic Intragastric Balloon Placement. Los Angeles, DDW.

Chapter 4

Laparoscopic Adjustable Gastric Banding

Gianni Segato, Nadey S. Hakim, Maurizio De Luca and Franco Favretti

Introduction

The laparoscopic application[1,2] of an adjustable gastric banding, introduced by Kuzmack in 1986,[3] is gaining more and more in consensus as a surgical procedure for the treatment of morbid obesity. In many countries it is the most common bariatric surgery procedure, and it is calculated that in the last seven years about 400,000 gastric bandings have been applied all over the world.

According to the register of the Italian Society for Obesity Surgery (SICOB), by December 2007, 8,000 gastric bandings had been put in place, making this the most common bariatric procedure. The advantages of surgery that preserves the integrity of the gastrointestinal tract and that can be carried out by laparoscopy are obvious.

The laparoscopic approach was perfected and standardized by our group since 1993 with the use of the Lap-Band® (INAMED Health, USA)[1,4] (Fig. 1). The standardization made it possible to reduce the rate of complications to a minimum and to obtain stable results over time.[5,6]

Indications and Contraindications

Many believe that adjustable gastric banding is the first-choice surgical procedure in the majority of morbidly obese patients.[2,5,7,8] In any case, the Body Mass Index (BMI) must be higher than 40 kg/m^2 or than 35 kg/m^2

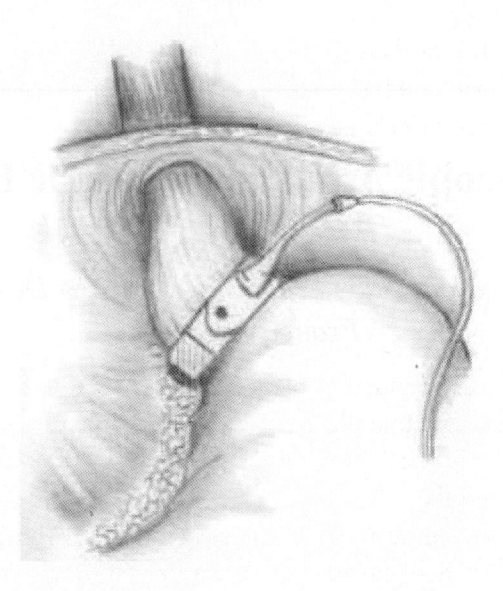

Figure 1. Gastric banding with Lap-Band®.

in the presence of co-morbidities. Surgery is indicated only in the failed conservative treatment of morbidly obese patients, such as long time controlled diets, physical activity programmes and behavioural alterations. The candidate patients for this kind of procedure must be committed to changing their dietary habits permanently and materially. The adjustable gastric banding is contraindicated in patients with:[9]

- diencephalic obesity;
- Prader–Willi syndrome;
- chronic gastrointestinal inflammatory diseases, gastroduodenal ulcer;
- severe cardiopulmonary failure;
- oesophageal/gastric varices;
- congenital or acquired gastrointestinal atresias or stenoses;
- pregnancy;
- alcohol or drug addiction;
- presence of infection, if there is a possibility of the prosthesis being contaminated;

- inability to accept the dietary restrictions required for the procedure;
- allergic reactions to the prosthetic materials;
- emotional instability that might affect the procedure;
- autoimmune diseases (lupus erythematosus, scleroderma).

Preparation for Surgery

Haematochemical tests should include a full blood count (in particular for the identification of polycythemia), count of serum electrolytes, glycaemia with blood glucose response curve, kidney and liver function tests and blood coagulation tests. If the patient's history shows evidence of thyroid and/or adrenal gland dysfunctions, a targeted hormonal study will also be necessary.

Moreover, routine tests should also include ECG, chest X-ray, liver sonography, oesophago–gastro–duodenoscopy (OGD) and spirometry.

Surgical Instruments

The commonly used surgical instruments for the adjustable gastric band (Lap-Band®) positioning by laparoscopy include:[1,4]

- One Veress needle;
- One optical trocar with five 10 mm sleeves;
- One 0° lens and one 30° lens;
- One Endo Retract™;
- One Endo Dissect™;
- One Endo Shear™;
- Articulating dissector for gastric band application (Greenstein);
- One Endo Babcock™;
- Two Endo Grasp™;
- One Endo Stitch™;
- Silk thread 2–0;
- (Tyco™ and STORZ™ equipment).

Of course, the corresponding reusable equipment can also be used.

Patient and Surgical Team Positioning

It is believed that the patient positioning procedures and the performance of the surgery itself are made easier if the patient is laid flat on his/her back on the operating table with the arms spread and legs abducted (Fig. 2). The operating table is inclined in a 30° anti-Trendelenburg position. Compression bandages or pneumatic equipment should be used on the legs, which should be laid straight and comfortably on pillows, for venous compression. The surgeons, anaesthesiologist and scrub nurses are positioned as shown in Fig. 3.

Procedural Steps

Perigastric technique

The procedure's key points, as defined and standardized in June 1995, are (Fig. 4):

- identification of the reference points for dissection (equator of the balloon containing 25 cc of air and left diaphragmatic pillar);
- creation of the retrogastric tunnel above the peritoneal reflection of the lesser sac;
- creation of a 'virtual' pouch;

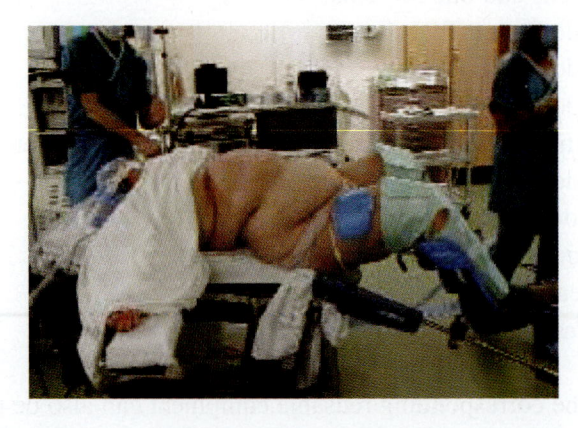

Figure 2. Patient positioning.

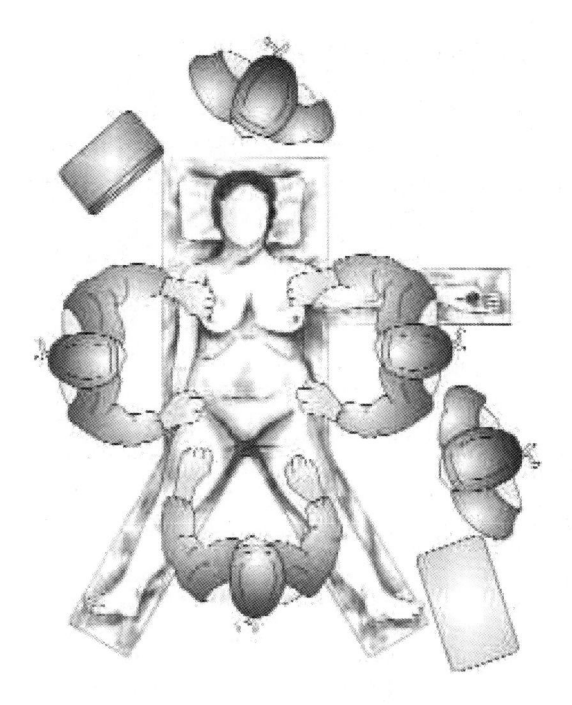

Figure 3. Positioning of the surgical team.

- retention sutures to avoid slippage.

The surgical technique can be schematized as follows:

Insufflation

A veress needle is inserted in the usual way in the supraumbilical area. This creates a pneumoperitoneum with a regulated 15 mm Hg intra-abdominal pressure.

Trocar and instruments positioning

Five trocars should be introduced in the following way:

- One 10 mm trocar for the 30° lens, at a distance of roughly six fingers below the sternum's xiphoid process;

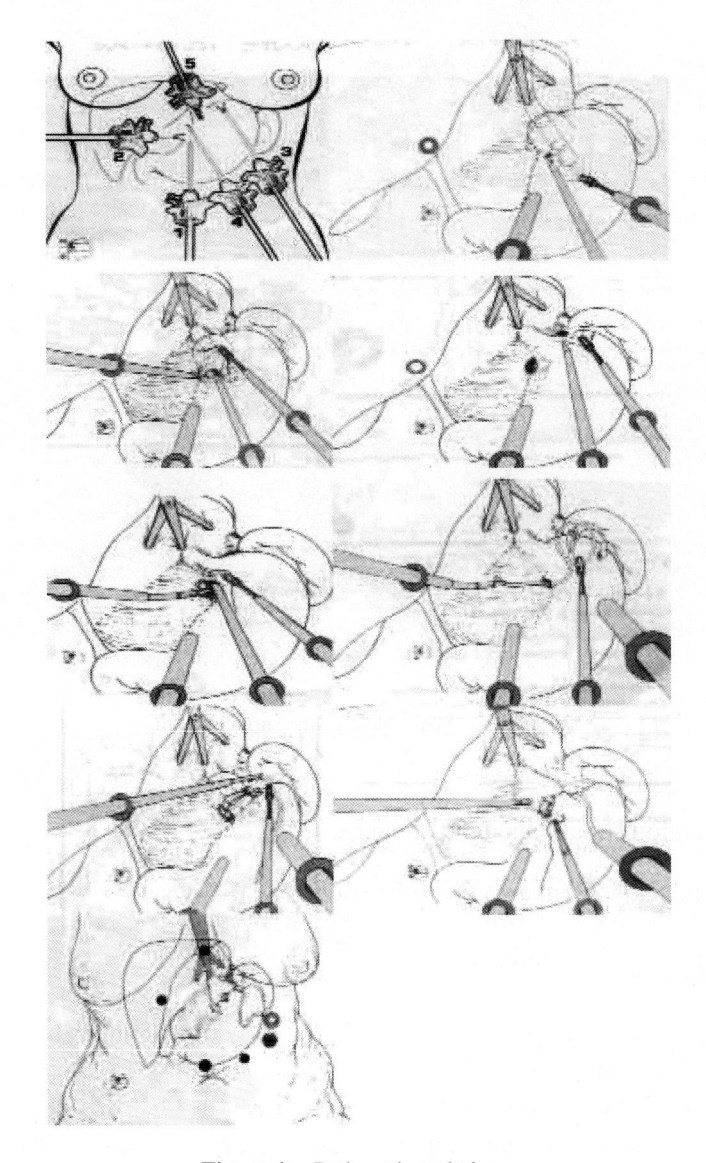

Figure 4. Perigastric technique.

- One 5 mm trocar for liver retraction in the subxiphoid area;
- One 5 mm trocar in the abdomen's upper right quadrant, for the grasper, the dissector and the tool used to close the Lap-Band®;

- One 10 mm trocar in the abdomen's left upper left quadrant for the electrocautery hook, the needle-holder and the grasper for the introduction of the Lap-Band® and tank positioning;
- One 5 mm trocar along the left anterior axillary line, just below the rib margin, for the use of the Endo Babcock™, the grasper and shears.

In order to minimize damage to the abdominal wall vessels and the intraperitoneal organs, optical trocars are usually positioned under direct vision (Visiport System, Covidien™).

Reference points

The anaesthesiologist should introduce a calibration tube with a balloon on the end into the stomach, through the mouth; the balloon should be inflated with about 25 cc of air and retracted into the oesophagus–gastric junction. The stomach should be retracted downwards. The bulge of the balloon makes it possible for the surgeon to decide where to place the initial dissection.

The dissection on the lesser curvature is made along the balloon's equator that is marked with the electrocautery hook. Therefore, the reference point on the lesser curvature is given by the balloon's equator, while on the greater curvature the reference point is given by the gastrophrenic ligament next to the left pillar of the diaphragm, or the angle of His. The identification of these two reference points is essential for the correct positioning of the bandage.

Lesser curvature dissection–perigastric technique

The dissection of the retrogastric tunnel starts about 2 cm below the cardia on the lesser curvature. Through the trocar, inserted in the right hypochondrium, the grasper is used to stretch the hepatogastric ligament and an Endo Babcock™ stretches the gastric wall through the leftmost trocar.

This technique stretches the peritoneum of the lesser curvature. The dissection is made as near as possible to the gastric wall, taking care not to damage it and to preserve the Latarjet's nerve. Under direct vision, a small narrow passage is created, clearly identifying and preserving the stomach's posterior wall. Tunnel dissection should have the same dimensions as the bandage, or be even smaller, in order to avoid slippage of the band.

During dissection on the gastric wall, the nasogastric tube will have to be retracted into the oesophagus in order to avoid injury to the stomach.

Retrogastric dissection

Retrogastric dissection, which is meant to connect the two previously identified reference points, must be carried out above the peritoneal reflection of the lesser sac. Indeed, if the band is positioned below the peritoneal reflection of the lesser sac, an unacceptable rate of complications ensues (stomach slippage).

Gastrophrenic ligament dissection

A grasper is used through the leftmost trocar to stretch the gastric fundus caudad, so as to place traction on the gastrophrenic ligament. A small window is then opened in this ligament with the electrocautery hook. The position of this window normally corresponds to the most prominent part of the left pillar of the diaphragm, very close to the angle of His. In many cases the angle of His and the gastrophrenic ligament are masked by the presence of a fat pad, sometimes a big one, called Belsey's fat pad.

The banding must be applied so as to exclude this fat tissue, lest it creates a stenosis and an upper occlusion immediately after surgery. Therefore, this fat pad needs to be excised and partially excluded, starting from the adhesions to the diaphragm and the gastric fundus and proceeding towards the oesophagus and the angle of His. In this way a perfect vision of the gastro-oesophageal angle is obtained.

Retrogastric tunnel

A special instrument with an articulating head is introduced into the trocar positioned in the right hypochondrium, and positioned under direct vision in the retrogastric tunnel. The distal part of the instrument is then bent, becoming quite visible in the dissection area of the gastrophrenic ligament, in front of the left diaphragmatic pillar.

The use of the electrocautery hook can help free the distal end of the instrument, so that it emerges in the left part of the retrogastric tunnel.

Introduction and positioning of the Lap-Band® gastric bandage

The adjustable gastric bandage (Lap-Band®) and its connecting tube are introduced in the abdominal cavity through the trocar in the left hypochondrium. The banding is then hooked to the articulating instrument already present in the retrogastric tunnel and slipped around the stomach along the dissection plane.

In order to introduce the gastric banding into the abdominal cavity, therefore, 15 mm or 18 mm diameter trocars are unnecessary. Simply remove the 10 mm trocar from the left hypochondrium and insert the Band following its path.

Band locking

The surgeon checks that the band is positioned correctly, using the calibration tube. The silicone band is locked around the sub-cardiac area.

Stabilization sutures

The anaesthesiologist extracts the calibration tube. Three to five sutures are sewn between the stomach's serous membrane proximally to and distally from the band, in order to prevent it from slipping. These sutures prevent band and/or stomach slippage and are applied in the seromuscular layer of the stomach just before and after the band. This anti-slippage suture needs to start as near to the greater curvature as possible, in order to immobilize the bandage.

If there is a gap on the lesser curvature, it must be closed by stitches applied distally from the bandage, between the lesser curvature and the hepatogastric ligament, paying attention not to damage the vagus nerve. In this way a 'virtual' proximal gastric pouch is created.

Port positioning

The connection tube is retracted through the port in the left hypochondrium. The port is then secured to the abdominal wall fascia in the left hypochondrium with four sutures. Thanks to this port it is possible to adjust the diameter of the new gastric stoma formed by the bandage.

Bandage adjustment

The bandage is adjusted repeatedly after surgery, under radiological control the first time and blindly after that. The calibre of the passage through the new gastric stoma is regulated according to the patient's needs, the weight loss and the radiological images.

Pars flaccida approach

In the last few years a new method, known as the *pars flaccida* approach, has been proposed for the creation of the retrogastric tunnel. This has rapidly gained consensus and is widely used, as it is considered easier to learn compared to the perigastric approach, and probably less conducive to complications (perforations and slippage); see Fig. 5.

Once the lesser omentum's *pars flaccida* has been divided up to the extragastric vagal fibres, which are preserved, the liver's caudate lobe and the right diaphragmatic pillar become visible. The pillar's anterior edge, next to the inflated intragastric balloon's equator (see above), is marked with the electrocautery hook. This is the starting point for the blunt dissection towards the angle of His, remaining in front of the plane of the diaphragmatic pillars, just as in fundoplication operations in cases of gastroesophageal reflux disease or hiatal hernia.

During dissection the balloon should be deflated and the calibration tube retracted inside the oesophagus, to avoid injury.

The level of this retrogastric tunnel is also high, as it is positioned quite close to the gastro–oesophageal junction. In order to avoid accessing the mediastinum and/or damaging the posterior gastric wall, it is advisable to check the position of the oesophagus and of the gastric wall, with the help of the calibration tube.

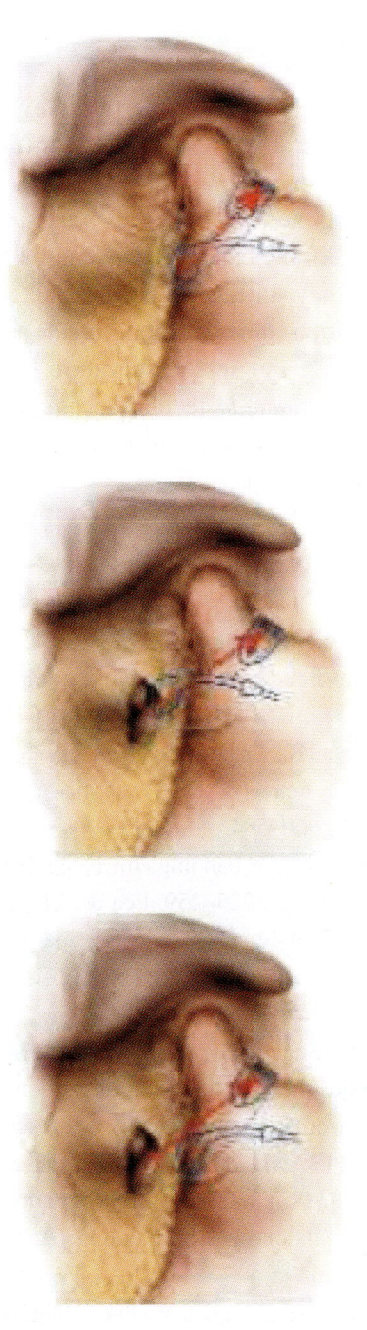

Figure 5. Perigastric, *pars flaccida* and mixed approaches.

Mixed technique

It is possible to use a combination of the two previous techniques, especially in the case of viscerally obese patients, to avoid too much tissue being included in the bandage.

The dissection starts according to the *pars flaccida* approach, and once the tunnel is created, the bandage tube can be positioned therein. At this point, the surgeon may shift to the perigastric technique and, near the equator of the calibration tube balloon, create an antero–posterior–perigastric opening along the lesser curvature until the tube, already positioned with the *pars flaccida* technique, is met, grasped and pulled through. Therefore, the bandage is positioned from the angle of His to the perigastric window (see Fig. 5).

References

1. Favretti, F., Cadière, G.B., Segato, G. *et al.* (1997). Laparoscopic adjustable gastric banding (Lap-Band®): how to avoid complications. *Obes Surg* 7: 352–358.
2. Favretti, F., Cadière, G.B., Segato, G. *et al.* (1998). Bariatric analysis and reporting outcome system (BAROS) applied to laparoscopic banding patients. *Obes Surg* 8: 500–504.
3. Kuzmack, L. (1986). Gastric banding. In: Deitel M. (ed.). *Surgery for the Morbidly Obese Patient,* pp. 225–259, Lea & Febbiger, Philadelphia.
4. Favretti, F., Segato, G., Ashton, D. (2007). Laparoscopic adjustable gastric banding in 1791 consecutive obese patients: 12-year results. *Obes Surg* 17: 168–175.
5. Busetto, L., Pisent, C., Segato, G. *et al.* (1997). The influence of a new timing strategy of band adjustment on the vomiting frequency and the food consumption of obese women operated with laparoscopic adjustable silicone gastric banding (LAP-BAND®). *Obes Surg* 7: 505–512.
6. Busetto, L., Valente, P., Pisent, C. *et al.* (1996). Eating pattern in the first year following adjustable silicone gastric banding (ASGB) for morbid obesity. *Obes Surg* 20: 539–546.
7. Belachew, M., Legrand, M., Vincent, V. *et al.* (1998). Laparoscopic adjustable gastric banding. *Obes Surg* 22: 955–963.

8. Busetto, L., Segato, G., De Marchi, F. *et al.* (2002). Outcome predictors in morbidly obese recipients of an adjustable gastric band. *Obes Surg* 12: 83–92.
9. National Institutes of Health Consensus Development Conference Statement (1991). *Gastrointestinal Surgery for Severe Obesity*, National Institutes of Health, Bethesda MD, 25–27 March.

Suggested Reading

Cadière, G.B., Bruyns, J., Himpens, J. *et al.* (1994). Laparoscopic gastroplasty for morbid obesity. *Br J Surg* 81: 1524–1525.

Cadière, G.B., Favretti, F., Bruyns, J. *et al.* (1994). Gastroplastie par coeliovideoscopie: Technique. *Le Journal de Celio-Chirurgie* 10: 27–41.

Chevallier, J.M., Zinzindohoue, F., Elian, N. *et al.* (2002). Adjustable gastric banding in a public university hospital: prospective analysis of 400 patients. *Obes Surg* 12: 93–99.

De Jong, I.C., Tan, K.G., Oostenbroek, R.J. (2000). Adjustable silicone gastric banding: a series with three cases of band erosion. *Obes Surg* 10: 26–32.

Dixon, J.B., Dixon, M.E., O'Brien, P.E. (2001). Pre-operative predictors of weight loss at 1-year after Lap-Band®surgery. *Obes Surg* 11: 200–207.

Fabry, H., Van Hee, R., Hendrickx, L. *et al.* (2002). A technique for prevention of port complications after laparoscopic adjustable silicone gastric banding. *Obes Surg* 12: 285–288.

Meir, E., Van Baden, M. (1998). Adjustable silicone gastric banding (ASGB) and band erosion (BE). *Obes Surg* 8: 385.

Meir, E., Van Baden, M. (1999). Adjustable silicone gastric banding and band erosion: personal experience and hypotheses. *Obes Surg* 9: 191–193.

Susmallian, S., Ezri, T., Charuzi, I. (2002). Laparoscopic repair of access port site hernia after LAP-BAND®system implantation. *Obes Surg* 12: 682–684.

Chapter 5

Long-Term Results in Laparoscopic Adjustable Gastric Banding (LAP-BAND®) for Obese Patients

Maurizio De Luca, Luca Busetto, Gianni Segato, Nadey S. Hakim and Franco Favretti

Introduction

A bariatric operation is currently the only effective treatment for morbid obesity in terms of inducing and maintaining satisfactory weight loss and decreasing weight-related co-morbidities. Laparoscopic access for bariatric operation has had a profoundly positive impact in terms of reducing recovery time and perioperative complications. Although laparoscopic Roux-en-Y gastric bypass (RYGB) is considered the gold standard in the United States, most European surgeons prefer a less invasive, reversible procedure, such as laparoscopic adjustable gastric banding (LAGB).

LAGB is the most commonly performed surgical procedure for morbid obesity in Europe, Australia and South America. To date, more than 300,000 of these bariatric procedures have been performed worldwide. LAGB has gained in popularity around the world as a first-choice surgical therapy for severely obese patients.[1]

LAGB is a purely restrictive operation that relies on decreased amount of intake as the mechanism for weight loss, and has less risk of malnutrition than with diversionary or bypass procedures. Adjustable gastric banding involves the surgical implantation of an inflatable silicone band around the uppermost part of the stomach, which is tightened according to individual weight loss and appetite.

Band tightening or adjustments are performed by percutaneously by accessing a subcutaneous reservoir port that is connected to the band, and injecting fluid into the system.

True judgment of any bariatric procedure requires sound data, not only with regard to the surgical technique and its related mortality, morbidity and weight loss, but also to the procedure's impact on baseline co-morbidities and life expectancy.

Such data can be provided only by studies that have a very high follow-up rate extended over the long-term. Short- and medium-term series have found the band to be both safe and effective. However, a paucity of large long-term follow-up studies has created uncertainty in some about the efficacy over time.

Laparoscopic Technique

Perigastric dissection

The key steps of the laparoscopic procedure, defined and standardized by our team[2] and by the Free University of Brussels in June 1995, are:

1) establishment of reference points for dissection (equator of the balloon inflated with 25 cc of air at the left crus);
2) creation of a retrogastric tunnel above the peritoneal reflection of the bursa omentalis;
3) creation of a 'virtual' pouch;
4) embedding of the band.

The main steps of the procedure we use, known as the 'perigastric technique', are summarized below.

After initiation of pneumoperitoneum, four 5 mm and one 10 mm ports are created. They are located at the junction of the upper third and second third of the xipho-umbilical line (5 mm), below the xiphoid (5 mm), in the left (10 mm) and right hypochondrium (5 mm) and on the left anterior axillary line below the rib cage (5 mm). All the ports are introduced by means of an optical port (Visiport™) or screw port (EndoTip™) in order to reduce the risk of damaging abdominal organs and abdominal wall vessels.

A calibrated balloon-tipped orogastric tube is inserted into the stomach. The balloon is inflated with 25 ml of air and withdrawn to the gastro-oesophageal (GO) junction. This allows clear visibility along the lesser curve and into the phreno-gastric ligament. These two sites correspond to the most bulging part of the balloon and are marked with the coagulating hook. The reference point on the lesser curvature is the equator of the balloon, which, on the phreno-gastric ligament on the greater curvature, corresponds to the left crus. The identification of these two points is essential to ensure correct positioning of the band. The left crus is dissected.

To avoid gastric wall injuries, the calibration tube must be withdrawn during dissection, which must be done perpendicularly so as not to enter the inferior mediastinum along the oesophagus.

A tunnel is created behind the stomach, joining the two dissected reference points. The bursa omentalis (lesser sac) should not be entered, and the dissection should be performed in the phreno-gastric ligament above the peritoneal reflection of the bursa omentalis. An articulating dissector (or equivalent instrument) is passed through the tunnel to grasp the tip of the band. The band is introduced through the path of the left subcostal port. The 10 mm port is removed, and its path is utilized. However, the manufacturer recommends that the band be passed into the abdominal cavity via a 15 mm or 18 mm trocar.

The calibration tube provided with the band is used to check the correct placement of the band prior to locking it. The inflatable balloon of the calibration tube is inflated to 15–25 ml and the tube is pulled up against the bottom of the GO junction. The band should be positioned over the bulge created by the balloon from the middle of the balloon on the lesser curve, to the top of the balloon at the angle of His. Gastric tissue should be clearly seen above the band. A 'virtual' pouch based on the 25 ml initial measurement is created. A loose fit can be evaluated by deflating the balloon and nearly locking the band over the calibration tube. There should be room for an instrument to pass bluntly under the band. If the band appears to be too tight, then loosen the band to allow for access to remove or incise excess omental tissue. Blunt dissection is recommended to avoid damaging the gastric wall. Re-check the 'fit' before proceeding. The band is then locked in place over the calibration tube, with a final confirmation of adequate space under the band. The band is left either empty or only slightly inflated to avoid post-operative obstruction. Next, retention sutures are applied to prevent band slippage and/or stomach slippage; these anti-slippage sutures are placed in the seromuscular layer of the stomach from proximal to distal to the band and should start as close as possible to the greater curvature, embedding the band. If there is a gap on the lesser curvature, it should be closed by applying one or two stitches distal to the band from the lesser curvature to the hepato-gastric ligament, taking care not to damage the vagus nerve. The reservoir (access port) is implanted on the left anterior rectus sheath just distal to the costal margin.

Pars flaccida dissection

As one of the first centres to utilize the LAP-BAND® System, proficiency was gained with the peri-gastric dissection technique. We continue to utilize this approach satisfactorily. However, in recent years there has been a shift in training towards a slightly different dissection path around the stomach, now known as the *pars flaccida* technique.[3] This approach is readily understood and adopted by new LAP-BAND® surgeons due to the similarities to the common approach for a Nissen fundoplication. It has also been reported to be associated with a reduced operative incidence of gastric perforation as well as post-operative incidence of erosion and slippage. Briefly, this dissection begins directly lateral to the equator of the calibration balloon in the avascular space of the *pars flaccida*. Once the caudate lobe of the liver is visible, blunt dissection is continued over to the angle of His (after the right crus, and then the left crus have been sighted).

Pars flaccida to perigastric dissection

Some surgeons use a combination of both of the above methods of dissection of the lesser curvature, called the *pars flaccida* to perigastric technique.[4] This dissection is made at the mid-point (equator) of the balloon near the stomach until the perigastric dissection intercepts the *pars flaccida* dissection. This second window does not require completion of the entire perigastric dissection. Creation of a simple path next to the lesser curve is required to 'pick up' the band tubing lying in the *pars flaccida* path. The band is then placed from the angle of His through to the perigastric opening. This method is especially valuable in very large men who may have excessive intra-abdominal adipose tissue which can result in the band being too tight in the early post operative period. Moving to the perigastric location brings the band closer to the stomach and avoids including the thick lesser omentum within the band in these patients.

Role of the Balloon

The rate of intraoperative complications is higher in the super-obese than in morbidly obese patients. In laparoscopic surgery, the creation and maintenance of the pneumoperitoneum is particularly worrisome in super-obese patients, and the operative field is frequently poorly visualized with a high rate of conversion to open surgery.

The BioEnterics® Intragastric Balloon System (BIB®) has been found to improve the conditions for laparoscopic surgery, reducing the rate of conversion to open surgery and the rate of intraoperative complications in super-obese patients during LAGB. Both the placement and the removal of the BIB® device are performed under deep sedation with anaesthesiological assistance. Under endoscopic control, the deflated balloon should be introduced through the mouth and positioned in the stomach cavity. The balloon should then be injected with 500–700 ml of saline and methylene blue (50:1). A modified liquid diet should be followed for the first two weeks. Continuous treatment with a proton pump inhibitor is recommended while the balloon is in place. Balloon removal can take place on an outpatient basis six months after placement. Under endoscopic control, the balloon is punctured with a sclerosis needle, deflated, grabbed and gradually extracted. In general, we suggest that the LAP-BAND® can be placed one month after the balloon removal.

The preoperative weight loss produced by the BIB® is associated with a reduced rate of conversion to open surgery and of intraoperative complications.[5] Operative time and hospital stay are also significantly shortened. It has been observed that in the first phase of weight loss following LAP-BAND® placement, a preferential reduction of visceral fat and a 12 per cent reduction of liver volume occurs. It is possible that similar variations in intra-abdominal anatomy can explain the positive impact of the preoperative weight loss on laparoscopic surgery provided by the intragastric balloon. It is obvious that these changes are related to the weight loss and not to the use of the BIB® *per se*. However, the weight loss obtained by the BIB® has been found to be higher than the weight loss obtained by diet only.

However, in a published study of our group, no significant differences between the two groups were observed at the following postoperative evaluations.[5] The weight loss attained by the two groups is very similar starting from one year after banding. Preoperative treatment with the intragastric balloon should not therefore be viewed as means to improve the long-term results of gastric banding.

Perioperative weight loss to reduce the surgical risk in these candidates for bariatric surgery is an established indication for use of the balloon. This sequential therapy should be considered in patients with extreme obesity.

Lap-Band® Series at Vicenza Regional Hospital, Padua

Methods

Our total series consists of 2,245 patients (September 1993–December 2007). We analysed a subset of 1,791 patients with a follow-up rate of 91 per cent.

From September 1993 through December 2005 1,791 consecutive patients underwent gastric banding surgery for morbid obesity at our institutions (Obesity Centres of Vicenza Regional Hospital and Padova University). All operations were performed by the same team of surgeons utilizing the LAP-BAND® Adjustable Gastric Banding System and all patients met the eligibility criteria for bariatric surgery according to the NIH Consensus Conference Statement of 1991.[6]

Outcomes measured over 12 years included mortality, complications, weight loss and resolution/improvement of co-morbidities. Life expectancy was evaluated in an adjunct study of LAP-BAND® versus medical therapy.

Preoperatively-recorded characteristics of 1,345 female (75.1 per cent) and 446 male (24.9 per cent) patients were: mean age 38.7 ± 10.9 years, mean height 1.66 ± 0.09 metres, mean weight 127.7 ± 24.3 kg, and mean BMI 46.2 ± 7.7.

Baseline co-morbidities were present in 71 per cent of our patients: 57.8 per cent suffered from osteoarthritis, 35.6 per cent hypertension, 31.4 per cent Obstructive Sleep Apnoea Syndrome (OSAS), 27.1 per cent dyslipidemia, 22.0 per cent type II diabetes, 21.2 per cent depression, 9.3 per cent hyperuricaemia, 8.7 per cent gallstones, 4.9 per cent amenorrhea, and 1.4 per cent heart failure.

Of 1,791 patients, 125 (7 per cent) underwent preoperative application of a BIB® (Bioenterics Intragastric Balloon) with the aim of reducing the surgical risk. Their mean age was 44.8 ± 11.8 years, mean height 1.68 ± 0.10 metres, mean weight 161.4 ± 30.1 kg and mean BMI 56.8 ± 9.1.

The perigastric dissection, as has been previously described,[2] was performed in 1,393 patients (77.8 per cent), the *pars flaccida* technique was used in 384 (21.5 per cent) and the combined approach in 14 (0.8 per cent). Table 1 shows the number of operations performed per year.

Table 1. Number of operations per year follow-up rate (mean follow-up 91 per cent).

Year	No. of operations	Total	Follow-up years	N. pts follow-up	Follow-up rate (per cent)
1993	4	4	12	4	100
1994	18	22	11	22	100
1995	59	81	10	74	91.3
1996	129	210	9	188	89.5
1997	130	340	8	311	91.4
1998	143	483	7	415	85.9
1999	168	651	6	588	90.3
2000	192	843	5	765	90.7
2001	133	976	4	895	91.7
2002	143	1119	3	1001	89.4
2003	201	1320	2	1198	90.7
2004	198	1518	1	1353	89.1
2005	273	1791	—	—	—

Patients were followed at 1, 3, 6 and 12 months post-operatively and yearly thereafter. All data concerning mortality, complications, reoperations, weight loss and co-morbidities were recorded during the follow-up visits. Band adjustments were performed with barium swallow under fluoroscopy.

The co-morbidities were specifically investigated in 830 consecutive patients, consisting of 647 women (77.9 per cent) and 183 men (22.1 per cent), from September 1993 until November 2005.[7] For this group of patients a complete cardiovascular risk factor profile was collected both before and 12–18 months after surgery (mean follow-up time: 15.3 ± 2.1 months).

Results

There was zero surgical mortality in our entire series of 1,791 patients. The follow-up rate at 12 years was 91 per cent.

The conversion rate was 1.7 of which 1.2 per cent was due to technical problems such as difficult perigastric dissection and giant left liver lobe hypertrophy, 0.5 per cent caused by intraoperative complications such as gastric perforation and bleeding.

The 125/1,791 patients who had a BIB® applied preoperatively lost 24.7 ± 11.7 kg, 8.7 points of BMI and a percentage EWL of 27.9 ± 11.8 at the time of LAP-BAND® placement.

This group of patients showed the same conversion and intraoperative complication rate as the rest of the series.

Major complications requiring reoperation occurred in 106 patients (5.9 per cent); see Table 2.

These included:

- Stomach slippage and pouch dilatation in 70 patients (3.9 per cent). The bands were removed in 20 patients (1.1 per cent) and repositioned in 50 patients (2.8 per cent).
- Erosion in 16 patients (0.9 per cent). The bands were removed.
- Psychological intolerance in 14 patients (0.7 per cent). The bands were removed.

Table 2. Major complications requiring reoperation (106/1,791 patients, September 1993 – December 2005).

Complications	Number	Rate of complications (per cent)	Reoperation	Number	Rate of reoperation (per cent)
Stomach slippage + pouch dilatation	70	3.9	• Removal • Repositioning	20 50	1.1 2.8
Erosion	16	0.9	Removal	16	0.9
Psychological intolerance	14	0.7	Removal	14	0.7
Miscellaneous (HIV, infections, microperforation)	5	0.27	Removal	5	0.27
Gastric necrosis	1	0.05	Gastrectomy	1	0.05
Total	**106**	**5.9**	**Total**	**106**	**5.9**
Unsatisfactory results (lack of compliance)	41	2.3	• BPD • Removal • "BandInaro"	5 12 24	0.27 0.7 1.3

- Miscellaneous (HIV, infection, microperforation) in five patients (0.27 per cent), whose bands were removed); gastric necrosis in one patient (0.05 per cent); a gastrectomy was performed.

If we exclude the 31 major complications of the learning curve period (the first 100 patients), the complication rate is reduced to 4.4 per cent.

Of the 41 patients (2.3 per cent) with unsatisfactory results, the band was removed in 12 (0.7 per cent). A classical biliopancreatic diversion was performed in 5 (0.27 per cent) and a biliopancreatic diversion with gastric preservation ('bandinaro') was done in 24 (1.3 per cent) (see Table 2).

Minor complications requiring reoperation occurred at the port site in 200 patients (11.2 per cent). The port was substituted in 182 (10.2 per cent), repositioned in 9 (0.5 per cent) and removed in 9 (0.5 per cent). (These port issues, almost entirely related to the port-tubing transition,

Table 3. Weight loss (kg, BMI, %EWL) of the entire series.

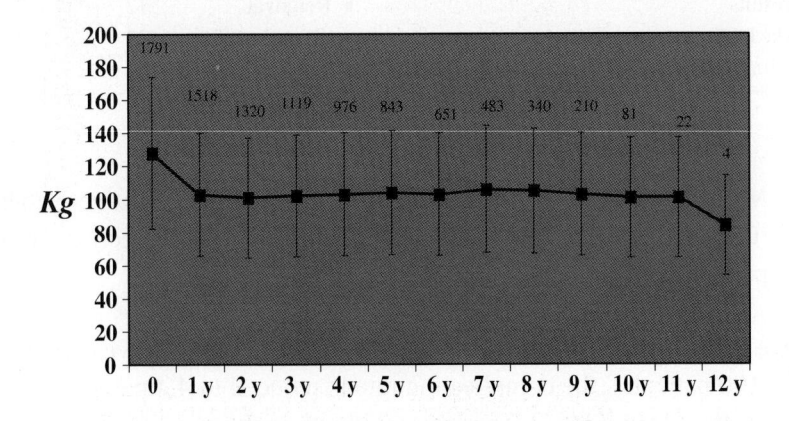

Time	Weight	BMI	%EWL
0	127.7 ± 24.3	46.2 ± 7.7	—
1 y	103.7 ± 21.6	37.7 ± 7.1	40.3 ± 19.7
2 y	101.5 ± 23.3	36.8 ± 7.6	43.7 ± 21.7
3 y	102.5 ± 22.5	37.2 ± 7.2	41.2 ± 23.2
4 y	104.1 ± 23.5	37.8 ± 7.5	38.6 ± 24.4
5 y	105.0 ± 23.6	38.1 ± 7.6	37.3 ± 25.3
6 y	105.3 ± 24.6	38.1 ± 8.1	37.4 ± 28.2
7 y	106.8 ± 24.3	38.5 ± 7.9	35.9 ± 26.7
8 y	105.0 ± 24.0	37.8 ± 7.9	37.7 ± 26.7
9 y	103.3 ± 26.2	37.5 ± 8.5	38.5 ± 27.9
10 y	101.4 ± 27.1	37.7 ± 9.1	35.4 ± 29.6
11 y	101.2 ± 31.9	38.1 ± 11.5	38.4 ± 32.8
12 y	84.0 ± 27.5	31.6 ± 8.5	49.2 ± 49.5

Figure 1. Weight loss (kg) of the entire series.

were more common early in our experience. With refinements to the placement technique and design improvements to the port tubing, these complications have been all but eliminated.)

Weight loss (kg, BMI, percentage EWL) for the entire series is represented in Table 3 and shown in Figs. 1–4. At ten years the average weight was 101.4 ± 27.1 kg (loss of 26.3 kg), the BMI 37.7 ± 9.1 (loss of 8.5 points) and the percentage EWL was 38.5 ± 27.9.

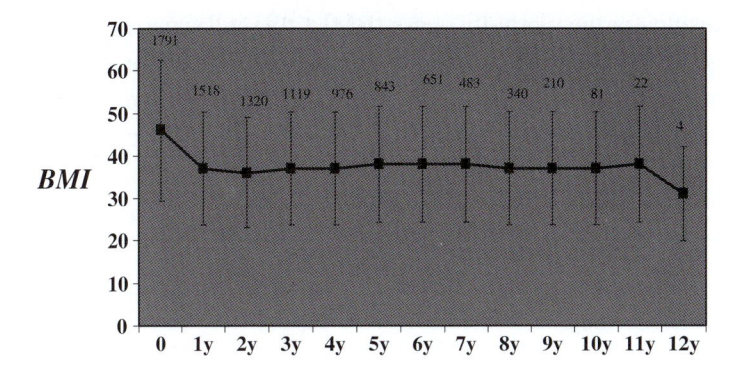

Figure 2. Weight loss (BMI) of the entire series.

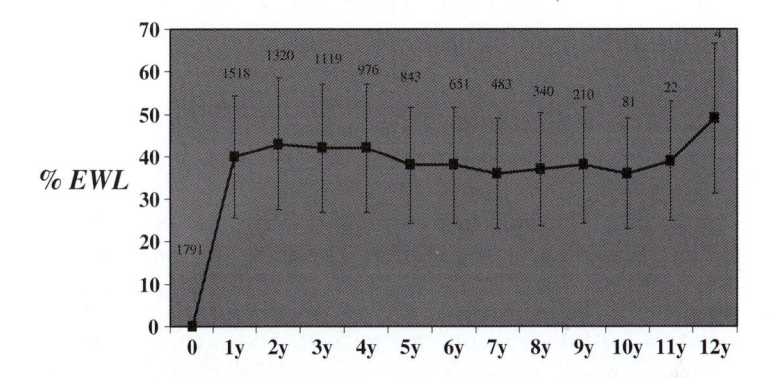

Figure 3. Weight loss (% EWL) of the entire series.

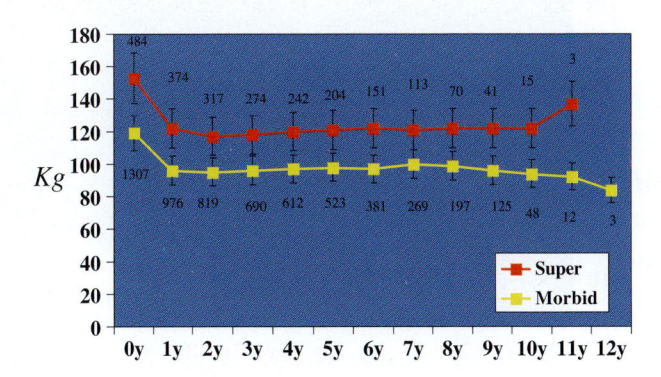

Figure 4. Weight loss (kg) in super and morbid obese patients.

Results for the morbidly obese (BMI ≤ 49) and super-obese (BMI ≥ 50) were separated into two groups for evaluation/comparison and weight loss in terms of kg and BMI is reported in Table 4 and shown in Fig. 5. At ten years the weight of the morbidly obese group was 94.6 ± 18.0 kg and was

Table 4. Weight loss (kg, BMI) in super and morbidly obese patients.

Time	n. Morbid	n. Super	Weight Morbid	Weight Super	BMI Morbid	BMI Super
0 y	1307	484	118.4 ± 16.9	152.8 ± 23.7***	42.6 ± 4.3	56.2 ± 5.8***
1 y	976	374	96.6 ± 16.3	122.1 ± 22.9***	34.8 ± 4.7	45.0 ± 7.0***
2 y	819	317	95.3 ± 20.2	117.4 ± 23.4***	34.3 ± 6.2	43.3 ± 7.3***
3 y	690	274	96.4 ± 18.1	118.0 ± 24.8***	34.7 ± 5.2	43.5 ± 7.7***
4 y	612	242	97.7 ± 18.7	120.3 ± 26.6***	35.2 ± 5.4	44.3 ± 8.1***
5 y	523	204	98.6 ± 18.9	121.3 ± 26.6***	35.6 ± 5.5	44.6 ± 8.4***
6 y	381	151	98.6 ± 19.4	122.3 ± 28.0***	35.4 ± 5.8	44.9 ± 9.1***
7 y	269	113	100.5 ± 19.8	121.8 ± 27.4***	35.8 ± 5.7	44.8 ± 8.7***
8 y	197	70	99.0 ± 19.1	122.0 ± 28.1***	35.4 ± 5.6	44.5 ± 9.4***
9 y	125	41	96.7 ± 18.2	123.6 ± 35.2***	35.0 ± 5.4	44.9 ± 13.9***
10 y	48	15	94.6 ± 18.0	123.2 ± 38.5**	35.2 ± 5.4	45.7 ± 13.5***
11 y	12	3	92.1 ± 20.3	137.7 ± 48.9*	34.4 ± 6.6	53.0 ± 16.2**
12 y	3	0	84.0 ± 27.5	—	31.6 ± 8.5	—

Student's t-test: * = $p < 0.05$; ** = $p < 0.01$; *** = $p < 0.001$.

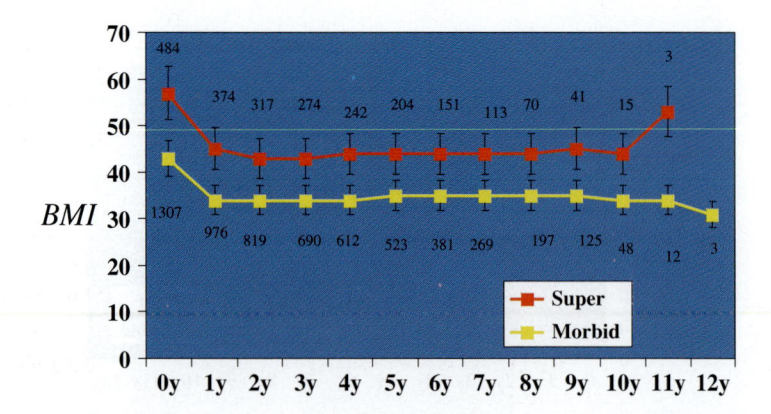

Figure 5. Weight loss (BMI) in super and morbid obese patients.

123.2 ± 38.5 kg in the super-obese group, indicating weight losses of 23.8 kg and 29.6 kg, respectively.

At ten years the BMI in the morbidly obese group was 35.2 ± 5.4 and 44.9 ± 13.9 in the super-obese group, down 7.4 and 11.3 points, respectively.

The percentage EWL in the morbidly and super-obese groups is reported in Table 5 and shown in Fig. 6. At ten years, percentage EWL was 40.3 ± 27.6 and 36.0 ± 30.2, respectively.

The effect of LAP-BAND® was specifically analysed in our first 830 consecutive patients.[7] The prevalence of diabetes at baseline was 11.2 per cent (17.7 per cent in men and 9.2 per cent in women; $p < 0.05$); 36.2 per cent of the patients with diabetes were treated with oral hypoglycaemic drugs and none with insulin. Hypercholesterolaemia was diagnosed in 53.9 per cent of patients (48.4 per cent in men and 55.4 per cent in women), low HDL-cholesterol in 13.1 per cent (18.8 per cent in men and 11.5 per cent in women) and hypertriglyceridaemia in 19.4 per cent (30.6 per cent in men and 16.0 per cent in women; $p < 0.01$ per cent). Finally, the prevalence of hypertension was 32.2 per cent (45.9 per cent in men

Table 5. Weight loss (% EWL) in super and morbidly obese patients.

Time	n. Morbid	n. Super	Weight loss Morbid	Weight loss Super	% EWL Morbid	% EWL Super
0 y	1307	484	—	—	—	—
1 y	976	374	21.7 ± 11.2	30.9 ± 15.6***	42.3 ± 20.4	35.1 ± 16.6***
2 y	819	317	23.2 ± 15.5	34.4 ± 16.9***	45.2 ± 25.5	39.8 ± 18.5**
3 y	690	274	21.8 ± 13.4	33.7 ± 18.0***	42.1 ± 20.4	39.1 ± 19.5*
4 y	612	242	20.5 ± 13.5	31.0 ± 19.2***	39.6 ± 25.5	36.2 ± 21.0*
5 y	523	204	19.8 ± 13.8	30.1 ± 19.6***	38.1 ± 26.5	35.1 ± 21.7
6 y	381	151	20.1 ± 15.1	29.1 ± 21.5***	38.7 ± 29.7	33.9 ± 23.9*
7 y	269	113	18.7 ± 13.5	29.0 ± 20.4***	36.6 ± 27.8	34.0 ± 23.9
8 y	197	70	19.9 ± 13.9	28.7 ± 20.5**	38.8 ± 27.2	34.5 ± 24.9
9 y	125	41	20.2 ± 13.9	26.1 ± 22.4	40.3 ± 27.6	32.9 ± 28.7
10 y	48	15	17.6 ± 14.2	29.2 ± 22.7	35.2 ± 29.7	36.0 ± 30.2
11 y	12	3	20.5 ± 18.6	25.7 ± 5.1	40.9 ± 36.1	28.3 ± 13.3
12 y	3	0	16.5 ± 14.6	—	49.2 ± 49.5	—

Student's t-test: * = $p < 0.05$; ** = $p < 0.01$; *** = $p < 0.001$.

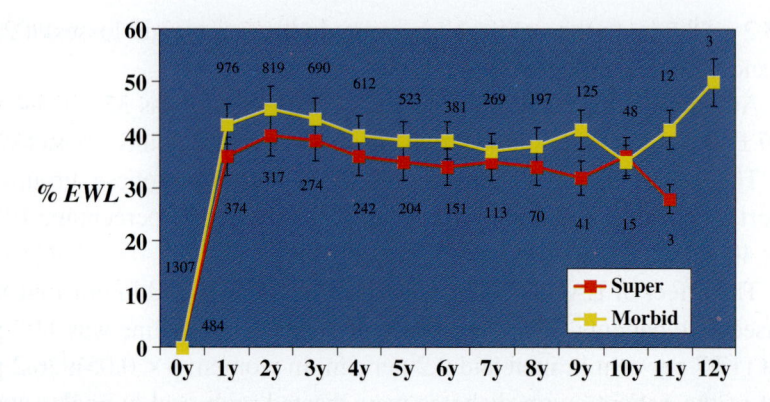

Figure 6. Weight loss (BMI) in super and morbid obese patients.

and 27.9 per cent in women; p < 0.001), with 60.6 per cent of hypertensive patients being treated pharmacologically.

Discussion

The conversion rate is 0.1–1.7 per cent which in most cases is due to technical problems such as difficult perigastric dissection and giant left liver lobe hypertrophy.

Of the major complications requiring reoperation (5.9 per cent), stomach slippage with pouch dilatation accounts for 2.3–3.9 per cent.[8–10]

One of the most appealing aspects of gastric banding is its total reversibility, which is important in cases of psychological intolerance of the prosthesis. In case of unsatisfactory results, due mainly to the patient's lack of compliance, a biliopancreatic diversion with gastric preservation can be offered.[11]

There is a 0.1 per cent of patients who require reoperation due to intra-abdominal haemorrhage from a trocar site, the same values discussed in any advanced laparoscopic surgery.

Minor complications requiring reoperation include those occurring at the port-site with an approximate occurrence of 11.2 per cent. In most cases, a leak can be detected and the port substitution required. In a minority of patients, the port has to be repositioned for pain (0.5 per cent) or removed because of infection (0.5 per cent). With the use of 'low-profile' ports the leakage rate has been greatly reduced.[12,13]

A mortality rate of 0 per cent in all major studies attests to the benign nature of the surgery.[14,15] The Australian Safety and Efficacy Register of New Interventional Procedures–Surgical systematic review of the worldwide literature found a significant difference in mortality between the RYGB, vertical banded gastroplasty and LAGB. The LAGB had one death in 2,000 (0.05 per cent), which is one-tenth the mortality seen with RYGB and one-sixth the mortality with vertical banded gastroplasty. In a study from a New York University programme, the LAGB had significantly fewer complications compared with RYGB and biliopancreatic diversion with duodenal switch (10 per cent versus 29.2 per cent versus 27.6 per cent).[16]

With regard to the weight loss curves, in the long term the average weight is expected to decrease an average of 26.3 kg with a decrease of 8.5 of BMI score. The curves are stable over time, with no statistically detectable rebound. Weight loss associated with the LAGB is slower compared with that seen with RYGB, progression is gradual over a two to four year period and then usually stabilizes at approximately 50–60 per cent, corresponding with that of RYGB in the same time frame.[14]

There was a difference in the results of the morbidly obese patients (BMI < 50) and super-obese patients (BMI > 50) with better results in the super-obese patients. After the fourth year no statistical difference between the value of the two curves has been proved and they tend to merge together. The weight loss that can be observed in morbidly obese patients in the first 12–18 months after gastric banding is associated with clinically significant improvements in multiple cardiovascular risk factors.[17]

However, only a low level of correlation can be observed between the degree of body weight reduction and the magnitude of cardiovascular risk improvement. In particular, a 10–11 per cent weight loss appeared to be associated with the maximal benefit in diabetic control, with no further gain being derived from more pronounced levels of body weight reduction.[18,19]

O'Brien et al. observed that after LAGB, patients experienced 74 per cent improvement or resolution of dyslipidemia, 94 per cent resolution of obstructive sleep apnoea, 55 per cent resolution of hypertension, 100 per cent improvement of asthma, and 76 per cent resolution with 14 per cent improvement in gastro-oesophageal reflux. Weight loss following LAGB surgery has a major impact on type II diabetes mellitus, with resolution or improvement of diabetes in 80.8 per cent of patients.[7,14,19]

Life Expectancy Study

Working with epidemiologists and internists of the Multisites Cohort of the Italian Study Group on Morbid Obesity, our group was able to conduct a case/control study on the effect of the LAP-BAND® on life expectancy (see also Chapters 12 and 13).[17,20]

In this study 821/1,791 of our LAP-BAND® patients were matched with 821 similar patients who received only medical treatment (Fig. 7). The five-year survival in the LAP-BAND®-treated group and in the medically-treated group is shown in Fig. 8, where a statistically significant difference in survival can be clearly seen in favour of the surgical group.

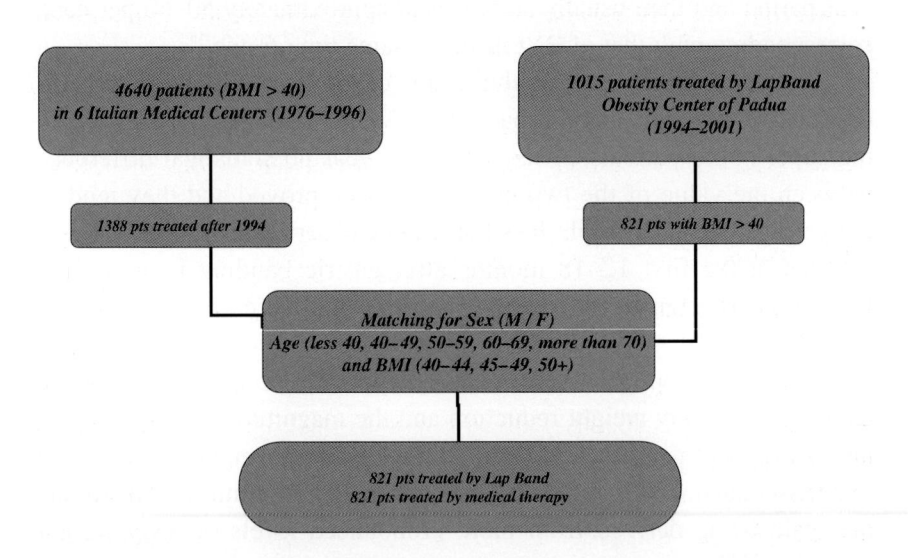

Figure 7. Case/control study involving 821 patients of our LapBand series and 821 patients treated by medical therapy in other Italian Medical Centers matching and selection of patients in the Case Group and Control Group.

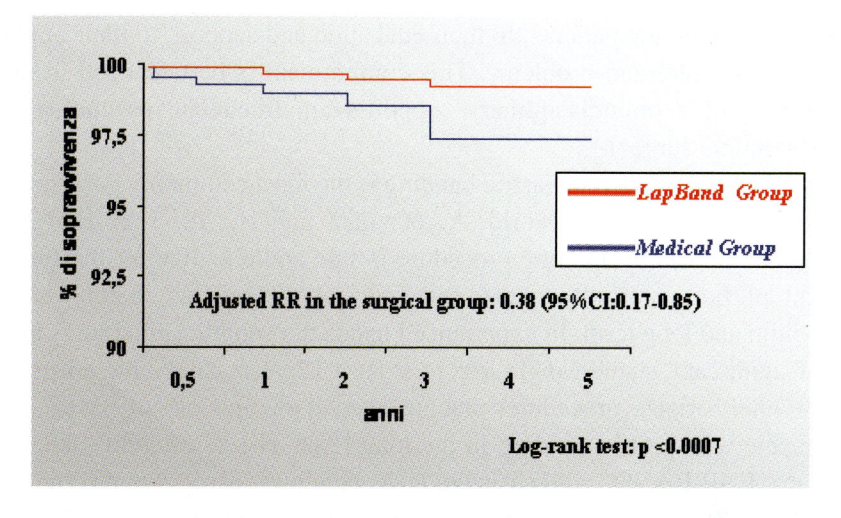

Figure 8. Five years survival in the lapband- and medical-treated groups.

Kaplan–Meier survival curves were calculated at six months and at one, two, three and five years and differences in survival between groups evaluated by logrank test. The survival rate was significantly higher in the LAP-BAND® group ($p < 0.0007$).

Relative risk of death after adjustment for sex, age and BMI in the surgical group was 0.38 (95 per cent CI: 0.17–0.85). So, the surgically-treated group is shown to have a 60 per cent reduction in total mortality.

Conclusion

LAP-BAND® System placement is proved to be a safe, effective, and gentle procedure which enables major and durable weight loss with improvement of a broad range of co-morbidities. It is quickly performed, well accepted by patients, with low mortality and mild complications which very rarely become lethal.

There are some clear requirements for the successful use of the LAP-BAND®. Though these requirements are not difficult or unusual, they are essential. The surgeon needs to have good laparoscopic skill and bariatric experience. Reasonable competence and experience can be achieved with good, specifically-oriented training and proctoring. There must be a commitment to the patients, to their education and support, to their ongoing routine care and problems. This commitment is best realized in the presence of a multidisciplinary support team (dietician, psychologist, internist and surgeon).

It is no accident that gastric banding is the most commonly performed bariatric surgery in the world. As our data indicate, the LAP-BAND® Adjustable Gastric Banding procedure is safe and effective for the treatment of both morbidly obese and super-obese patients in the short, medium and long term. In experienced hands the complication rate is low and significant, stable weight loss to at least 12 years can be the norm.

Other bariatric procedures that are fixed at the time of surgery cannot compete with gastric banding in the long-term. The adjustability feature of the LAP-BAND® allows patients to continue losing weight and to maintain lost weight over time. Of course, intensive follow-up and regular stoma adjustments must be a strictly enforced part of the process as they are integral to the patients' success.

References

1. Buchwald, H. (2005). Consensus Conference Statement — bariatric surgery for morbid obesity: health implications for patients, health professionals and third-party payers. *Surg Obes Relat Dis* 1: 371–381.
2. Favretti, F., Cadière, G., Segato, G. *et al.* (2002). Laparoscopic banding: selection and technique in 830 patients. *Obes Surg* 12: 385–390.
3. Fielding, G., Allen, J. (2002). A step-by-step guide to placement of the lap-band adjustable gastric banding system. *Am J Surg* 184(Suppl): 26S–30S.
4. Weiner, R., Engert, R., Weiner, S. *et al.* (2003). Outcome after laparoscopic adjustable gastric banding – 8 years experience. *Obes Surg* 13: 427–434.
5. Busetto, L., Segato, G., De Luca, M., *et al.* (2004). Preoperative weight loss by intragastric balloon in super-obese patients treated with laparoscopic gastric banding: a case-control study. *Obes Surg* 14: 671–676.
6. National Institutes of Health Consensus Development Conference Draft Statement (1991). Gastrointestinal surgery for severe obesity. *Obes Surg* 1: 257–266.
7. Busetto, L., Sergi, G., Enzi, G.I. *et al.* (2004). Short term effects of weight loss on the cardiovascular risk factors in morbidly obese patients. *Obes Res* 12(8): 1–8.

8. Dargent, J. (2004). Surgical treatment of morbid obesity by adjustable gastric band: the case for a conservative strategy in the case of failure — a 9-year series. *Obes Surg* 14: 986–990.
9. Chevallier, J.-M., Zinzindohoue, F., Douard, R. et al. (2004). Complications after laparoscopic adjustable gastric banding for morbid obesity: experience with 1,000 patients over 7 years. *Obes Surg* 14: 407–414.
10. Parikh, M.S., Fielding, G.A., Ren, C.J. (2005). U.S. experience with 749 laparoscopic adjustable gastric bands: intermediate outcomes. *Surg Endosc* 19(12): 1631–1635.
11. Cadière, G.B., Favretti, F., Himpens, J. (2001). Anneau gastrique et derivation bilio-pancreatique par laparoscopie. *J Coelio-Chir* 38: 32–35.
12. Ponce, J., Paynter, S., Fromm, R. (2005). Laparoscopic adjustable gastric banding: 1,014 consecutive cases. *J Am Coll Surg* 201(4): 529–535.
13. Favretti, F., Cadière, G., Segato, G. et al. (1997). Laparoscopic adjustable silicone gastric banding (LAP-BAND ®): how to avoid complications. *Obes Surg* 7: 352–358.
14. O'Brien, P., Dixon, J. (2002). Weight loss and early and late complications — the international experience. *Am J Surg* 184(Suppl): 42S–45S.
15. Belachew, M., Belva, P.H., Desaive, C. (2002). Long-term results of laparoscopic adjustable gastric banding for the treatment of morbid obesity. *Obes Surg* 12(4): 564–568.
16. Parikh, M., Laker, S., Weiner, M. et al. (2006). Objective comparison of complications resulting from laparoscopic bariatric procedures. *J Am Coll Surg* 202: 252–261.
17. Favretti, F., Segato, G., Ashton, D. et al. (2007). Laparoscopic adjustable gastric banding in 1,791 consecutive obese patients: 12-year results. *Obes Surg* 17: 168–175.
18. O'Brien, P.E., Dixon, J.B., Laurie, C. et al. (2005). A prospective randomized trial of placement of the laparoscopic adjustable gastric band: comparison of the perigastric and *pars flaccida* pathways. *Obes Surg* 15(6): 820–826.
19. Goldstein, D.J. (1992). Beneficial health effects of modest weight loss. *Int J Obes Relat Metab Disord* 16(6): 397–415.
20. Busetto, L., Mazza, M., Mirabelli, D. et al. (2006). Total mortality in morbid obese patients treated with laparoscopic adjustable gastric banding: a case-control study. *Obes Metab* 2(Suppl): 365 (abst).

Chapter 6

Laparoscopic Adjustable Gastric Banding (LAP-BAND®): Diagnosis, Prevention and Treatment of Complications

Maurizio De Luca, Luca Busetto, Gianni Segato, Nadey S. Hakim and Franco Favretti

Introduction

Laparoscopic adjustable gastric banding using the LAP-BAND® (Allergan Inc., Irvine, CA, USA) has been performed in our institution since 1993.[1,2]

In the past ten years the procedure has gained widespread acceptance and is now the most frequently performed bariatric procedure in many countries of the world.

Laparoscopic adjustable gastric banding brings many advantages to patient and surgeon. The procedure is completely reversible as it does not require the opening of the gastrointestinal tract or rerouting of the anatomy and it does not rely on cutting or stapling of the stomach so the patient does not suffer from the resultant, sometimes serious complications. Laparoscopic adjustable gastric banding (LAGB) has the distinction of being the *only* bariatric operation designed to be performed laparoscopically (the operation is laparoscopically accomplished in > 98 per cent of all cases). LAP-BAND® therefore allows patients to leave the hospital much earlier than more drastic open bariatric procedures, and subjects can return to work and normal activity much sooner.[2–8]

Complications with LAP-BAND® are unavoidable; they can be treated by laparoscopy in most cases and are rarely life-threatening if managed appropriately.

It is worthwhile noting that as techniques for placement have evolved, complication rates with the LAP-BAND® have declined. Surgeons and patients should adopt strategies that will help avoid complications and be sensitive to any indications of their emergence.[9–17]

In this chapter we report the long-term outcome of a large group of morbidly obese patients treated with the LAP-BAND®. We focus on the complications that required revisional surgery and present our methods of diagnosis, prevention and treatment.

Lap-Band® Series at Vicenza Regional Hospital, Padua

Our total series consisted of 2,225 patients between September 1993 and November 2007; we analyzed a subset of 1,800 patients with a follow-up rate of 91 per cent.

Between September 1993 and December 2005, the same surgical team performed LAP-BAND® procedures on 1,800 consecutive patients (75.1 per cent women, mean age 38.7 years, mean body weight (BW) 127.7 ± 24 kg, mean body mass index (BMI) 46.2 ± 7.7). Perigastric dissection was used in 77.8 per cent of the patients while *pars flaccida* was used in 21.5 per cent and a mixed approach in 0.8 per cent. Patients' data were analysed according to co-morbidities, conversion, short and long term complications and weight loss. Fluoroscopy-guided adjustments were performed and patients received intensive follow-up.[1]

Most common baseline co-morbidities were hypertension (35.6 per cent), osteoarthritis (57.8 per cent), diabetes (22 per cent), dyslipidaemia (27.1 per cent), obstructive sleep apnoea syndrome (OSAS) (31.4 per cent), depression (21.2 per cent), sweet eating (22.5 per cent) and binge eating (18.5 per cent). Conversion to open surgery was 1.7 per cent, of which 1.2 per cent was due to technical difficulties and 0.5 per cent to intraoperative complications. Together with the positioning of the band additional surgery was performed in 11.9 per cent of the patients: hiatal hernia repair (2.4 per cent), cholecystectomy (7.8 per cent) and other procedures (1.7 per cent). The mortality rate was 0 per cent. The follow up rate is 91 per cent. Band related complications, not all requiring reoperation, occurred in 230 patients. (12.8 per cent): pouch dilation 132 (11.7 per cent), slippage 77 (4.3 per cent), erosion 20 (1.1 per cent), infection 1 (0.1). Reoperations were required for 123 patients (6.8 per cent): band removal 69 (3.9 per cent) and band repositioning 54 (3.0 per cent). Port related complications occurred in 200 patients (11.2 per cent).

The BW (kg) was 103.7 ± 21.6, 102.5 ± 22.5, 105.0 ± 23.6, 106.8 ± 24.3, 103.3 ± 26.2 and 101.4 ± 27.1 at 1, 3, 5, 7, 9, 11 years after surgery. The BMI, at the same intervals, was 37.7 ± 7.1, 37.2 ± 7.2, 38.1 ± 7.6, 38.5 ± 7.9, 37.5 ± 8.5 and 37.7 ± 9.1.[1]

Complications

The LAP-BAND® operation is not without complications, but these occur on a smaller scale and have a much lower risk profile compared to other methods currently used in obesity surgery. It is important to note that complications can usually be corrected and that the LAP-BAND® appears to be the lowest risk operation currently available for the treatment of morbid obesity. Another important aspect of this kind of surgery, even though it requires advanced laparoscopic experience, is that most of the complications can be corrected by laparoscopy.

The following are the most common complications of LAP-BAND®:

1. Gastric perforation;
2. Stomach slippage;
3. Stoma obstruction;
4. Oesophageal and gastric pouch dilatation;
5. Erosion;
6. Gastric necrosis;
7. Tubing/access port problems;
8. Lack of compliance/unsatisfactory result.

Gastric perforation

The stomach may be perforated during surgery, mainly at the creation of the retrogastric tunnel. This step can be difficult in patients with very high BMI, visceral obesity and especially in males.[16–18]

Causes

The relationship of this 'gastric perforation' to the surgical procedure is evident and emergency surgery is indicated.

Incidence

Most surgeons have reported one or two stomach perforations, primarily during the learning curve period with a gastric perforation rate ranging from 0.2 to 3.5 per cent.

Symptoms

Gastric perforation is characterized by free leakage of gastric contents into the peritoneum similar to when perforation of the gastric lining leads to peritonitis.

Diagnosis

This complication can be detected easily during surgery by inflating the stomach with a methylene blue solution once the band tubing has been pulled into the retrogastric tunnel. Utilizing the methylene blue *after* the band has been positioned and locked could be useless. In fact, the band might completely fill the perforation and not show any leakage. An upper GI X-ray series with gastrographin, done routinely on the first postoperative day, can show the perforation.

How to avoid it

During the creation of the retrogastric tunnel there is in any patient a 'blind area'. If we want to avoid this complication, the area can be reduced by a wider downward exposition of the left crus and by a wider dissection along the lesser curvature. This is a consideration if the 'perigastric' dissection path is utilized. To avoid gastric wall injuries the calibration tube must be withdrawn during dissection and should be undertaken perpendicularly so as not to enter the inferior mediastinum along the oesophagus. We have found that the Articulating Dissector (Automated Medical Products Corp., Edison, NJ, USA) is atraumatic enough to avoid damaging the gastric wall. Good surgical technique with adequate exposure and use of appropriate instruments can reduce the incidence of this serious complication.

If the retrogastric dissection turns out to be risky, a very valuable option is the video-hand-assisted technique. The right hand of the surgeon is introduced into the abdomen through a mini-laparotomy. The perigastric dissection is undertaken digitally using the in-place calibration tube as a reference. The articulating instrument is put in place, the mini-laparotomy is closed and the rest of the operation is completed, usually by laparoscopy.

Treatment

If the perforation is detected at surgery and if it occurs at a location distant from the band, some surgeons have repaired the stomach laparoscopically and placed the band successfully. But, if the exposure is not satisfactory it is advisable to postpone the placement of the band, suture the stomach wall, drain the area and have a naso-gastric tube in place. If the perforation is detected post-operatively, and gross contamination has already occurred causing peritonitis and subsequent emergency surgery, the band has to be removed and traditional surgical approaches have to be implemented.

Stomach slippage

Stomach slippage is the post-operative development of an overly-large upper gastric pouch. Often referred to as gastric prolapse and often confused with pouch dilatation, this complication can occur anteriorly and/or posteriorly.[16,17,19]

Causes

Posterior gastric slippage is the most common type. The posterior gastric wall moves through the band resulting in the creation of a large posterior pouch. The band rotates to a vertical position, or even rotates beyond vertical, with the inferior aspect of the band lying more to the left. This problem is principally a consequence of placing the band across the apex of the lesser sac rather than through the tissue above the lesser sac.

Anterior gastric slippage results from failure of the anterior fixation (retention sutures). The band moves to a horizontal position and the enlarged proximal stomach overlies the left side of the band. The sutures may be placed in a way that fails to fix the lateral (greater curvature) aspect. They may be insufficient in number to give full fixation or they may be inserted above the band into the fat pad overlying the oesophago-gastric junction rather than into the upper gastric wall, so they subsequently tear out. Both posterior and anterior pouch dilatation lead to excessive stomach tissue inside the band and to obstruction between the upper pouch and the lower stomach.

Incidence

This is the most frequent complication associated with the LAP-BAND® procedure. Its incidence has been dramatically reduced over the years (from as high as 22 per cent down to less than 5 per cent by a better understanding of the anatomy of the gastro-oesophageal junction and by the evolution of the surgical technique).

Three techniques for the positioning of the LAP-BAND® have been described:

1. the perigastric method (Fig. 1);
2. the *pars flaccida* method (Fig. 2);
3. the *pars flaccida* to perigastric technique (Fig. 3).

Of these the perigastric technique may have the highest rate of slippage, probably because it is more difficult to master. But in fact the perigastric technique, properly performed, has a very low incidence of slippage, 10 per cent in our series, of which 1.9 per cent required reoperation.

Symptoms

Stomach slippage should be suspected when patients who have had a normal post-operative period begin to experience changes in their eating

Peri-Gastric Technique

The dissection starts directly on the lesser curve at the mid-point (equator) of the calibration balloon. Dissection is completed behind the stomach towards the angle of His under direct visualization. Avoidance of the lesser sac is important. Retro-gastric suturing is an option.

Red = Direction of dissection
Blue = The LAP-BAND® System placement

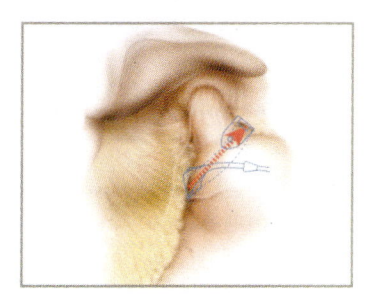

Figure 1. Peri-gastric technique. The dissection starts directly on the lesser curve at the mid-point (equator) of the calibration balloon. Dissection is completed behind the stomach towards the angle of His under direct visualization. Avoidance of the lesser sac is important. Retro-gastric suturing is an option.

Red = direction of dissection; blue = LAP-BAND® System placement

Pars Flaccida Technique

Dissection begins directly lateral to the equator of the calibration balloon in the avascular space of the Pars Flaccida. After seeing the caudate lobe of the liver, blunt dissection is continued under direct visualization until the right crus is seen, followed immediately by the left crus over to the angle of His.

Red = Direction of dissection
Blue = The LAP-BAND® System placement

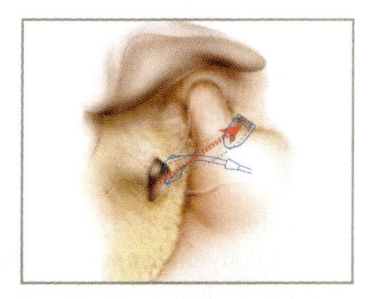

Figure 2. *Pars flaccida* technique. Dissection begins directly lateral to the equator of the calibration balloon in the avascular space of the *pars flaccida*. After seeing the caudate lobe of the liver, blunt dissection is continued under direct visualization until the right crus is seen, followed immediately by the left crus over to the angle of His.

habits. The symptoms of slippage are those of partial or complete obstruction and of fluid stasis in the lower oesophagus and upper distended gastric pouch. They include:

- heartburn;
- vomiting;
- free reflux of fluid into the mouth;

Pars Flaccida to Peri-Gastric (Weiner) Technique

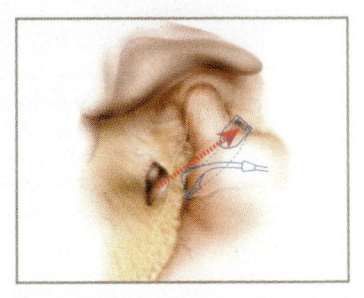

Figure 3. *Pars flaccida* to peri-gastric (Weiner) technique. Dissection begins with the *pars flaccida* technique. A second dissection is made at the midpoint (equator) of the balloon near the stomach until the peri-gastric dissection intercepts the *pars flaccida* dissection. The band is then placed from the angle of His through to the peri-gastric opening.

Red = direction of dissection; blue = the LAP-BAND™ System placement

- dysphagia;
- coughing and choking spells (particularly at night);
- wheezing;
- ability to tolerate only fluids.

The problem is usually chronic. Nevertheless, the patient can develop significant dehydration with electrolyte imbalance and ischemia of the upper stomach. Ischemic lesions are particularly dreadful since they can lead to gastric necrosis.

Diagnosis

Investigation and management depend on the severity and acuteness of symptoms. No patient should have the aforementioned symptoms as a 'normal' part of the post LAP-BAND® process. Therefore the onset of these symptoms indicates that either the band has been set too tightly or there is some slippage present. An upper gastrointestinal (GI) X-ray series is diagnostic (Fig. 4).

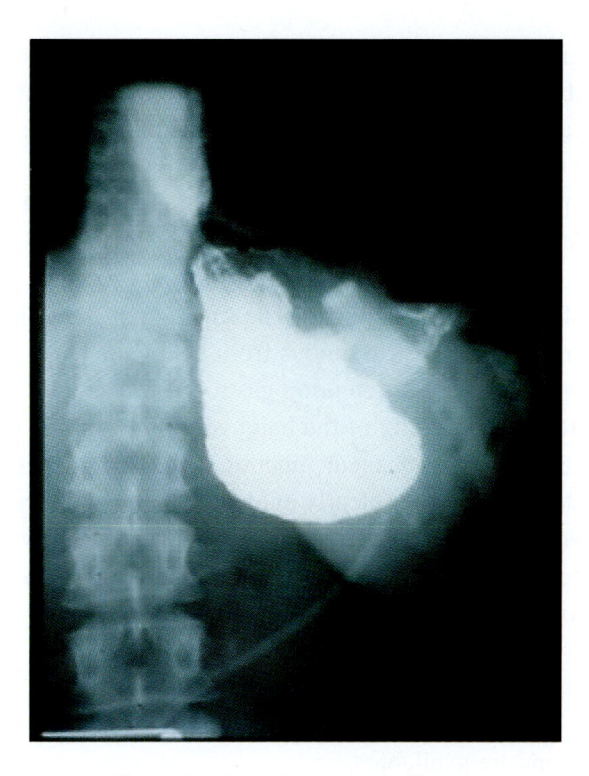

Figure 4. Posterior stomach slippage.

How to avoid it

In order to avoid this complication it is important to correctly select the sites for dissection along the lesser curvature and into the phreno-gastric ligament. A reliable reference point for dissection is the equator of the balloon (calibration tube inflated with 25 cc of air and withdrawn to the gastro-oesophageal junction) which, on the phreno-gastric ligament, corresponds to the left crus.

The retrogastric tunnel is created by joining the reference points. The dissection has to be perpendicular and has to aim at the left crus. The bursa omentalis should not be entered and the dissection has to be performed into the phreno-gastric ligament above the peritoneal reflection of the bursa omentalis. Once the LAP-BAND® has been positioned, an anterior 'embedment' is carried out with a few retention sutures applied from the greater towards the lesser curvature. Following these steps it is unlikely that either the band or the stomach walls can slip.

It is unquestionable that the lower reported incidence of stomach slippage is due to:

a) The creation of a 'virtual' pouch. The smaller pouch has less ability to stretch and pull the gastric fundus from below the band.
b) The sound placement of retention gastro-gastric sutures.
c) The posterior positioning of the band very high and in close proximity to the gastro-oesophageal junction. This anatomic tendency for high posterior position is clearly evident in the *pars flaccida* and combined *pars flaccida* to perigastric techniques. However, surgeons experienced with the perigastric technique have always recommended a high posterior position as well.

Treatment

Different options are available:

a) Deflation: The band system is deflated via the access port and an upper GI X-ray series is performed. This is the only way to positively establish the cause of the symptoms, and to establish whether any passage for the fluids exists through the band. In most cases the pouch returns to normal size and motility. After one month the band is gradually inflated with no more than 1.0 cc at a time. After deflation, if an upper GI series still shows slippage and/or the contrast passes with difficulty through the band, band removal or repositioning must be performed. True stomach slippage (as opposed to gastric pouch dilatation) does not respond to the above conservative measures and indicates the need for urgent laparoscopic or open exploration of the abdomen, especially in case of epigastric pain.
b) Removal: The LAP-BAND® System can be removed by laparoscopy. To reach the site of the band, which is usually covered by adhesions, it is advisable to follow the connecting tube and pull it. The buckle of

the band is easily identified and cut along the side of the buckle, allowing the withdrawal and removal of the device. In this case another surgical procedure could be offered to the patient.

c) Pull through technique: In the case of anterior gastric wall slippage, first the band must be deflated and exposed. At this point it is feasible to reduce the slippage by carefully pulling the gastric wall through the band. Retention sutures are applied. If the stomach above the band has become oedematous or hypertrophied to the extent that reduction is not possible, the band needs to be divided and a new band placed above the enlarged gastric pouch. Of course the position of the band on the lesser curvature and the location of the retrogastric tunnel have to be checked. If they are not correct, a repositioning has to be done.

d) Repositioning: Posterior stomach slippage is treated by removal of the band and placement of a new band higher up. The removal of the band requires just enough dissection to give access to the part of the band directly to the left of the buckle. The reference points for dissection have to be identified again to be sure that the retrogastric tunnel will be above the peritoneal reflection of the bursa omentalis. If the usual 'perigastric' technique for dissection and creation of the retrogastric tunnel is not possible due to local adhesions, the *'pars flaccida'* technique can be easily utilized. The *pars flaccida* pathway has not been previously dissected and is therefore easy to access. In this case dissection begins directly lateral to the equator of the calibration balloon in the avascular space of the *pars flaccida*. After seeing the caudate lobe of the liver, blunt dissection is continued under direct visualization until the right crus is seen, followed immediately by the left crus over to the angle of His.

Stoma obstruction

Stoma obstruction is defined as an obstruction to the passage of food from the gastric pouch to the rest of the stomach.

Incidence

It can happen any time, early or late in the postoperative period.

Symptoms

These include:

- sialorrhoea;
- vomiting;
- dysphagia;
- epigastric/retrosternal and chest pain;
- inability to swallow;
- new onset of reflux;
- repeated aspiration and pulmonary complications in severe cases.

Causes

Stoma obstruction in the early postoperative period has a number of possible causes all of which serve to narrow the stoma and simulate the effect of an over-tight band:

a) After band placement using the *'pars flaccida'* approach, stoma obstruction is most often associated with smaller bands applied over a thick gastro-oesophageal junction area or too distal from the GOJ.
b) After band placement using the 'perigastric' or the *'pars flaccida* to perigastric' approach, stoma obstruction is usually caused by the incorporation of too much tissue inside the band. In most of the cases, in fact, the band is positioned too distally from the GOJ causing a large amount of fundus and stomach wall to be encompassed by the band. Because the circumference of the band is fixed, obstruction results.
c) In other cases, especially in heavy male patients with thick GOJ areas the 9.75 or 10 cm bands may be placed around too much tissue. The surgeon can perform a delicate dissection, thinning out the area where the band is to be placed.
d) If a band still appears too tight just prior to locking, then consider using the 'two step dissection' option. When the *'pars flaccida'* technique has been used and when a band appears to be too tight just prior to locking the buckle, then stop, un-thread the band tubing and back

the band out of the retrogastric space. Leave the tubing in position behind the stomach and inflate the calibration tube to 25 cc. Pull the tube back so the balloon is firmly stopped against the bottom of the GOJ. Select a point at the equator (midline) of the inflated balloon on the edge of the lesser curve (as would be done to start the perigastric dissection). Deflate the balloon and pull the calibration tube back into the oesophagus. Bluntly dissect straight down access port alongside the lesser curve. Do not follow the stomach wall behind the stomach, just dissect straight downward until the band tubing is found in the *pars flaccida* pathway. Pull the band tubing up through the new perigastric window and re-thread the buckle. Just before locking all the way, confirm that the band now fits loosely. If not, excise fat tissue on the anterior gastric wall as needed to avoid being over-tight.
e) Post-operative oedema of the area incorporated by the band due to haematoma or post-operative reaction.

Late stoma obstructions are usually related to:

- gastric pouch dilation;
- stomach slippage;
- erosion;
- pouchitis and/or oesophagitis caused by bad eating habits.

Diagnosis

In most of the above-mentioned cases a post-operative contrast study with gastrographin (which must always be done on the first post-operative day) often reveals complete obstruction or near complete obstruction with minimal flow from the oesophagus and gastric pouch to the portion of the stomach below the band (Fig. 5). Tertiary oesophageal contractions (uncoordinated contractions) are usually evident.

Treatment

In many cases deflation of the band, a few days of liquid diet and medical treatment with pump inhibitors can prove salutary. For patients with

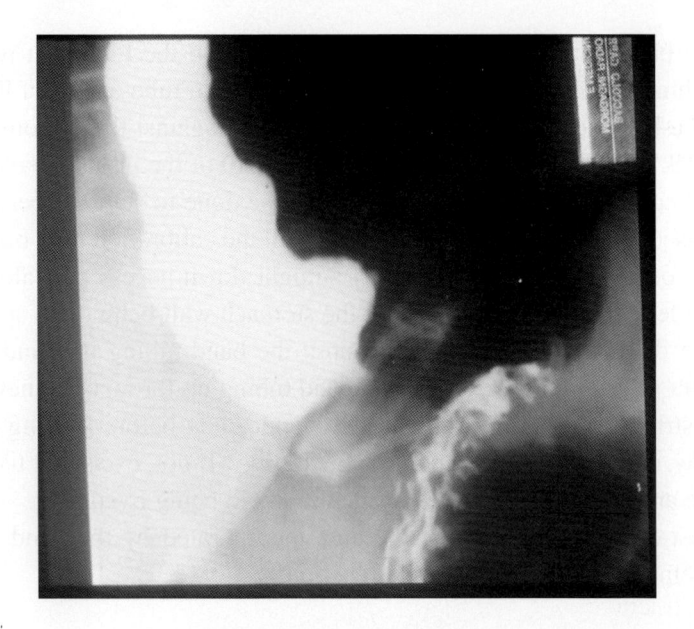

Figure 5. Stoma obstruction.

near-complete or partial obstruction, initial treatment can be conservative consisting of rehydration and reassurance in an inpatient setting. If patients do not improve clinically and radiologically within a few days they can be managed with exploratory laparoscopy as described earlier. If the stoma obstructions are caused by stomach slippage, pouch dilatation or erosion they are treated accordingly.

Oesophageal and gastric pouch dilatation

Oesophageal and gastric pouch dilatation without stomach slippage have been reported.[16-18]

Incidence

Oesophageal dilatation is a debatable complication having been observed and reported at essentially only one site in the U.S. Food and Drug Administration (FDA) clinical trial. In our series of 830 patients, 92 cases

(11 per cent) of oesophageal and gastric pouch dilatation were reported. Of these 92 cases, 83 (90 per cent) were caused by gastric slippage and 9 (0.9 per cent) by malposition of the band. It is our observation that oesophageal dilatation is a transient clinical 'finding' indicative of an overtightened band or a chronic outlet obstruction due to band malposition or slippage.

Causes

Even though the two entities, stomach slippage and gastric pouch dilatation, are different from an etiopathogenic point of view, they sometimes overlap; in a few cases the actual cause could be debatable. When this type of pouch enlargement occurs it is most likely caused by:

- over-inflation of the band resulting in a mechanically severe outlet obstruction;
- creation of an oversized pouch during surgery (band placed too low or malpositioned);
- patient's lack of compliance regarding oral intake (inappropriate food intake, insufficient chewing of food and overeating causing vomiting).

All these factors can stress and stretch the new small gastric pouch. Eventually the pouch and even the oesophagus may dilate as occurs in other restrictive procedures. Failure to address the issue will result in an atonic pouch and large atonic oesophagus.

Symptoms

These are indistinguishable from those previously described for stomach slippage.

Diagnosis

Periodic oesophageal imaging may help detect dilatation and therefore should be conducted at least once in the first post-operative year and/or at the time of adjustment (Fig. 6).

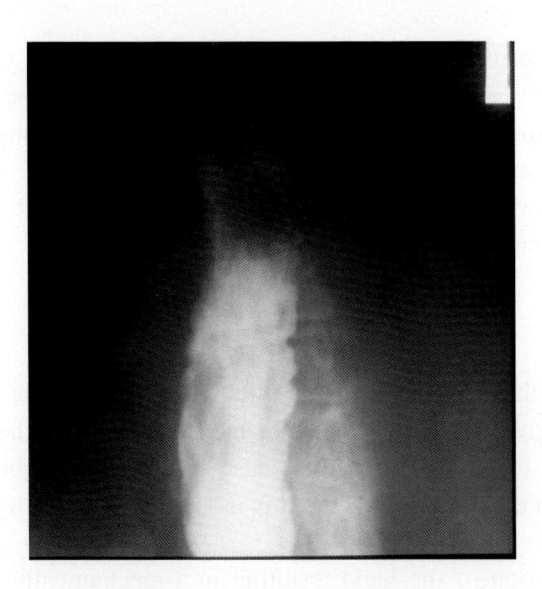

Figure 6. Oesophageal dilation.

How to avoid it

Creating a small upper pouch (15 ml or, even better, 'virtual') has been demonstrated to be vital to the success of surgery. There is a dramatic decrease in pouch enlargement problems when the initial pouch size is no more than 15 ml or 'virtual'. The size of the pouch and the dissection points for the retrogastric passage of the band have to be accurately determined with the use of the calibration tube/balloon supplied with each LAP-BAND® System.

Apart from the cases caused by an over-inflated band, we believe most of the reported cases are due either to stomach slippage (see above) or to malpositioning of the band. We avoid this complication by respecting the reference points for dissection and carrying out the retrogastric dissection as previously described. While creating the pouch, avoid any cul de sac that could be a recipe for further enlargement of the pouch leading to 'food intolerance'. The cul de sac is avoided by removing the calibration tube and by applying the retention sutures from below upwards. To reduce the incidence of early food intolerance we recommend that the LAP-BAND® stoma initially be kept large (band un-inflated) after surgery. A more open stoma may help accommodate any post-operative oedema or patient difficulty in compliance while learning new eating habits.

Treatment

Its management involves complete deflation of the band and, after two to three months, slow re-inflation with the surgeon being careful not to reach the previous point of over-inflation. If, after deflation, an upper gastrointestinal X-ray series shows a persisting oesophageal/gastric pouch enlargement with difficult passage of the contrast medium through the deflated band, the surgeon is probably dealing either with stomach slippage or with malpositioning of the band. In both cases the device is encompassing too much gastric tissue. Removal or repositioning of the band is usually required in these cases (see treatment of stomach slippage).

Erosion

Band erosion, defined as the partial or complete movement of a synthetic band into the gastric lumen of the stomach, is also known as migration, gastric incorporation and gastric inclusion. It exists as a possible complication following bariatric surgical procedures in which synthetic materials (silicone, Marlex®, Dacron® etc.) are used to create the gastric stoma. Band erosion may occur following vertical banded gastroplasty and gastric bypass as well as after LAP-BAND® System surgery. The occurrence of this complication renders any weight loss procedure ineffective and requires removal of the band, generally via surgery.[20-24]

Incidence

This complication occurred in 1 per cent of the patients of the LAP-BAND® FDA clinical trial. Omitting series in the international literature which include a large number of revision procedures and those performed during the learning curve, the LAP-BAND® System erosion rate is well below 1 per cent.

Causes

The level of laparoscopic expertise and the extent of LAP-BAND® System experience affect the surgeon's ability to avoid complications. The incidence of erosion is attributed to one or to a combination of the following:

- small, undetected injuries to the gastric wall that occur during band placement;
- necrosis due to pressure of the band;
- access port infection.

There is some disagreement among surgeons regarding the actual evolution of this process. While some believe that first the access port becomes infected, then the infection travels down the tubing to the band causing erosion, most believe that the infection of the port is a symptom of an already present erosion.

Symptoms

Most symptoms of erosion are of benign nature, non-urgent, non-life-threatening. Ileus or sepsis are rarely found in association with the onset of erosions. Erosions may go unnoticed for a considerable period of time because the capsule seals off the band from the peritoneal cavity and the band gradually transitions into the lumen without leakage or sepsis developing. Surgeons have observed a variety of (usually clinically benign) symptoms which may serve as indicators of band erosion. Many of these may be seen in combination and patients may present with:

- weight gain without apparent cause;
- feeling of lack of restriction/satiety;
- ineffectiveness of band adjustments;

- passage of contrast medium through and around then band shown on X-ray;
- chronic and persistent port infection (port site infection may be the first symptom of erosion, usually due to migration of bacteria from the stomach to the port site area along the tubing).

Diagnosis

An erosion can be diagnosed by an upper GI X-ray series, by OGDS and by fistulography (Fig. 7).

How to avoid it

A meticulous, gentle and careful operative dissection may avoid at least some of these erosion problems. If the surgeon suspects that an injury to or perforation of the lumen has occurred during surgery the injury should be addressed and serious consideration should be made as to whether placement should proceed at that time. During surgery, placement of

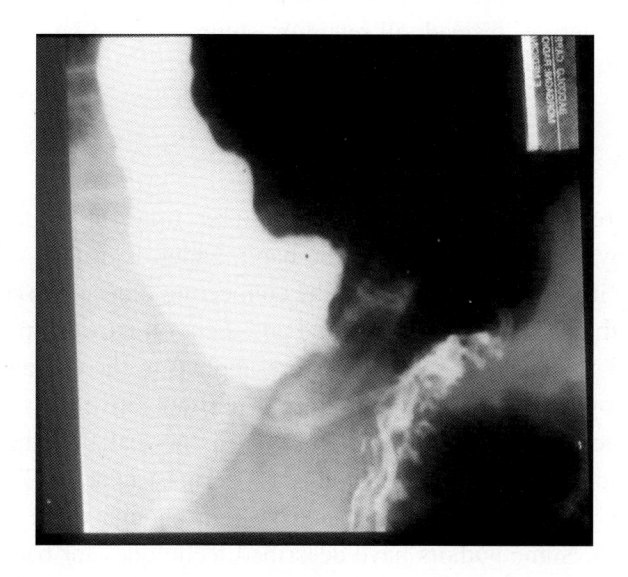

Figure 7.

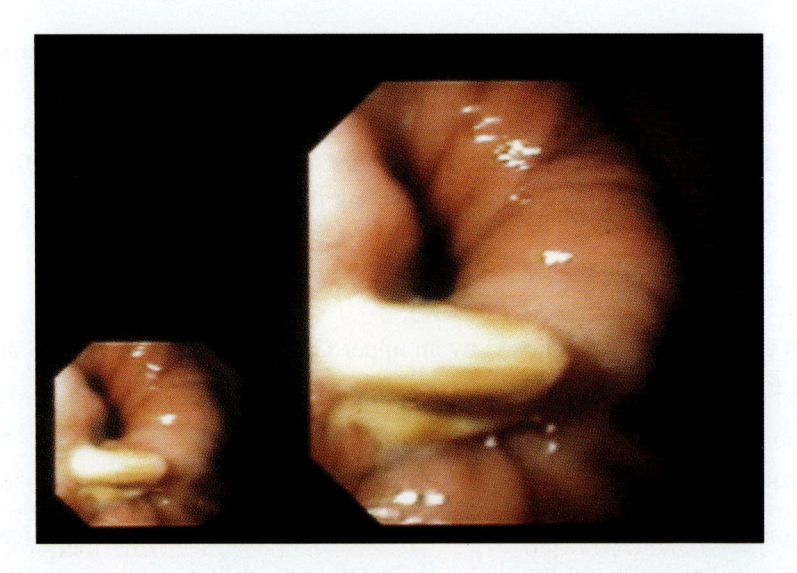

Figure 8.

gastro-gastric sutures over the locking mechanism (buckle) should be avoided. This area protrudes and can cause pressure necrosis to the gastric wall that covers it. Instead, all retention sutures should be placed to the left side of the locking mechanism.

Treatment

The occurrence of this complication requires removal of the band by laparoscopy. To reach the site of the band, which is usually covered by adhesions, it is advisable to follow the connecting tube and to pull it. The buckle of the band is easily identified and a cut on its weak part permits removal of the band. A few stitches are applied to the damaged gastric wall (gastrography). We usually perform a peri-operative gastroscopy and a methylene blue test to confirm that there is no leak. We then insert a naso-gastric tube for decompression and a perigastric drain. The surgical approach is the same even if erosion is high enough to be considered oesophageal. Some authors have described techniques for band removal (usually bands other than LAP-BAND®) with an oral endoscope regardless of whether or not the band is contained completely within the gastric lumen.

Gastric necrosis

By gastric necrosis we mean the necrosis of the upper gastric pouch.[17,18]

Incidence

Necrosis is very rare. In one series of 400 patients only one case (0.25 per cent) was reported. In our own series of 1,292 patients we recently experienced our first case as well. This patient, complaining of symptoms suggesting either gastric slippage or a gastric pouch dilatation, was hospitalized in a distant local hospital. Despite our suggestions about the need for referral and for prompt appropriate treatment she was kept there for a number of days under conservative treatment. Finally, due to the onset of exacerbating abdominal tenderness and peritonitis, she underwent exploratory laparotomy and gastric resection.

Causes

Gastric necrosis may occur early in the post-operative period or later when it is likely to be the result of a long-term undetected stomach slippage. Stomach slippage or gastric pouch dilatation can cause the band to exert continuous pressure against the gastric wall, which, in turn, may decrease the blood supply to the fundus. This pressure may also result from over-inflation of the band. The combination of decreased blood supply and continuous pressure may lead to necrosis of the gastric wall. Even in the absence of stomach slippage, an over-distended gastric pouch by itself can impair blood supply and progressively lead to gastric wall necrosis. The theoretical link between stomach slippage and necrosis is the reason stomach slippage should be considered a surgical emergency.

Symptoms

We have to consider that stomach slippage and pouch dilatation, if not diagnosed and treated accordingly, can lead to gastric necrosis. The typical symptoms are abdominal tenderness and peritonitis. Abdominal pain is a herald; a sign that must be responded to immediately.

Diagnosis

If the symptoms are not considered diagnostic an upper GI X-ray series with gastrographin and an OGDS can be done.

Treatment

Repair of gastric necrosis requires exploratory laparotomy and implementation of traditional surgical approaches.

Tubing/access port problems

The access port is an essential component of the LAP-BAND® System and its placement requires careful attention.[17,18,25]

Incidence

In our own series we had tubing and port problems in 11 per cent of the cases. The complication is fairly common in most series.

Causes

In part these problems can be linked to design features at the interface between the access port and the tubing, and in part to the method of placement of the port.

Symptoms

The patient can be fully asymptomatic or he can complain of some discomfort at the port site or there can be difficulties in accessing the port for adjustment. Often the patient complains of a sudden loss in sensation of satiety and of an increase in body weight.

Diagnosis

Absence of fluid in the system indicates that something is wrong. There should be no 'normal' loss of fluid. A plain X-ray of the abdomen is appropriate to see if there has been complete detachment of the tubing with movement of the proximal end back into the abdomen. When in doubt, injection of contrast medium (Conray™) into the system will show the leakage in most cases. Very small leaks in the tubing, especially those due to needle sticks, may not be obvious. Contrast media can flow along the tubing and pool around the band.

How to avoid it

The access port should be placed lateral to the trocar opening. A pocket must be created for the port so it is placed far enough from the trocar path to avoid abrupt kinking of the tubing. Alternatively a smooth arching path without sharp turns or bends may be created either with a 5 mm trocar or a haemostat to provide a gradual entry path into the abdominal cavity or creating a subcutaneous tunnel so that the tubing enters the abdomen through a second trocar path. The port is usually positioned in the left hypochondrium, sutured to the rectus fascia with 4 Prolene® suture (Figs. 9 and 10).

Treatment

If the port has to be replaced and repositioned it can be scheduled as a day surgery procedure. If the proximal end of the tubing is into the abdominal cavity, laparoscopy and recovery of the tubing are needed as part of the repair. Sometimes a lengthening of the tubing has to be made at the same time. With the recently improved access port design we have had minimal tubing problems since 2004.

Lack of compliance/unsatisfactory results

In case of lack of compliance or unsatisfactory results we offer the patient the 'bandinaro' procedure as a second choice or as remedial surgery. This

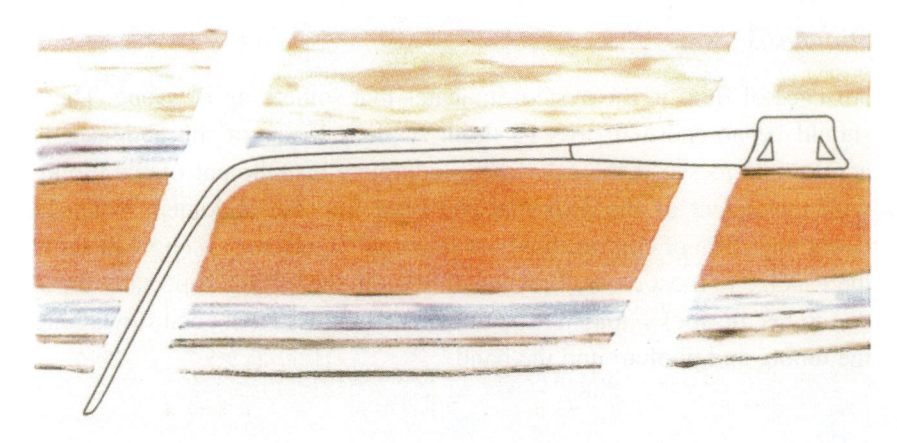

Figure 9. Creating a sub-Q tunnel so that the tubing enters the abdomen through a second trocar path.

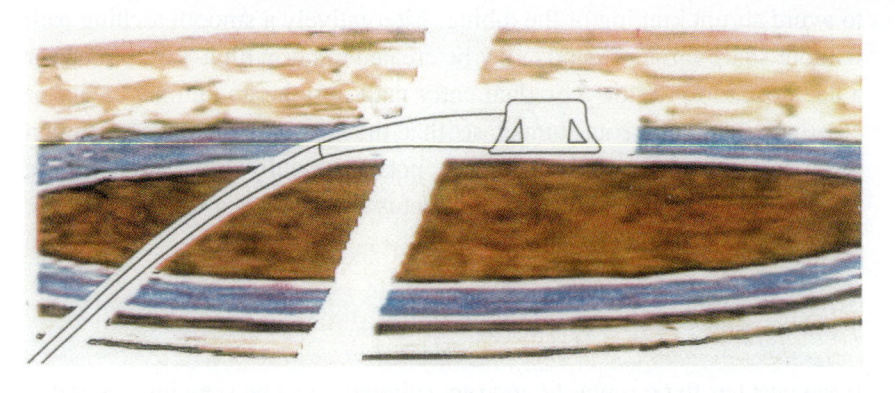

Figure 10. A smooth, arching path, without sharp turns or bends in the tubing, is optimal. A tubing path can be created with a 5 mm trocar or a haemostat (e.g. Kelly) to provide a gradual entry path into the abdominal cavity.

second stage consists in the addition of a biliopancreatic diversion duodenal switch (BPD DS) to the previous LAP-BAND® (gastric preservation). BPD DS has a 200 cm alimentary channel and a 50 cm common channel (Fig. 11).[1-18]

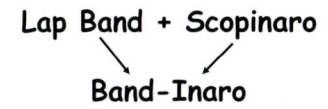

Lap Band + Scopinaro
Band-Inaro

☐ Digestive loop = 200 cm.

☐ Common loop = 50 cm

☐ Bilio-pancreatic loop = remainder of small intestine

Band Inaro

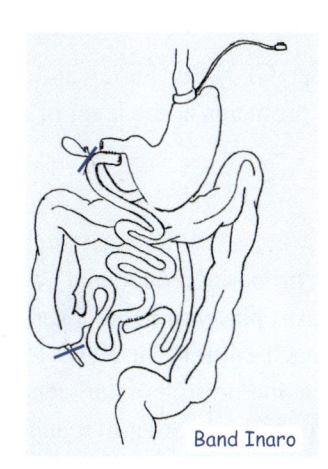

Figure 11. LAP-BAND® + Scopinaro = Band-Inaro (Bandinaro). Digestive loop = 200 cm; common loop = 50 cm; bilio-pancreatic loop = remainder of small intestine.

Incidence

Failure to maintain long-term weight loss in adjustable gastric banding™ is estimated at 25 per cent.

Causes

Once the presence of slippage, pouch enlargement, erosion and tubing/port problems have been excluded, the main reason for unsatisfactory results is the patient's lack of compliance with the LAP-BAND® System.

Symptoms

The patient is asymptomatic, apart from the unsatisfactory weight loss, a couple of years after the original LAP-BAND® procedure. The patient has been not able to change his eating habits according to the new gastric restrictive situation.

Diagnosis

An Upper GI X-ray Series and an OGDS have to be done in order to exclude problems at the level of the band.

Rationale

Vassallo proposed a duodenal switch by laparotomy in addition to a transitory gastroplasty or to an absorbable band of polydioxanone, preserving the stomach entirely, in 1997. In this series the patients experienced no diarrhoea and/or protein deficiency. Sleeve gastrectomy was added to the duodenal switch in order to reduce the marginal ulcer incidence and to add some sort of restriction. Thanks to the work of De Meester we are well aware that the preservation of 3–4 cm of viable duodenum is enough to greatly reduce the incidence of marginal ulcers. Moreover a restriction can be achieved by applying a LAP-BAND®, therefore avoiding a sleeve gastric resection with its irreversibility, risk of bleeding, leakage and stenosis. This procedure, being a fusion of the LAP-BAND® plus Scopinaro's BPD, is known as 'Bandinaro'.

Results

From March 2001 to August 2007 the total series of patients undergoing sequential treatment (restrictive as the first step and malabsorptive as the second step) was 84. The malabsorptive procedure was performed laparoscopically in the last 58 cases.

At the time of the first LAP-BAND® operation of the series of 84 patients, mean weight was 139.3 ± 26.8; at the time of duodenal switch operation mean weight was 118.1 ± 24.3 kg and percentage EWL 17.2 ± 11.3; at two years mean weight was 60 kg and percentage EWL 80.3 ± 10.4; at five years mean weight was 57.3 kg and percentage EWL 83.1.

We registered one case of mortality for malignant hypertemia, one case of gastro-colic bleeding requiring reoperation and two cases of duodenal-ileal fistulas not requiring reoperation.

Conclusions

The LAP-BAND® has proven to be remarkably safe. Given the anaesthetic and operative risk status of these patients it is difficult to think of any surgical procedure for them that could have a better safety record than LAP-BAND® placement. The minimally invasive nature of the procedure — no cutting, stapling or alteration of the anatomy — tends to keep the complication rate down, especially for serious complications.

There are some clear requirements for the successful use of the LAP-BAND®. Though these are not difficult or unusual, they are essential. The surgeon needs to have good laparoscopic skill and bariatric experience. Reasonable competence and experience can be achieved with good, specifically-oriented training and proctoring. There must be a commitment to the patients, to their education and support, to their ongoing routine care and problems. This commitment is best realized in the presence of a multidisciplinary support team (dietician, psychologist, internist and surgeon).

Because of the ability to adjust the degree of restriction, the weight loss is achieved in a gentle way. Ideally it occurs slowly over two or more years and should not be associated with symptoms of severe restriction or vomiting, but rather with a sense of satiety before eating and an early sense of fullness after eating small amounts.

The LAP-BAND® is the only bariatric surgical procedure that is entirely reversible. Patients are not trapped permanently into a state of distorted anatomy that can only be undone with difficulty. It is comforting for both the patient and the surgeon that, should the need arise, the band can easily be removed and the stomach allowed to return to normal.[1,2,7-9]

Most LAP-BAND® complications are not life-threatening and, when they do occur, many can be remedied laparoscopically.

The evolution of the procedure, with modifications to the device and to the technique, has served to greatly reduce the incidence of complications. And, of course, avoiding complications in the first place is always the best complications management strategy.[19,26,27]

We hope to have offered here a good overview of the potential complications of the LAP-BAND® placement, their causes, symptoms, prevention strategies and possible remedies. Equipped with the knowledge that can be provided by the extensively experienced surgeons at our centre and others, newer LAP-BAND® surgeons will no doubt see the learning curve for this procedure substantially reduced and the already low complication rates diminished even further.

References

1. Favretti, F., Segato, G., Ashton, D. et al. (2007). Laparoscopic Adjustable Gastric Banding in 1791 consecutive obese patients: 12-year results. *Obes Surg* 17: 168–175.
2. Favretti, F., Cadière, G.B., Segato, G. et al. (2002). Laparoscopic banding: selection and technique in 830 patients. *Obes Surg* 12: 385–390.
3. Belva, P.H., Takieddine, M., Lefebvre, J.C. et al. (1998). Laparoscopic LAP-BAND gastroplasty: European results. *Obes Surg* 8: 364.
4. Dargent, J. (1999). Laparoscopic adjustable gastric banding: lessons from the first 500 patients in a single institution. *Obes Surg* 9: 446–452.
5. Biesheuvel, T.H., Sintenie, J.B., Pels Rijcken, T.H. et al. (1998). Laparoscopic adjustable silicone gastric banding for treating morbid obesity in the centre of Amsterdam. *Obes Surg* 8: 360.
6. Vertruyen, M. (2002). Experience with LAP-BAND system up to 7 years. *Obes Surg* 12: 569–572.
7. Belachew, M., Legrand, M.J., Defechereux, T.H. et al. (1994). Laparoscopic adjustable silicone gastric banding in the treatment of morbid obesity, a preliminary report. *Surg Endosc* 8: 1354–1356.
8. Chevallier, J.M., Zinzindohoue, F., Elian, N. et al. (2002). Adjustable gastric banding in a public university hospital: prospective analysis of 400 patients. *Obes Surg* 12: 93–99.
9. Forestieri, P., Meucci, L., De Luca, M. et al. (1998). Two years of practice in adjustable silicone gastric banding (LAP-BAND): evaluation of variations of body mass index, percentage ideal body weight and percentage excess body weight. *Obes Surg* 8: 49–52.
10. O'Brien, P., Brown, W., Smith, A. et al. (1998). The LAP-BAND provides effective control of morbid obesity — a prospective study of 350 patients followed for up to 4 years. *Obes Surg* 8: 398.
11. Belachew, M., Belva, P.H., Desaive, C. (2002). Long-term results of laparoscopic adjustable gastric banding for the treatment of morbid obesity. *Obes Surg* 12: 564–568.

12. Cadière, G.B., Himpens, J., Vertruyen, M. et al. (2000). Laparoscopic gastroplasty (adjustable silicone gastric banding). *Semin Laparosc Surg* 7: 55–65.
13. Fielding, G., Allen, J. (2002). A step-by-step guide to placement of the LAP-BAND adjustable gastric banding system. *Am J Surg* 184: 26S–31S.
14. Fielding, G.A., Rhodes, M., Nathanson, L.K. (1999). Laparoscopic gastric banding for morbid obesity: surgical outcome in 335 cases. *Surg Endosc* 13: 550–554.
15. Cadière, G.B., Favretti, F., Bruyns, J. et al. (1994). Gastroplastie par coelio-videoscopie: technique. *J Coelio-Chir* 10: 27–31.
16. Chelala, E., Cadière, G.B., Favretti, F. et al. (1997). Conversions and complications in 185 laparoscopic adjustable silicone gastric banding cases. *Surg Endosc* 11: 268–271.
17. Spivak, H., Favretti, F. (2002). Avoiding postoperative complications with the LAP-BAND system. *Am J Surg* 184: 31S–37S.
18. Favretti, F., Cadière, G.B., Segato, G. et al. (1997). Laparoscopic adjustable silicone gastric banding (LAP-BAND®): how to avoid complications. *Obes Surg* 7: 352–358.
19. Niville, E., Dams, A. (1999). Late pouch dilation after laparoscopic adjustable gastric and esophagogastric banding: incidence, treatment and outcome. *Obes Surg* 9: 381–384.
20. Carbajo Caballero, M.A., Del Olmo, J.C.M., Blanco Alvarez, J.I. et al. (1998). Intragastric migration of laparoscopic adjustable gastric band (Lap-Band) for morbid obesity. *J Laparoendosc Adv Surg Tech* 8(4): 241–244.
21. Meir, E., Van Baden, M. (1998). Adjustable silicone gastric banding (ASGB) and band erosion (BE). *Obes Surg* 8: 385.
22. Meir, E., Van Baden, M. (1999). Adjustable silicone gastric banding and band erosion: personal experience and hypotheses. *Obes Surg* 9: 191–193.
23. Mittermair, R.P., Weiss, H., Nehoda, H. et al. (2002). Uncommon intragastric migration of the Swedish adjustable gastric band. *Obes Surg* 12: 372–375.
24. Baldinger, R., Mluench, R., Steffen, R. et al. (2001). Conservative management of intragastric migration of the Swedish adjustable gastric band by endoscopic retrieval. *Gastrointest Endosc* 53: 98–101.
25. Fabry, H., Van Hee, R., Hendrickx, L. et al. (2002). A technique for prevention of port complications after laparoscopic adjustable silicone gastric banding. *Obes Surg* 12: 285–288.

26. Weiner, R., Bockhorn, H., Rosenthal, R. *et al.* (2001). A prospective randomized trial of different laparoscopic gastric banding techniques for morbid obesity. *Surg Endosc* 15: 63–68.
27. Belachew, M., Zimmermann, J.-M. (2002). Evolution of a paradigm for laparoscopic adjustable gastric banding. *Am J Surg* 184: 21S–25S.

Chapter 7

Roux-en-Y Gastric Bypass

Bruno Dillemans and Sebastiaan Van Cauwenberge

Introduction

Overweight and obesity are widespread in industrialized and rich nations and the incidence is growing at an alarming rate. The World Health Organization (WHO) has now coined the term globesity (global obesity) to highlight the growth of this worldwide problem.

With respect to durable weight reduction, bariatric surgery is the most effective long-term treatment for obesity with the greatest chances for amelioration and even resolution of obesity-associated complications.

Roux-en-Y gastric bypass (RYGB) usually is considered to be the standard bariatric surgical procedure. Excellent sustained weight loss and profound improvement in medical co-morbidities can dramatically change the lives of patients.

In this chapter we will focus first of all on the history of the procedure and explain its working mechanism. The preoperative assessment of the patient undergoing RYGB surgery will be discussed. Afterwards we will describe some technical issues regarding the operative technique. Since complications are inherent to surgery, we explain the most frequently encountered problems and side effects after RYGB and their management.

Background and history of gastric bypass surgery

Gastric bypass was first performed by Mason and Ito in 1966.[1] In this variation, a horizontal distal gastrectomy was performed to create a gastric reservoir to which a loop of jejunum was anastomosed.

In 1977, Alden *et al.* created a stapled pouch without dividing the stomach. The same year, Griffen *et al.* reported Roux-en-Y gastric bypass (RYGB). Since then, there have been ongoing innovations in the technique, especially in the restrictive component.[2,3] Torres *et al.* applied a vertical gastric pouch, Linner *et al.* reinforced the gastrojejunal anastomosis with a band, Salmon combined vertical gastroplasty with distal bypass, and Fobi introduced the silastic ring proximal to the divided vertical gastrojejunostomy.[4-7]

Current variations in the surgical technique include the method by which the gastric pouch is created, the technique of gastrojejunostomy, and the configuration and length of the alimentary and biliopancreatic limbs. Those issues will be discussed below in the section *Technical aspects of the laparoscopic RYGB* (LRYGB) *procedure*. With the increase in the performance of the LRYGB, first popularized by Wittgrove and Clark, the effect of these alterations on outcomes has been studied extensively.[8]

Another type of gastric bypass is the laparoscopic mini-gastric bypass (LMGBP), first reported by Rutledge.[9] In this procedure a gastric pouch is created and a point selected on the small bowel about 200 cm distal to the ligament of Treitz. The jejunal loop is brought up antecolic, and a stapler is used to anastomose the stomach and the small bowel at this point.

Comparing the five-year trend from 2003 to 2008 regarding the evolution of RYGB surgery, markedly different trends were found for Europe and USA/Canada. In Europe, RYGB increased from 11.1 per cent to 39.0 per cent, whereas in USA/Canada, RYGB decreased from 85.0 per cent to 51.0 per cent.[10]

Physiology of the Roux-en-Y Gastric Bypass

Body weight is the result of complex physiologic mechanisms that control food intake and energy expenditure. Regulation of body weight involves several systems such as the adipose tissue, the hypothalamus and the adrenal glands, which are linked by neural and hormonal signals. Recent investigations have identified several key molecules that regulate food intake, including ghrelin, neuropeptide Y (NPY) and melanocortins, and have focused on the relationship between obesity and leptin levels.[11]

It is commonly believed that the RYGB induces weight loss through a combination of mechanisms, including decreasing the capacity of the stomach, restricting the rate of emptying of the pouch, prohibiting the intake of high osmolar foods, and causing selective malabsorption of fat. Although convincing data of the relation between gastric pouch or stomal size and achieved weight loss are lacking, the restriction of food is considered as the major causative factor of successful weight loss after the gastric bypass. Moreover, the majority of patients with weight regain after an initial good success of their gastric bypass, do complain of a loss of restriction and satiety when eating, explaining an increased caloric intake. The malabsorptive component of the gastric bypass is believed to be less important than the restrictive part; at least in the proximal type of gastric bypass. Studies have showed that the serum albumine and faecal fat are not altered after a gastric bypass, and no major malabsorption of anticancer agents after a gastric bypass has been reported yet.[12] The hormonal effect of the gastric bypass is probably more important, although not fully understood yet. By enabling salivary secretions and meals going directly into the distal jejunum, RYGB might stimulate the release of gut hormones, which inhibit the brain appetite centre or cause the feeling of nausea. The observation that RYGB induces resolution of type 2 diabetes mellitus prior to the occurrence of weight loss further suggests that the mechanism of action of this operation might involve some endocrine effects.[11]

A number of peptides released from the gastrointestinal tract have recently been shown to regulate appetite and food intake, effecting both orexigenic and anorexic outcomes through actions on the hypothalamic arcuate nucleus. Ghrelin, a hormone produced from the stomach in the preprandial state, increases expression of the orexigenic hypothalamic NPY and stimulates food intake in rodents and humans. In contrast, peptide YY (PYY), released postprandially from the distal gastrointestinal tract, acts within the arcuate nucleus to inhibit the release of NPY. Intravenous PYY$^{3-36}$ infusions into humans and intraperitoneal injections into rodents induce satiety and reduce food intake. Glucagon-like peptide 1 (GLP-1) acts mainly as an incretin, promoting postprandial insulin release and improving pancreatic β-cell function, and has also been reported to inhibit food intake in humans. Pancreatic polypeptide (PP) has recently been shown to inhibit appetite and food intake and promotes energy expenditure.[13]

Le Roux *et al.* demonstrated a pleiotropic endocrine response to bariatric surgery, which might account for the appetite reduction that leads to long-term changes in body weight. They have shown that following RYGB, patients have increased postprandial PYY and GLP-1 favouring enhanced satiety to a meal. Furthermore, RYGB patients experience early and exaggerated insulin responses, potentially mediating the improved glycaemic control in patients with type 2 diabetes mellitus. None of these effects were observed in patients losing similar weight through gastric banding (GB), suggesting that the hormonal changes are not secondary to weight loss alone. They further demonstrated in a rodent model of intestinal bypass that elevated PYY may have a causative role in mediating reduced food intake.[13]

The authors propose that the higher postprandial PYY response after gastric bypass surgery due to the altered intestinal anatomy may contribute to the patients' increased satiety and weight loss. RYGB is thought to be significantly more effective than restrictive procedures such as vertical banded gastroplasty for weight loss in morbid obesity, especially for patients addicted to sweets. The banding patients did not have an exaggerated PYY response. There are no direct comparisons of satiety between RYGB and GB, although reports indicate that patients do experience sensations reported as enhanced satiety after GB and RYGB.

In both rodent and human studies, high GLP-1 was observed in parallel with PYY. GLP-1 is produced from the same entero-endocrine cells (L cells) as PYY and acts as an incretin, releasing insulin and improving pancreatic β-cell function in rodents. Reduction in food intake has also been reported. Previously, increased GLP-1 concentrations have been shown following intestinal bypass. Consistent with previous RYGB studies, the study of le Roux found no difference in fasting GLP-1 levels but demonstrates an exaggerated GLP-1 response following a 420 kcal meal in gastric bypass subjects. The increased GLP-1 response may contribute as a satiety signal and incretin. Glycaemic control in type 2 diabetes mellitus patients improves following RYGB surgery and often before significant weight loss occurs.[13]

Ghrelin was initially associated with appetite reduction following gastric bypass. The reduced appetite following gastric bypass was explained by the failure of ghrelin to show the expected rise observed in diet-induced weight loss. However, a series of publications have since shown inconsistent ghrelin changes after RYGB and GB. These studies have recently been reviewed, and the heterogeneity of the findings makes it unlikely that ghrelin has a major role in the weight loss after RYGB. In the study of le Roux *et al.*, both bypass and banding patients had lower fasting ghrelin levels compared with lean control subjects, although these levels were similar to those of the obese control subjects. In agreement with the majority of studies, the authors did not find an anticipated compensatory rise in ghrelin among surgical subjects.

Patients treated for obesity with gastric bypass therefore have alterations of several peripheral signals that potentially contribute to their reduced appetite and enhanced glucose homeostasis. An exaggerated postprandial PYY and GLP-1 might combine to enhance satiety, leading to a long-term reduction in calorie intake, while increased GLP-1 and insulin might contribute to immediate improvements in glycaemic control.[13]

Preoperative Evaluation

Morbidly obese patients undergoing gastric bypass have multiple issues regarding their co-morbidities and as in many centres, require a multidisciplinary team approach. The preoperative evaluation is similar for all bariatric procedures. The components include determining a patient's indications for surgery, identifying issues which may interfere with the success of the surgery and assessing and treating co-morbid diseases. Typical assessment includes nutritional evaluation, medical assessment and psychological testing.[14]

Nutritional evaluation

The dietician is an integral part of the multidisciplinary bariatric team and will be responsible for nutritional assessment, diet education regarding postoperative eating behaviours and preoperative weight loss efforts.[15] Preoperative very-low-calorie diet for six weeks has been shown to reduce liver volume by 20 per cent and to improve access to the upper stomach during laparoscopic surgery, with 80 per cent of the volume change occurring in the first two weeks.[15,16] It has been shown that patients who are able to achieve 10 per cent EBWL preoperatively have shorter hospitalization and more rapid weight loss.[17] No evidence-based, standardized dietary guidelines exist for either pre- or postoperative nutritional management of the bariatric patient. Further studies and clinical trials are required to help define the role of the dietician in the bariatric team.

Medical Evaluation

Laparoscopic RYGB for obesity is a major procedure and can have severe postoperative complications, hence a thorough history and physical examination with systematic review is used to identify co-morbidities that may complicate the surgery. Consultation with a medical subspecialist is often necessary to optimize medical conditions to reduce peri- and postoperative risk. Routine laboratory evaluation typically includes complete blood count, metabolic profile, coagulation profile, lipid profile, thyroid function tests and ferritin. Vitamin B12, and fat-soluble vitamin levels may be evaluated if considering a malabsorptive procedure. Cardiovascular evaluation includes electrocardiogram and possible stress test to identify occult coronary artery disease. Respiratory evaluation may include chest X-ray, arterial blood gas and pulmonary function tests. Sleep apnoea, if suspected on the basis of Epworth score, may be diagnosed by sleep study and the patient started on continuous positive airway pressure prior to surgery. Upper endoscopy may be used if suspicion of gastric pathology exists. If *Helicobacter pylori* infection is present, preoperative therapy is advised.[18] The liver may be assessed by hepatic profile and ultrasound. In cases of suspected cirrhosis, biopsy may be indicated. Ultrasound may be used to detect gallstones, allowing the surgeon to decide on concomitant cholecystectomy.[19]

Psychological Evaluation

Patients referred for bariatric surgery are more likely than the overall population to have psychiatric problems such as social phobia, obsessive–compulsive disorder, substance abuse/dependency, binge-eating disorder, post-traumatic stress disorder, generalized anxiety disorder and depression.[20] Patients with psychiatric disorders may have a suboptimal outcome after bariatric surgery. However, no consensus recommendations exist regarding preoperative psychological evaluation.[21] It is not certain which psychosocial factors predict success following bariatric surgery, yet many surgeons exclude patients who are illicit drug abusers, have active uncontrolled schizophrenia or psychosis, severe mental retardation, heavy alcohol use, or lack of knowledge about the surgery.[22]

Technical Aspects of the Laparoscopic RYGB Procedure

Various techniques of laparoscopic RYGB have been described. In general the procedure consists of partitioning the stomach with surgical stapling devices in order to create a small gastric pouch. This pouch is the restrictive part of the construction. The pouch is then connected with a loop of small bowel that has been transected 30–50 cm below Treitz. The small bowel limb is measured at a certain length and reconstructed in a Roux-en-Y fashion to restore the continuity. This 'alimentary limb' is responsible for the malabsorptive part of the procedure.

Some technical key-steps have been the subject of extensive discussion. These debates focus on:

- Construction and size of the gastric pouch;
- Construction of the gastrojejunostomy (handsewn, linear or circular stapled);
- Antecolic versus retrocolic placement of the alimentary limb;
- Length of the alimentary limb;
- Construction and closure of the jejuno-jejunostomy;
- Closure versus non-closure of the mesenteric defects.

Construction and size of the gastric pouch

The restriction imposed by a small pouch size is one of the most important aspects of RYGB. The goal of most bariatric surgeons has been to construct small volume pouches in the proximal stomach to restrict the intake of food. To date, a gastric pouch with a volume of 20–30 ml is generally accepted as the standard volume.

Construction of the gastrojejunostomy

A variety of surgical techniques has been developed for the establishment of the gastrojejunostomy such as the circular-stapled anastomosis, the linear-stapled anastomosis, and the totally hand-sewn anastomosis.

In the circular technique the anastomosis is performed with a circular stapler with a diameter of 21 or 25 mm. The anvil of the circular stapler can be introduced either transabdominally or transorally (e.g. the Orvil method).

In the linear stapled gastrojejunostomy, a stab opening is made in the gastric pouch and one in the jejunum that has been pulled up. A 45 mm linear stapler is then introduced with one jaw in the stomach and one jaw in the jejunum to perform the anastomosis. The common stab opening is then closed with a resorbable suture. After this step one has to transect the proximal small bowel to complete the anastomosis.

The hand-sewn anastomosis is usually performed in a standard 2-layer fashion with resorbable sutures, running and interrupted, and sized with an intraluminal 32 Fr tube.

Strictures at the gastrojejunostomy, leading to vomiting, dysphagia, nausea, solid food intolerance, or even severe dehydration, are a well-known complication following RYGB. Different stricture rates have been described for the three techniques ranging from 0.8 to 33 per cent, depending on the diameter of the anastomosis and the learning curve. While in circular-stapled anastomosis, the inner diameter of the gastrojejunostomy is well defined, in hand-sewn anastomosis or in linear-stapled anastomosis, in the absence of a calibration tube, the inner gastrojejunostomy diameter might differ, although it is assumed to be larger than in circular-stapled anastomosis.[23]

Antecolic versus retrocolic placement of the alimentary limb

The alimentary limb can be pulled up to the level of the gastric pouch in two ways. In the first method the small bowel is pulled over the transverse colon (antecolic). In most cases division of the greater omentum is then necessary to facilitate the positioning of the alimentary limb and to limit traction on the gastro-jejunal anastomosis. Another technique is to make an opening in the mesentery of the transverse colon to pull up the jejunum through this opening (retrocolic). The small bowel limb might then be positioned either antegastric or retrogastric (i.e. in relation to the excluded stomach). The retrocolic retrogastric pathway is considered as the most traction-less method as this is the shortest anatomical distance to the gastric pouch.

Intestinal obstruction has been reported following RYGB surgery depending on the position of the alimentary limb. There is controversy about whether the alimentary limb should be placed in the retrocolic or antecolic position.

In a study of 754 patients, a greater incidence of intestinal obstruction and internal hernia was observed in the retrocolic technique group than in the antecolic technique group undergoing LRYGB. The results of this study have shown that the use of the retrocolic technique is a risk factor for intestinal obstruction after LRYGB.[24]

Length of the alimentary limb

The ideal length of the gastric bypass limbs is debated. RYGB that is performed with a long Roux limb seems to result in greater weight loss than shorter Roux limb procedures in super-obese patients (BMI > 50 kg/m^2). Conversely, longer Roux limb procedures do not provide greater weight loss in less obese (BMI < 50 kg/m^2) patients.[25–27] The definition of a long and short Roux limb varies however according to the different authors; with a long limb mostly counting around 150 cm and a short one around 75 cm. Modest elongation of the Roux limb in the range of 150–200 cm does not result in more frequent nutritional sequelae compared with shorter Roux limb procedures. Conversely, RYGBs, in which the Roux or the biliopancreatic limb is very long with anastomosis to the mid or distal ileum (very, very long), usually results in more metabolic problems than RYGBs in which the Roux limb measures up to 150 cm and the biliopancreatic limb is short.[28]

Construction and closure of the jejuno-jejunostomy

Many surgeons utilize a single stapling technique and subsequently close the enterotomy with a running suture. Others utilize a double or even a triple stapling technique to anastomose and close the small bowel.

Closure versus non-closure of the mesenteric defects

There are three sites where an internal hernia after RYGB may occur:

1. through the transverse mesocolon defect;
2. through the entero-enterostomy mesenteric defect;
3. through the space between the mesentery of the Roux limb and transverse mesocolon (the so-called Petersen's space).

The increased incidence of internal hernia after LRYGB has been primarily attributed to the reduced formation of postoperative adhesions following laparoscopy. Another technical feature recognized as having a possible role in the occurrence of internal hernia is the placement of the Roux limb. There is evidence that the majority of internal hernias (69 per cent) occur at the transverse colon mesenteric defect. The hypothesis that the antecolic RYGB is followed by a lower incidence of internal hernias compared to the retrocolic counterpart is confirmed in a lot of scientific reports.

Even though accurate closure of all mesenteric defects does not avoid this complication, closure is recommended because it resulted in a reduced incidence of internal hernias in several studies.[29] We have completely standardized Fully Stapled Laparoscopic Roux-en-Y gastric bypass (FS-LRYGB) to minimize its sometimes substantial morbidity and mortality.[30]

In the next section we describe our technique in detail.

Operative Technique of the Fully Stapled Laparoscopic Roux-en-Y Gastric Bypass

Patient positioning and trocar placement

The patient is placed in the supine position, split-leg with reverse Trendelenburg position. All patients get a flexion of the hips to help

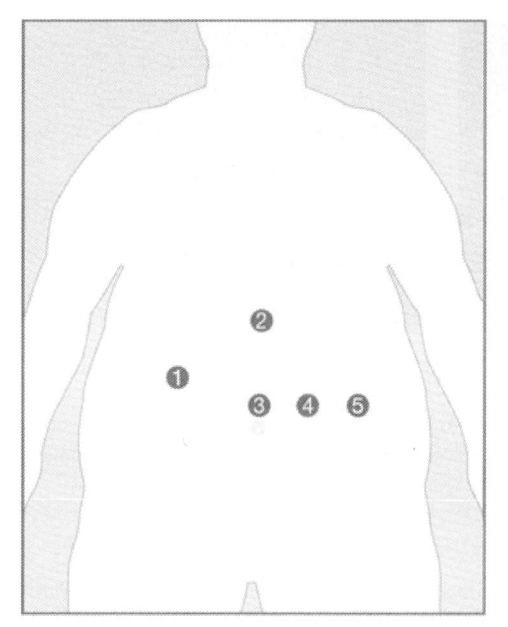

Trocars	Instruments
1 (12 mm)	Liver Retractor Graspers Linear Stapler
2 (5mm)	Graspers
3 (10mm)	Scope
4 (12mm)	Graspers Harmonic Suction Linear Stapler Scissors
5 (12mm)	Graspers Scissors Linear Stapler Circular Stapler

Figure 1. Trocar port sites for fully stapled laparoscopic Roux-en-Y gastric bypass.

increase surgical abdominal workspace.[31] The surgeon stands between the legs. A video monitor is positioned at the level of the patient's head. A 30° angle scope is used. Abdominal insufflation with carbon dioxide (CO_2) is achieved using a Veress needle. Intra-abdominal pressures are maintained at 15 mmHg.

A five-port technique is employed: a 10 mm port 10–15 cm below the xiphoid process, a 5 mm port high epigastric on the midline, a 12 mm port in the right upper quadrant and two 12 mm ports in the left upper quadrant. The latter two ports are placed on the same line as the 10 mm port, while the 12 mm port in the right upper quadrant, somewhat higher above the same line (sub costal) (Fig.1).

Creation of the gastric pouch

A small window is made between the lesser omentum and the lesser curvature of the stomach, entering the lesser sac 5–6 cm below the gastro-oesophageal junction (Fig. 2a). At this point a linear stapler (Endo GIA™

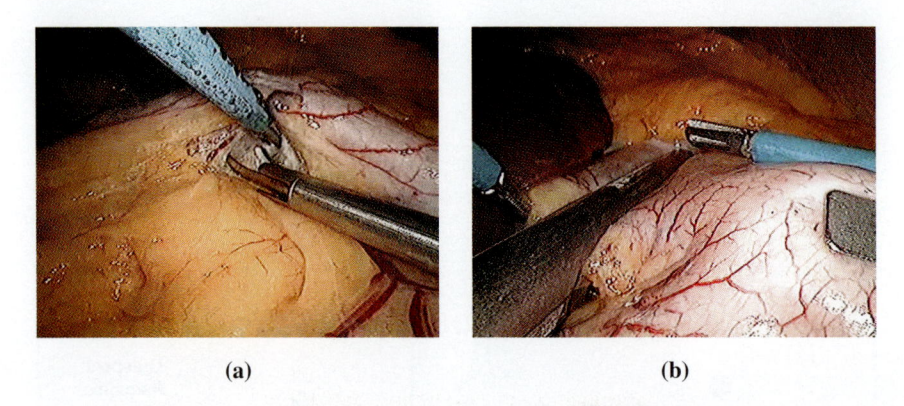

Figure 2. Creation of the gastric pouch. (**a**) Start of the dissection at the lesser curvature 5–6 cm below the gastro-oesophageal junction. (**b**) The first linear stapler cuts the stomach horizontally.

Universal Stapler System, Covidien, USA or Echelon™ 60 Endopath Stapler, Ethicon, USA), usually with a blue cartridge, is introduced through this window and the stomach cut horizontally over a distance of 50 mm (Fig. 2b).

A second linear 60 mm stapler is then introduced and fired to vertically transect the stomach using a 34 Fr. orogastric tube as a guide (Fig. 3a). The next step consists of dissection and opening of the angle of His (Fig. 3b). Posterior to the stomach the dissection is completed to create a window at the angle of His. Finally, the pouch is completed by vertically firing one or two more 60 mm cartridges in the direction of and through the latter created window, along the gastric tube (Fig. 3c).

Creation of the gastro-jejunostomy

A small opening is made in the lower left corner of the pouch (Fig. 4a), the opening stretched and a purse-string suture is sewn using an absorbable monofilament suture (PDS* II 3/0, Ethicon, USA) (Fig. 4b).

A 25 mm Premium Plus CEEA™ (Covidien, USA) is then introduced intra-abdominally via the most left lateral, manually-dilated trocar opening. The anvil is brought into the gastric pouch opening and the purse-string tied (Fig. 5).

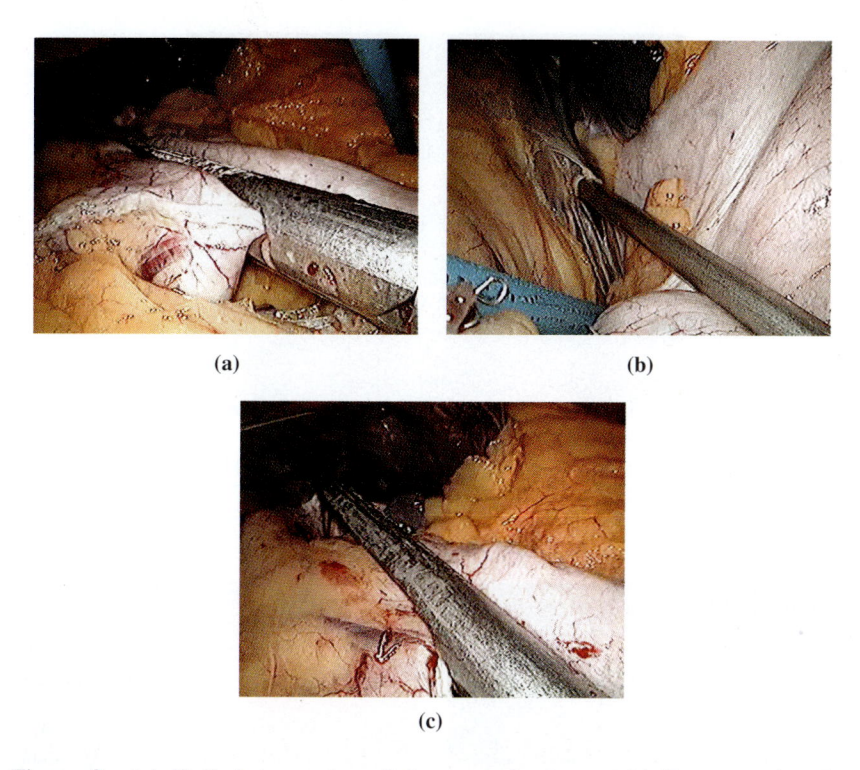

Figure 3. (a) Vertical transection of the stomach along a 34 Fr. orogastric tube. (b) Opening of the angle of His. (c) Final stapling at the angle of His.

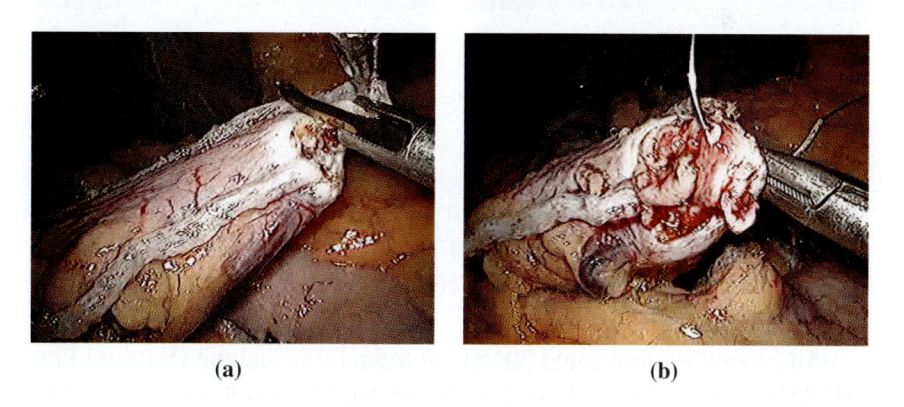

Figure 4. Creation of the gastrojejunostomy. (a) Opening of the gastric pouch in the lower left corner. (b) Purse-string suturing with PDS 3/0.

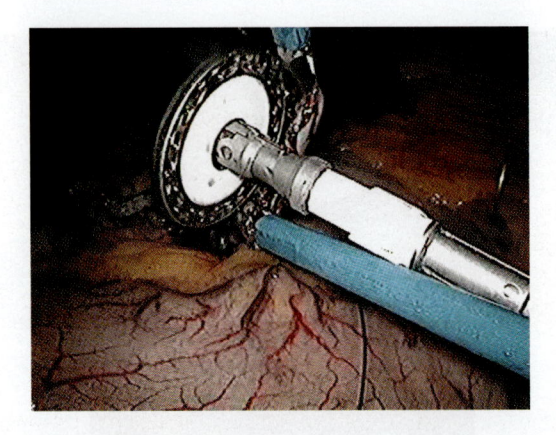

Figure 5. Introduction of the anvil of the circular stapler and tying of the pursestring.

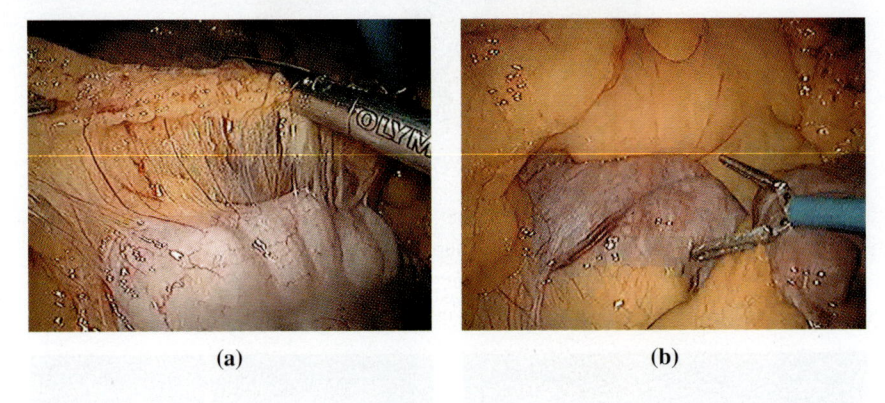

Figure 6. (**a**) Division of the greater omentum. (**b**) Identification of the ligament of Treitz.

Thereafter, the greater omentum is lifted and divided up to the left side of the transverse colon (Fig. 6a). Next the ligament of Treitz is identified and a loop of jejunum is antecolically pulled up from this point to the gastric pouch (Fig. 6b).

An enterotomy is created 30–50 cm from Treitz and the Premium Plus CEEA™ introduced over 5–6 cm in the jejunal loop via this opening in the distal direction (Fig. 7a). We then perforate the jejunum under slight traction with the spike, remove the spike and connect the stapler to the anvil (Fig. 7b).

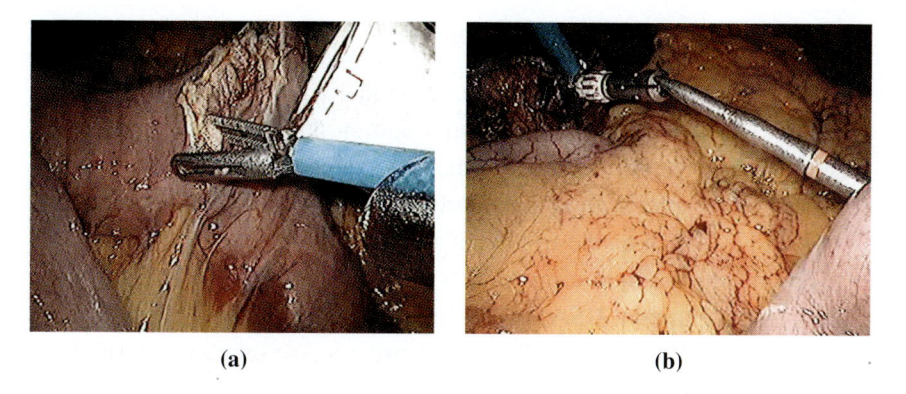

Figure 7. (**a**) Enterotomy 30–50 cm from the angle of Treitz. (**b**) Antimesenteric perforation of the jejunum with the spike after introduction of the circular stapler.

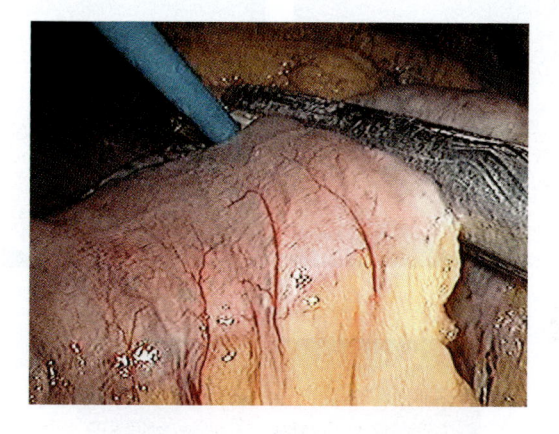

Figure 8. Finalization of the anastomosis by transection of the remaining small bowel 1 cm proximal to the gastrojejunostomy.

The anastomosis is completed by closing and firing the instrument. The remaining small bowel loop with the previously created opening is then resected 1 cm proximal to the gastrojejunostomy using a linear stapler with a 60 mm white cartridge so as to avoid a long blind loop of jejunum (Fig. 8).

Creation of the jejuno-jejunostomy

The length of the alimentary limb is a standard 130 cm. In patients with BMI > 50 kg/m^2, 200 cm is measured and an antimesenteric opening is created both in the alimentary and the biliopancreatic limb (Fig. 9a, b). A linear 60 mm stapler with a white cartridge is introduced in both openings in order to establish a side-to-side anastomosis (Fig. 9c).

The resulting enterotomy defect is lifted by three holding stitches (PDS* II 4/0, Ethicon, USA) and then longitudinally closed using a similar stapler (Fig. 10a). The final step is transecting the remaining blind loop of the biliopancreatic limb, also with a similar linear stapler, and removal of the piece of bowel (Fig. 10b).

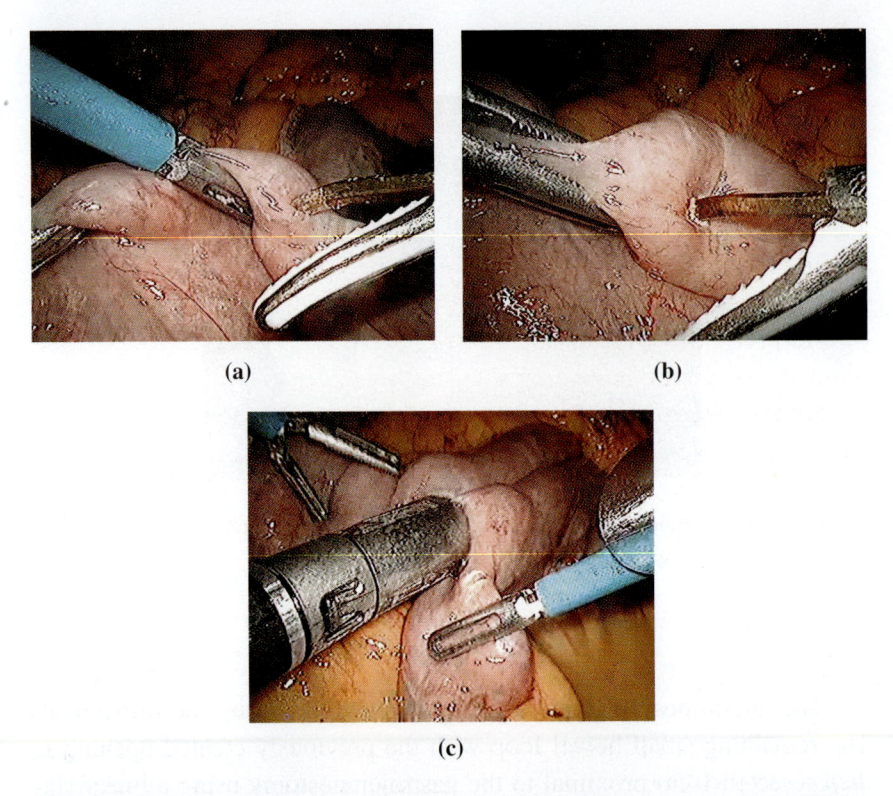

Figure 9. Creation of the jejuno-jejunostomy. (**a**) Antimesenteric opening in the alimentary limb. (**b**) Antimesenteric opening in the biliopancreatic limb. (**c**) Side-to-side anastomosis with a linear 60 mm stapler.

(a) **(b)**

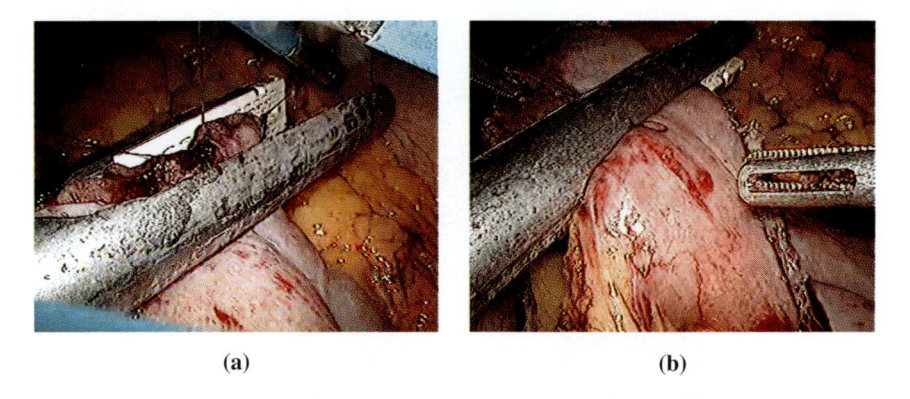

Figure 10. Creation of the jejuno-jejunostomy. (**a**) Closure of the enterotomy defect using three stay sutures. (**b**) Transection of the remaining blind loop of the biliopancreatic limb.

Testing of the gastro-jejunostomy

A leakage test is done by forcefully injecting methylene blue through the orogastric tube at the level of the gastrojejunostomy anastomosis. The gastrojejunostomy is reinforced if necessary with some additional stitches of an absorbable monofilament suture (PDS* II 4/0, Ethicon, USA) (Fig. 11).

To prevent postoperative bleeding all staple lines are inspected under an elevated systolic arterial pressure above 140 mmHg.[28]

The left lateral trocar port site, which was enlarged to introduce the Premium Plus™ CEEA, is closed with the help of the Endo Close™ trocar site closure device (Covidien, USA) to prevent 'lateral entrapment' or herniation (Fig. 12).

Complications of Roux-en-Y Gastric Bypass

Laparoscopic gastric bypass has a similar spectrum of complications in comparison to any other major laparoscopic procedure. The two most important independent risk factors in relation to complications are male gender and patient size. Age has also been reported to be a risk factor. Though bariatric surgery can be performed on older patients, there is a higher morbidity and mortality rate if complications were to occur.

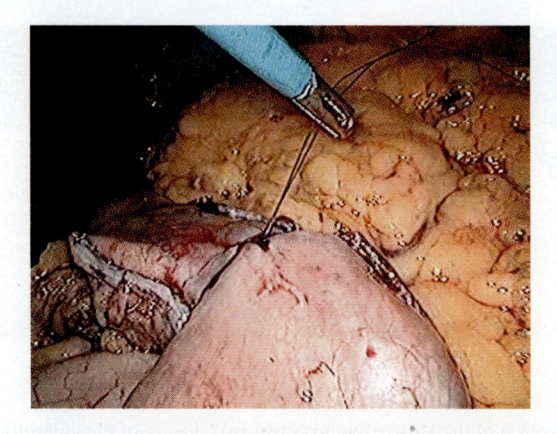

Figure 11. Additional reinforcement stitch at the level of the gastrojejunostomy.

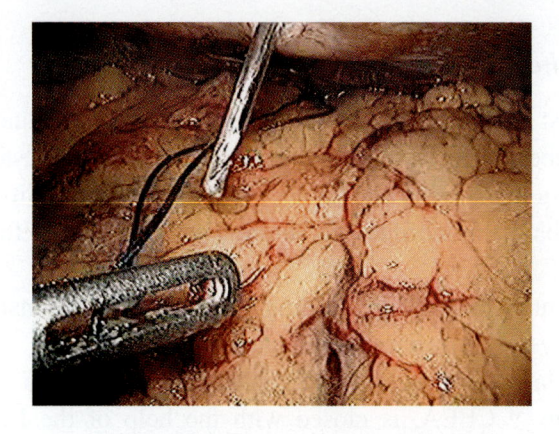

Figure 12. Closure of the left lateral trocar port site with the Endo Close™ trocar site closure device.

Similarly patients with oxygen dependent hypoxia and atherosclerotic cardiovascular disease are at a higher risk.

Mortality

Mortality is uncommon, ranging from 0 to 1.5 in various reports. The mortality rate seems to be slightly higher in the open than in the laparoscopic RNY bypasses, but this may be the result of patient selection.[32–34]

In the two meta-analyses published by Buchwald *et al.* the mortality in the subgroup of gastric bypasses dropped from 0.5 per cent (2004) to 0.16 per cent in 2007.[35,36] The major reasons for mortality were leaks and pulmonary embolisms.

In autopsy series, leaks were responsible for approximately 50 per cent of deaths.[37]

Anastomotic leaks

Leakage rates

The reported leak rate following gastric bypass is between 0 and 5.6 per cent, with the average leak rate between 2 and 3 per cent.[38–41] The most common site of a leak is the anastomosis at the gastrojejunostomy, but in addition other leaks secondary to staple line failure in the divided gastric pouch or excluded stomach are also commonly reported as 'anastomotic leaks'.

Age, gender and BMI were associated with gastrointestinal leaks after laparoscopic Roux-en-Y gastric bypass procedures. Others had also found that leaks are more common in men and in those patients with higher BMI. Revisional surgery, age and diabetes mellitus have been noted to produce higher leak rates.[41]

Aetiology of leakage

The aetiology of anastomotic leaks is multifactorial. Ischaemia, excessive tension on the anastomosis, infection and surgeon's experience are implicated in its aetio-pathogenesis.[42] There is no significant difference in leak rates between the open and laparoscopic approach, neither between the different types of gastrojejunostomy or jejunojejunostomy construction. Reinforcement of anastomotic staple/suture lines with either bovine pericardial strips or fibrin glue may decrease the frequency of leaks.[43,44]

Diagnosis

Early symptoms of a leak are sometimes subtle and require clinical vigilance for signs such as tachycardia, respiratory distress and low-grade fevers.[45]

A leak may be radiographically confirmed by upper gastrointestinal series with gastrografin swallow, but its sensitivity is reported to be low (22 per cent).[45] Computed tomography scans should be done with the administration of contrast materials (intravenous and oral). In order to increase the sensitivity of the study, patients should take 30–60 cc of oral contrast material immediately before the study to opacify the gastric pouch and its connection to the Roux limb. The CT scan renders a better assessment of the proximal portion (excluded stomach) (100 per cent), proximal efferent Roux limb (99 per cent) and gastric pouch (96 per cent) than the distal portion jejunostomy (67 per cent) of the Roux-en-Y gastric bypass anatomy.[46]

Management of leakage

Because of the rapid progression to sepsis in these patients with co-morbidities, prompt exploratory surgery is warranted. Furthermore surgeons should have a low threshold for operative management in patients who exceed weight limitations for adequate radiological evaluation. In patients for whom the diagnosis is unclear, a diagnostic celiotomy or laparoscopy is an integral part of the treatment algorithm of suspected anastomotic leaks. The mainstay of treatment of leaks is operative, with the specific goals of achieving wide and adequate drainage, correcting the underlying defect and accessing the excluded stomach.[47]

Pulmonary embolus

Pulmonary embolus (PE) remains one of the leading causes of early mortality following gastric bypass and was the second most important cause (30 per cent) in autopsy series.[37] In the same study, 80 per cent had silent pulmonary emboli despite prophylaxis. The frequency of PE and deep vein thrombosis (DVT) is approximately 0–3.3 per cent with laparoscopic bypasses[38,39] and 0.3–1.9 per cent with open bypasses.[48,49] Though there is no optimal strategy for preventing DVT/PE, most bariatric surgeons use both pneumatic compression devices in conjunction with subcutaneous low molecular weight heparin. Diagnosis is made by nuclear lung scan, CT-angiography and lower extremity duplex scan; but immediate anticoagulation is prescribed for patients for whom there is a high level of clinical suspicion. Low molecular weight heparin (LMWH) is prescribed in most centres for an extended period after discharge from the hospital.

Bleeding

Bleeding after gastric bypass has been described in 0.6–4.0 per cent of patients.[38,40,50] Early bleeding typically occurs from one of the surgical anastomotic and/or staple lines, and may be intra- or extra-luminal, although it is most commonly intra-luminal. Patients frequently present with tachycardia, a decreased haematocrit and melena.[51] Such bleeding typically resolves without surgical intervention, but may require transfusion of blood products and reversal of anticoagulation. Careful endoscopic examination and therapy is appropriate for on-going bleeding with transfusion requirements. Surgery is reserved for haemodynamic instability or continued bleeding despite restoration of normal coagulation status.[50,51] Late bleeding from the gastric remnant is typically secondary to peptic ulcer disease and can be a diagnostic and therapeutic dilemma.

Gastric remnant distension

Gastric remnant distension is a rare but potentially lethal complication following gastric bypass.[52] The gastric remnant is a blind pouch and may become distended if paralytic ileus or distal mechanical obstruction occurs postoperatively. Iatrogenic injury to vagal fibres along the lesser curvature may also contribute, possibly by leading to impaired emptying of the bypassed stomach. Progressive distension can ultimately lead to rupture, spillage of massive gastric contents and subsequent severe peritonitis.[53] The combination of the large size of inoculum (litres) and the injurious contents (acid, bile, pancreatic enzymes and bacteria) makes this complication more serious than leakage occurring at the gastrojejunostomy. Clinical features include pain, hiccups, left upper quadrant tympany, shoulder pain, abdominal distension, tachycardia or shortness of breath. Radiographic assessment may demonstrate a large gastric air bubble.

Treatment consists of emergent operative decompression with a gastrostomy tube or percutaneous gastrostomy.[54] Immediate laparotomy and decompression is required if percutaneous drainage is not feasible or if perforation is suspected.

Wound infection

Rates of wound infection are significantly greater with open (10–15 per cent) than laparoscopic (3–4 per cent) gastric bypass procedures.[39,55] The incidence of wound infections can be decreased by prophylactic perioperative administration of antibiotics (e.g. co-amoxiclav).

Stomal stenosis

In gastric bypass, the pouch is constructed with a capacity of 20–30 ml, and gastrojejunostomy should have a diameter of 10–12 mms. Stomal stenosis has been described in 6–20 per cent of patients who have undergone RYGB.[33] Several technical factors such as size of anastomosis, the retrocolic or antecolic positioning of the roux limb, tissue ischaemia or increased tension are known to be responsible for the stomal stenosis. The rate of anastomotic stricture was significantly lower using the 25 mm circular stapler than the 21 mm.[56] Patients typically present several weeks after surgery with nausea, vomiting, dysphagia, gastro-oesophageal reflux and eventually an inability to tolerate oral intake. The diagnosis is usually established by endoscopy or with an upper gastrointestinal series. Gastroscopic balloon dilation is usually successful.[57,58] Repeat dilation sessions may be required for some patients. The complication rate for dilation is approximately 3 per cent. Surgical revision (required in less than 0.05 per cent of patients) is reserved for those who have persistent stenosis despite repeated dilations.[59]

Marginal ulcers

Marginal ulcers develop in 0.6–16 per cent of patients.[58,60] Causes of marginal ulcers include:[61,62]

- Larger pouch size, poor tissue perfusion due to tension or ischemia at the anastomosis;

- Presence of foreign material, such as staples or nonabsorbable suture (stitch ulcers);
- Excess acid exposure in the gastric pouch due to gastrogastric fistulas;
- Nonsteroidal anti-inflammatory, steroid drug use;
- Helicobacter pylori infection;
- Smoking, alcohol;
- Critical illness, burns.

Diagnosis of a marginal ulcer is usually established by upper endoscopy. Initial medical treatment consisting of gastric acid suppression with or without the addition of sucralfate is successful in the majority of patients (95 per cent).[58] Nonsteroidal anti-inflammatory drugs should be discontinued and patients should be encouraged to stop smoking. Observational studies have shown that patients with *H. pylori* colonization have a higher incidence of marginal ulcer formation.[63–65] Furthermore, in one study, preoperative testing and treatment of *H. pylori* significantly reduced the incidence of postoperative marginal ulcers (2.4 versus 6.8 per cent in unscreened patients).[65] Therefore, preoperative *H. pylori* screening should continue, especially in geographically high-prevalence areas.[66]

Surgical treatment for marginal ulcers is indicated if persistent pain or recurrent bleeding occurs, despite maximal medical management. Surgical revision is rarely required.[58] Truncal vagotomy at the time of revision has been described.[67] Post operative proton pump inhibitors should be given empirically in high risk groups and a zero tolerance policy towards NSAIDs in gastric bypass patients.

Cholelithiasis

Without prophylaxis, cholelithiasis develops in as many as 38 per cent of patients within six months of surgery, and up to 41 per cent of such patients become symptomatic.[68] Rapid weight loss contributes to the development of gallstones by increasing the lithogenicity of bile. Obesity itself is also a risk factor. Some surgeons recommend performing cholecystectomy at the time of bypass if a patient has symptomatic gallstones preoperatively. The surgical opinion about asymptomatic gallstones is more divided, and studies have failed to demonstrate a benefit for simultaneous cholecystectomy for incidental gallstones at the time of RYGB. Further investigations in the form of randomized, prospective studies are necessary to clearly define the indications for cholecystectomy at the time of weight loss surgery.[68]

Uncommonly, patients develop choledocholithiasis (stones in the common bile duct). Diagnosis of choledocholithiasis can be confirmed by ultrasound or magnetic resonance cholangiopancreatography (MRCP); however, endoscopic retrograde cholangiopancreatography (ERCP) with cannulation of the papilla can be difficult because of the relative inaccessibility to the duodenum due to the altered anatomy of the Roux-en-Y configuration. Thus, patients may require laparoscopic assisted transgastric access to the common bile duct or transhepatic percutaneous access.[69] Placement of a gastrostomy tube into the bypassed stomach at the time of gastric bypass,[70] with the addition of a radiopaque marker to facilitate future percutaneous access to the gastric remnant has been described. More recently, successful therapeutic ERCP through a double balloon enteroscopy has been reported, obviating the need for surgery in the majority of patients with choledocholithiasis after RYGB.[71]

Ventral incisional hernia

Ventral incisional hernias occur with a frequency of 0–1.8 per cent in laparoscopic series and as high as 24 per cent in open series, highlighting a clear advantage of the laparoscopic approach in this regard. Many surgeons postpone a formal repair until significant weight loss occurs (> 1 year). Indications for early surgical repair include significant pain, bowel obstruction and rapid enlargement of the hernia.[72]

Internal hernias

Laparoscopic GBP does offer distinct advantages over traditional open surgery, such as fewer wound complication, superior cosmesis, better visualisation and fewer post operative adhesions. Adhesions, however are required for fixation of roux limb to prevent its displacement and to close mesenteric defects that allow postoperative herniation of the bowel and subsequent complications.[73] Incidence of internal herniation in laparoscopic gastric bypass in the literature has been reported to be 3–4.5 per cent.[74] Postoperative weight loss typically occurs some months after surgery, resulting in loss of intraperitoneal fat which, in turn, leads to larger mesenteric defects. Internal hernias on average present clinically on average 14 months after surgery. Paroz *et al.*[75] noted mean loss of 14.5 BMI units between primary operation and hernia presentation. Patients usually present with intermittent post prandial colicky abdominal pain and nausea. Higa *et al.*,[76] in their series on 2,000 consecutive patients, reported that 20 per cent of symptomatic patients with internal hernia had completely normal contrast studies. The location of internal hernia has been documented with transverse colon hernias to be commonest followed by enteroenterostomy and then Peterson's space hernias. The use of antecolic anastomosis eliminates transverse mesocolic hernia thus reducing the overall incidence of internal hernias. Even accurate closure of all mesenteric defects does not avoid this complication.

The antecolic approach for the Roux-limb, the division of the greater omentum and the systematic closure of the defects with tight non absorbable running sutures are recommended.[77] A high index of suspicion is required for patients presenting with symptoms of intermittent small bowel obstruction, which warrants prompt non-invasive investigations and laparoscopy if the findings of contrast studies are equivocal.

Side Effects of Roux-en-Y Gastric Bypass

Postoperative hypoglycaemia

A small number of patients develop blackouts and seizures after weight loss surgery due to a severe form of recurrent hyperinsulinemic hypoglycaemia.[43] Pancreatic nesidioblastosis has been proposed as a mechanism for the pathologic finding of beta islet hypertrophy in these patients, although a few cases of insulinomas have been found.[44,78] Gastric bypass-induced weight loss may unmask an underlying beta cell defect or contribute to pathological islet hyperplasia.[44]

A wide variety of clinical approaches have been proposed to address severe hypoglycaemia after gastric bypass. We suggest beginning with simpler and safer interventions:

- Patients with symptomatic hypoglycaemia respond well to dietary modification (low carbohydrate diet).[79] Those patients that are refractory to a low carbohydrate diet can be treated with the alpha-glucosidase inhibitor acarbose.
- Based on the theory that severe, disabling hypoglycaemia after gastric bypass surgery occurs in patients with loss of gastric restriction, with resultant rapid food passage and absorption, restoration of gastric restriction can be therapeutic. Z'graggen *et al.* surgically placed a silastic ring or an adjustable gastric band around the pouch, and in their series resolved symptoms in 11 of 12 patients with this approach.[80]
- Subtotal pancreatectomy or total pancreatectomy has been recommended by some surgeons to control hypoglycaemia but should be used as last resort.[64]

Dumping

Symptoms of dumping syndrome are similar to those of hypoglycaemia, but dumping occurs early (within one hour after eating), is not associated with hypoglycaemia and is presumed to be caused by contraction of the plasma volume due to fluid shifts into the gastrointestinal tract. Dumping syndrome is commonly seen in post-gastric bypass patients when high levels of sugar and/or fat are ingested, and may contribute to weight loss in part by causing the patient to modify his/her eating habits. Patient's preoperative nutritional status influenced the presence of clinical manifestations. Adequate dietary management reduced the presence of dumping symptoms in 53 per cent of the patients, during a short-term follow-up period.[81] Monthly administration of a long acting repeatable octreotide may also improve symptoms and quality of life in patients with postoperative dumping.[82]

Nutritional deficiencies

Micronutrient and mineral deficiencies can occur after bariatric surgery, particularly after gastric bypass, both because of inadequate intake of nutrients and because of alterations in the digestive anatomy due to the surgery.

In addition to calcium and vitamin D deficiency leading to metabolic bone disease, gastric bypass patients also have decreased absorption of iron, vitamin B12, fat soluble vitamins (A, D, E, K), thiamine and folate.

After Roux-en-Y gastric bypass, the food stream bypasses most of the stomach. This results in various alterations that can lead to vitamin B12 deficiency, and can be corrected by supplements.[83] Peripheral neuropathy resulting from chronic vitamin B12 deficiency may not be reversible, and must be prevented by diligent laboratory monitoring and adequate replacement.

Absorption of dietary iron is also reduced due to lower acid content in the gastric pouch and the bypass of its main sites of absorption (the duodenum and proximal jejunum). Iron deficiency anaemia is more commonly seen in menstruating women following gastric bypass.[84] Prophylactic iron supplementation has been shown to lower the incidence of iron deficiency and subsequent anaemia.[85]

The following supplementation is recommended:

- Patients should receive intramuscular injections of 1,000 mcg of vitamin B12 every three months for life or take 1,000–2,000 mcg sublingual vitamin B12 daily. The dose may be reduced if long-term monitoring shows elevated vitamin B12 levels.
- Patients should take a daily multivitamin containing B vitamins and vitamin C, fat-soluble vitamins and minerals. Some patients require a liquid vitamin preparation because the pills are not tolerated by the stomach pouch. Patients should be transitioned to an adult pill supplement when possible.
- Vitamin D deficiency is a concern after gastric bypass and 800 IU is recommended daily. Most multivitamin supplements contain 400 IU of vitamin D. Additional supplementation is recommended by taking a second multivitamin, or ingesting a second supplement containing calcium and vitamin D.
- Patients should take calcium supplements that provide 1,200–1,500 mg of calcium daily. Calcium citrate may be better absorbed than calcium carbonate after gastric bypass.

- Patients at risk for iron deficiency (e.g. menstruating women, those intolerant to iron-containing foods) should take iron supplements prophylactically, and those who develop iron deficiency anaemia should receive 640 mg/day of supplemental iron. Iron absorption is improved when iron is administered along with vitamin C.
- Patients should be encouraged to eat fruits and vegetables.

Patients with persistent vomiting or other causes of inadequate nutrient intake should receive 50 mg thiamine daily. Two-year nutritional investigation is especially recommended because of its long-term predictive value.[86]

Secondary hyperparathyroidism

Morbid obesity is associated with vitamin D deficiency and secondary hyperparathyroidism even in patients who have not undergone bariatric surgery.[87] The vitamin D deficiency is speculated to be due to decreased sun exposure, insufficient intake, and reduced bioavailability of vitamin D from sequestration in fat.

While vitamin D levels may decrease after gastric bypass,[88] dietary calcium is best absorbed in the duodenum where the highest concentration of calcium transporters are present. After gastric bypass, however, ingested food does not pass through the duodenum and this may result in calcium deficiency.[89] This can be further exacerbated by low intake of vitamin D in the diet. Thus, secondary hyperparathyroidism can develop or persist postoperatively.[90]

Chronic poor calcium absorption combined with inadequate supplementation can lead to secondary hyperparathyroidism. Affected patients will show elevated levels of parathyroid hormone and normal to low serum calcium. One study in 193 women in the United States found that postmenopausal women, African–American women, and those with a higher BMI were at increased risk of developing secondary hyperparathyroidism after gastric bypass.[91]

Osteopaenia and metabolic bone disease after RYGB have been reported.[92] Post-gastric bypass patients are maintained on 1,200–1,500 mg calcium and 800 IU vitamin D daily to avoid metabolic bone disease.

Hyperoxaluria and nephrolithiasis have been reported following Roux-en-Y gastric bypass surgery.[91]

After laparoscopic Roux-en-Y gastric bypass, vitamin D deficiency and hyperparathyroidism commonly occur. Body mass index and Roux limb length are not associated with these two conditions, but racial differences do exist. There is a weak inverse correlation between vitamin D and parathyroid hormone (PTH). Further research is needed to elucidate the causes, treatments, and significance of hyperparathyroidism after LGB.[93]

Weight Evolution After RYGB

Weight loss after RYGB

Weight loss following gastric bypass surgery has been studied extensively. Favourable results are published in short-term as well as long-term follow-up studies.

Mean EWL after open RYGB ranges from 57 to 65 per cent at one year.[94] Schauer *et al.* found that EWL following laparoscopic RYGB was 68 per cent at one year and 83 per cent at two years.[95] In a meta-analysis, Buchwald *et al.* found that patients lose between 56.7 and 66.5 per cent excess weight within the first 24 months after gastric bypass.[35]

In the SOS study, RYGB produced the greatest long-term weight loss (25 per cent ± 11 per cent), followed by vertical banded gastroplasty (16.5 per cent ± 11 per cent) and fixed or variable banding procedures (13.2 per cent ± 13 per cent).[96] Fobi *et al.*, using the transected banded gastric bypass followed 22 of 51 patients for ten years and reported a mean of 72 per cent excess weight loss.[97]

The stability of the postoperative weight after RYGB was clearly demonstrated by Pories *et al.*[32] Their study of 608 patients with a 97 per cent follow-up showed a 58 per cent loss of excess weight after five years and a BMI of 33.7. After ten years, the excess weight loss was 55 per cent and the BMI was 34.7 (range, 22.5–64.7). At 14 years (ten patients), the EWL was 49 per cent and the BMI 34.9 (range, 25.9–54.6).

Insufficient weight loss or weight regain after RYGB

The course of excess weight loss after bariatric surgery continues to be a subject of investigation. Bariatric surgeons recognize that a certain weight regain occurs after obesity surgery compared to the lowest weight observed between 18 and 24 months after surgery, a period characterized by higher excess weight loss. Apparently, this regain mainly occurs between two and five years after gastric bypass.[98]

Brolin *et al.* reported a 33 per cent failure rate in super-obese patients seven years after surgery.[99] Capella *et al.* demonstrated an average excess weight loss of 77 per cent and failure because of excess weight loss less than 50 per cent in 7 per cent of the patients after five years of follow-up.[100] MacLean *et al.* demonstrated an excess weight loss less than 50 per cent in 7 per cent of morbidly obese patients over three years of follow-up and in 43 per cent of super-obese patients.[101]

Weight regain after RYGB can be due to increased volume intake from gastric pouch dilation, gastrojejunostomy dilation or presence of gastro-gastric fistulas.

It can also be caused by an inadequate length of the alimentary limb resulting in reduced malabsorption, and by changes in eating behaviour such as sweet-eating, grazing or polyphagia and volume eating or hyperphagia.

Gastric pouch dilatation or dilatation of the gastrojejunostomy can be treated with endoluminal techniques such as StomaphyX™ and Endocinch™. In the case of weight regain caused by volume eating or hyperphagia, a possible treatment can be offered by surgical revision aiming at restoring restriction. Additional restriction can be obtained by placing an adjustable or non-adjustable band around the gastric pouch (Fig. 13).[102,103] Lengthening of the alimentary limb by conversion to distal RYGB seems to result in unacceptable malnutrition.

Change of the patient's alimentary behaviour remains an extremely difficult aspect. Some patients start eating sweets because they are no longer affected by the dumping syndrome; others become grazers by eating too frequently (polyphagia). Due to these dietary flaws, patients can increase their caloric uptake and consequently gain weight.[104]

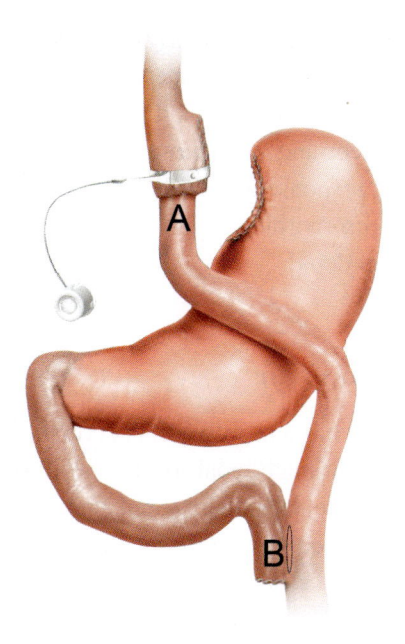

Figure 13. Adjustable banded gastric bypass (picture after Dr B. Dillemans).

Resolution of co-morbidities after RYGB

Morbidly obese patients have been identified as being at high risk for the metabolic syndrome comprising a combination of hypertension, dyslipidemia, glucose intolerance and obesity. If left untreated, the progression to cardiovascular disease has been documented in these patients. Weight loss is critical to the treatment of this condition, and one year postoperatively metabolic syndrome can be reversed in up to 98 per cent of patients.[105]

Diabetes, hypertension, hypercholesterolemia, and obstructive sleep apnoea are among the commonly reported co-morbid conditions which tend to improve significantly or resolve completely following RYGB. A meta-analysis of more than 136 studies, totalling more than 22,000 patients, was undertaken by Buchwald *et al*. Diabetes mellitus and glucose intolerance demonstrated concomitant improvement in haemoglobin A1C levels and fasting glucose in 83 per cent of affected patients. Hypertension resolved completely in 67.5 per cent of affected patients and improved in up to 87 per cent. Similarly, hyperlipidemia (96.9 per cent improvement), obstructive sleep apnoea (94.8 per cent resolution or improvement), gastroesophageal reflux disease, pseudotumor cerebri, urinary stress incontinence, and other co-morbid conditions demonstrated variable, but positive, response to RYGB.[35] In the chapter on the effect of bariatric surgery on co-morbidities all these conditions are discussed separately and more in detail.

Health-related quality of life

Because morbid obesity has a negative impact on health-related quality of life (HRQoL),[106] the ultimate goal of bariatric surgery is improved HRQoL through adequate weight loss and cure or amelioration of co-morbidities. As a consequence, divergent dimensions of quality of life (QoL) have been widely accepted as important health outcomes after surgical intervention.[107,108]

In general, QoL substantially improves following bariatric surgery,[109] especially within the first two postoperative years,[110] but also after long follow-up duration,[111] and even within six months[112] or as soon as two to three weeks after surgery.[113] Most studies suggest that HRQoL normalizes following bariatric surgery,[113,114] but according to others, improvements lag behind HRQoL of reference groups.[109] This may not be surprising, given that most patients are still obese.

QoL seems to be closely related to the patient's level of satisfaction with the results of the operation.[106,115,116] Most patients report satisfaction with the surgery, with some studies reporting >90 per cent satisfaction rates.[106,116] However, after some time a slight decline may occur, which can be explained by the slow-down of weight reduction or the occurrence of first complications.[117] It is important to note that up to 20 per cent of patients are dissatisfied, partly due to psychosocial problems, surgical complications and the surgery not meeting their expectations.[111,118]

However, almost all patients say they would undergo the operation again;[119] they appear to achieve most of their goals, even though not all of them obtain their desired weight loss.[120]

Hell et al. conducted a trial to compare the effects and outcomes of three different bariatric procedures: RYGB, VBG and AGB. In this prospective comparative study with 30 matched patients from each group, patients were followed to assess post-operative improvement in health status and quality of life, to compare the three different techniques. The Bariatric Analysis and Reporting Outcome System (BAROS) as described by Oria and Moorehead[121] has been used for evaluation.

The observation time was at least three years (three to eight years) in each individual case. A significant increase in quality of life and health status in 75 per cent of the surgically-treated patients was observed when compared with a non-operated control group of morbidly obese patients. By utilizing BAROS it has been found possible to compare the results of different procedures done by different surgeons with different techniques, utilizing patients from different cultures and with different languages. The results of this comparative study favour the standard gastric bypass for the treatment of morbid obesity. This operation is superior to purely gastric restrictive procedures in weight loss and improvement of quality of life.[122]

Long-term mortality after RYGB

Adams et al. examined the records of patients who had undergone gastric bypass surgery to determine their long-term risk of death, as compared with that of a population control group in which weight was self-reported. In this retrospective cohort study, the authors determined the long-term mortality among 9,949 patients who had undergone gastric bypass surgery and 9,628 severely obese persons who applied for driver's licences. From these subjects, 7,925 surgical patients and 7,925 severely obese control subjects were matched for age, sex and body-mass index. They determined the rates of death from any cause and from specific causes with the use of the National Death Index. During a mean follow-up of 7.1 years, adjusted long-term mortality from any cause in the surgery group decreased by 40 per cent, as compared with that in the control group (37.6 versus 57.1 deaths per 10,000 person-years, $P < 0.001$); cause-specific mortality in the surgery group decreased by 56 per cent for coronary artery disease (2.6 versus 5.9 per 10,000 person-years, $P = 0.006$), by 92 per cent for diabetes (0.4 versus 3.4 per 10,000 person-years, $P = 0.005$) and by

60 per cent for cancer (5.5 versus 13.3 per 10,000 person-years, P < 0.001). However, rates of death not caused by disease, such as accidents and suicide, were 58 per cent higher in the surgery group than in the control group (11.1 versus 6.4 per 10,000 person-years, P = 0.04). Despite certain limitations, these findings indicate that patients who undergo gastric bypass surgery have decreased long-term mortality from any cause and from disease-specific causes but have increased mortality from non-disease causes, as compared with control subjects. The study provides useful data for patients considering gastric bypass surgery, for medical professionals serving the severely obese population, and for insurance carriers making decisions about whether to cover this procedure.[123]

Conclusion

RYGB is nowadays considered as the 'gold standard' surgical weight loss procedure. It not only results in excellent weight loss, but also resolves or improves associated co-morbidities such as type 2 diabetes. Moreover, quality of life after RYGB seems to be superior to the restrictive type of bariatric procedures.

Acknowledgements

We would like to thank Dr. Girish Bapat for his contribution to the review of the literature on RYGB.

References

1. Mason, E.E., Ito, C. (1996). Gastric bypass in obesity, 1967. *Obes Res* 4(3): 316–319.
2. Alden, J.F. (1977). Gastric and jejunoileal bypass. A comparison in the treatment of morbid obesity. *Arch Surg* 112(7): 799–806.
3. Griffen, W.O., J., Young, V.L., Stevenson, C.C. (1977). A prospective comparison of gastric and jejunoileal bypass procedures for morbid obesity. *Ann Surg* 186(4): 500–509.
4. Torres, J.C., Oca, C.F., Garrison, R.N. (1983). Gastric bypass: Roux-en-Y gastrojejunostomy from the lesser curvature. *South Med J* 76(10): 1217–1221.

5. Linner, J.R., Drew, R.L. (1986). New modification of Roux-en-Y gastric bypass procedure. *Clin Nutr* 5: 33–34.
6. Salmon, P.A. (1988). Gastroplasty with distal gastric bypass: a new and more successful weight loss operation for the morbidly obese. *Can J Surg* 31(2): 111–113.
7. Fobi, M. (1991). Why the operation I prefer is silastic ring vertical gastric bypass. *Obes Surg* 1(4): 423–426.
8. Ali, M.R., Fuller, W.D., Choi, M.P. *et al.* (2005). Bariatric surgical outcomes. *Surg Clin North Am* 85(4): 835–852, vii.
9. Rutledge, R. (2001). The mini-gastric bypass: experience with the first 1,274 cases. *Obes Surg* 11(3): 276–280.
10. Buchwald, H., Oien, D.M. (2009). Metabolic/Bariatric surgery worldwide 2008. *Obes Surg* 9(12): 1605–1611.
11. Rubino, F., Gagner, M., Gentileschi, P. *et al.* (2004). The early effect of the Roux-en-Y gastric bypass on hormones involved in body weight regulation and glucose metabolism. *Ann Surg* 240(2): 236–242.
12. Brolin, R.E. (2002). Bariatric surgery and long-term control of morbid obesity. *JAMA* 288: 2793–2796.
13. le Roux, C.W., Aylwin, S.J., Batterham, R.L. *et al.* (2006). Gut hormone profiles following bariatric surgery favor an anorectic state, facilitate weight loss, and improve metabolic parameters. *Ann Surg* 243(1): 108–114.
14. Bauchowitz, A.U., Gonder-Frederick, L.A., Olbrisch, M.E. *et al.* (2005). Psychosocial evaluation of bariatric surgery candidates: a survey of present practices. *Psychosom Med* 67(5): 825–832.
15. Colles, S.L., Dixon, J.B., Marks, P. *et al.* (2006). Preoperative weight loss with a very-low-energy diet: quantitation of changes in liver and abdominal fat by serial imaging. *Am J Clin Nutr* 84(2): 304–311.
16. Lewis, M.C., Phillips, M.L., Slavotinek, J.P. *et al.* (2006). Change in liver size and fat content after treatment with Optifast very low calorie diet. *Obes Surg* 16(6): 697–701.
17. Still, C.D., Benotti, P., Wood, G.C. *et al.* (2007). Outcomes of preoperative weight loss in high-risk patients undergoing gastric bypass surgery. *Arch Surg* 142(10): 994–998.
18. Csendes, A., Burgos, A.M., Smok, G. *et al.* (2007). Endoscopic and histologic findings of the foregut in 426 patients with morbid obesity. *Obes Surg* 17(1): 28–34.

19. Collazo-Clavell, M.L., Clark, M.M., McAlpine, D.E. et al. (2006). Assessment and preparation of patients for bariatric surgery. *Mayo Clin Proc* 81(10 Suppl): S11–S17.
20. Scharrer, E. (1999). Control of food intake by fatty acid oxidation and ketogenesis. *Nutrition* 15(9): 704–714.
21. van Hout, G.C., Verschure, S.K., van Heck, G.L. (2005). Psychosocial predictors of success following bariatric surgery. *Obes Surg* 15(4): 552–560.
22. Buchwald, H., Buchwald, J.N. (2002). Evolution of operative procedures for the management of morbid obesity 1950–2000. *Obes Surg* 12(5): 705–717.
23. Bohdjalian, A., Langer, F.B., Kranner, A. et al. (2009). Circular- versus linear-stapled gastrojejunostomy in laparoscopic Roux-En-Y gastric bypass. *Obes Surg* 20(4): 440–446 (Epub 2009 Oct 24).
24. Escalona, A., Devaud, N., Perez, G. et al. (2007). Antecolic versus retrocolic alimentary limb in laparoscopic Roux-en-Y gastric bypass: a comparative study. *Surg Obes Relat Dis* 3(4): 423–427.
25. Choban, P.S., Flancbaum, L. (2002). The effect of Roux limb lenghts on outcome after Roux-en-Y gastric bypass: a prospective, randomised clinical trial. *Obes Surg* 12(4): 540–545.
26. MacLean, L.D., Rhode, B.M., Nohr, C.W. (2001). Long- or short-limb gastric bypass? *J Gastrointest Surg* 5(5): 525–530.
27. Gleysteen, J.J. (2009). Five-year outcome with gastric bypass: Roux limb makes a difference. *Surg Obes Relat Dis* 5(2): 242–247.
28. Brolin, R.E. (2005). Long limb Roux en Y gastric bypass revisited. *Surg Clin North Am* 85(4): 807–817, vii.
29. Iannelli, A., Facchiano, E., Gugenheim, J. (2006). Internal hernia after laparoscopic Roux-en-Y gastric bypass for morbid obesity. *Obes Surg* 16(10): 1265–1271.
30. Dillemans, B., Sakran, N., Van Cauwenberge, S. et al. (2009). Standardization of the fully stapled laparoscopic Roux-en-Y gastric bypass for obesity reduces early immediate postoperative morbidity and mortality: a single center study on 2606 patients. *Obes Surg* 19(10): 1355–1364.
31. Mulier, J.P., Dillemans, B., Luyten, A. (2008). Horizontal positioning of the trunk and maximal leg flexion increases the laparoscopic workspace for bariatric surgery. *Obes Surg* 18: 442–442.
32. Pories, W.J., Swanson, M.S., MacDonald, K.G. et al. (1995). Who would have thought it? An operation proves to be the most effective therapy for adult-onset diabetes mellitus. *Ann Surg* 222(3): 339–350.

33. Schneider, B.E., Villegas, L., Blackburn, G.L. et al. (2003). Laparoscopic gastric bypass surgery: outcomes. *J Laparoendosc Adv Surg Tech A* 13(4): 247–255.
34. Sugerman, H.J., Londrey, G.L., Kellum, J.M. et al. (1989). Weight loss with vertical banded gastroplasty and Roux-Y gastric bypass for morbid obesity with selective versus random assignment. *Am J Surg* 157(1): 93–102.
35. Buchwald, H., Avidor, Y., Braunwald, E. et al. (2004). Bariatric surgery: a systematic review and meta-analysis. *JAMA* 292(14): 1724–1737.
36. Buchwald, H., Estok, R., Fahrbach, K. et al. (2007). Trends in mortality in bariatric surgery: a systematic review and meta-analysis. *Surgery* 142(4): 621–32; discussion 632–635.
37. Melinek, J., Livingston, E., Cortina, G. et al. (2002). Autopsy findings following gastric bypass surgery for morbid obesity. *Arch Pathol Lab Med* 126(9): 1091–1095.
38. Wittgrove, A.C., Clark, G.W. (2000). Laparoscopic gastric bypass, Roux-en-Y 500 patients: technique and results, with 3–60 month follow-up. *Obes Surg* 10(3): 233–239.
39. Schauer, P.R., Ikramuddin, S., Gourash, W. et al. (2000). Outcomes after laparoscopic Roux-en-Y gastric bypass for morbid obesity. *Ann Surg* 232(4): 515–529.
40. Higa, K.D., Boone, K.B., Ho, T. (2000). Complications of the laparoscopic Roux-en-Y gastric bypass: 1,040 patients — what have we learned? *Obes Surg* 10(6): 509–513.
41. Fernandez, A.Z.J., DeMaria, E.J., Tichansky, D.S. (2004). Experience with over 3,000 open and laparoscopic bariatric procedures: multivariate analysis of factors related to leak and resultant mortality. *Surg Endosc* 18: 193–197.
42. Almahmeed, T., Gonzalez, R., Nelson, L.G. et al. (2007). Morbidity of anastomotic leaks in patients undergoing Roux-en-Y gastric bypass. *Arch Surg* 142(10): 954–957.
43. Service G.J., Thompson, G.B., Service, F.J. et al. (2005). Hyperinsulinemic hypoglycaemia with nesidioblastosis after gastric-bypass surgery. *N Engl J Med* 353(3): 249–254.
44. Patti, M.E., McMahon, G., Mun, E.C. et al. (2005). Severe hypoglycaemia post-gastric bypass requiring partial pancreatectomy: evidence for inappropriate insulin secretion and pancreatic islet hyperplasia. *Diabetologia* 48(11): 2236–2240.

45. Hamilton, E.C., Sims, T.L., Hamilton, T.T. *et al.* (2003). Clinical predictors of leak after laparoscopic Roux-en-Y gastric bypass for morbid obesity. *Surg Endosc* 17(5): 679–684.
46. Yu, J., Turner, M.A., Cho, S. *et al.* (2004). Normal anatomy and complications after gastric bypass surgery: helical CT findings. *Radiology* 231: 753–760.
47. Gonzalez, R., Nelson, L.G., Gallagher, S.F. *et al.* (2004). Anastomotic leaks after laparoscopic gastric bypass. *Obes Surg* 14: 1299–1307.
48. Hall, J.C., Watts, J.M., O'Brien, P.E. *et al.* (1990). Gastric surgery for morbid obesity. The Adelaide Study. *Ann Surg* 211(4): 419–427.
49. Fobi, M.A., Lee, H., Holness, R. *et al.* (1998). Gastric bypass operation for obesity. *World J Surg* 22(9): 925–935.
50. Nguyen, N.T., Rivers, R., Wolfe, B.M. (2003). Early gastrointestinal hemorrhage after laparoscopic gastric bypass. *Obes Surg* 13(1): 62–65.
51. Mehran, A., Szomstein, S., Zundel, N. *et al.* (2003). Management of acute bleeding after laparoscopic Roux-en-Y gastric bypass. *Obes Surg* 13(6): 842–847.
52. Sugerman, H.J. (1997). Gastric surgery for morbid obesity. In: Zinner, M.J., Maingot, S. (eds). *Abdominal operations*, pp. 1057–1079, Appleton & Lange, Stamford, CT.
53. Papasavas, P.K., Yeaney, W.W., Caushaj, P.F. *et al.* (2003). Perforation in the bypassed stomach following laparoscopic Roux-en-Y gastric bypass. *Obes Surg* 13(5): 797–799.
54. Gagner, M., Gentileschi, P., de Csepel, J. *et al.* (2002). Laparoscopic reoperative bariatric surgery: experience from 27 consecutive patients. *Obes Surg* 12(2): 254–260.
55. Nguyen, N.T., Goldman, C., Rosenquist, C.J. *et al.* (2001). Laparoscopic versus open gastric bypass: a randomized study of outcomes, quality of life, and costs. *Ann Surg* 234(3): 279–289.
56. Suggs, W.J., Kouli, W., Lupovici, M. *et al.* (2007). Complications at gastrojejunostomy after laparoscopic Roux-en-Y gastric bypass: comparison between 21- and 25-mm circular staplers. *Surg Obes Relat Dis* 3(5): 508–514.
57. Barba, C.A., Butensky, M.S., Lorenzo, M. *et al.* (2003). Endoscopic dilation of gastroesophageal anastomosis stricture after gastric bypass. *Surg Endosc* 17(3): 416–420.
58. Sanyal, A.J., Sugerman, H.J., Kellum, J.M. *et al.* (1992). Stomal complications of gastric bypass: incidence and outcome of therapy. *Am J Gastroenterol* 87(9): 1165–1169.

59. Go, M.R., Muscarella, P., Needleman, B.J. *et al.* (2004). Endoscopic management of stomal stenosis after Roux-en-Y gastric bypass. *Surg Endosc* 18(1): 56–59.
60. Sapala, J.A., Wood, M.H., Sapala, M.A. *et al.* (1998). Marginal ulcer after gastric bypass: a prospective 3-year study of 173 patients. *Obes Surg* 8(5): 505–516.
61. Dallal, R.M., Bailey, L.A. (2006). Ulcer disease after gastric bypass surgery. *Surg Obes Relat Dis* 2(4): 455–459.
62. Rasmussen, J.J., Fuller, W., Ali, M.R. (2007). Marginal ulceration after laparoscopic gastric bypass: an analysis of predisposing factors in 260 patients. *Surg Endosc* 21(7): 1090–1094.
63. Csendes, A., Burgos, A.M., Smok, G. *et al.* (2007). Endoscopic and histologic findings of the foregut in 426 patients with morbid obesity. *Obes Surg* 17(1): 28–34.
64. Ramaswamy, A., Lin, E., Ramshaw, B.J. *et al.* (2004). Early effects of *Helicobacter pylori* infection in patients undergoing bariatric surgery. *Arch Surg* 139(10): 1094–1096.
65. Schirmer, B., Erenoglu, C., Miller, A. (2002). Flexible endoscopy in the management of patients undergoing Roux-en-Y gastric bypass. *Obes Surg* 12(5): 634–638.
66. Hartin, J.W., Remine, D.S., Lucktong, T.A. (2009). Preoperative bariatric screening and treatment of *Helicobacter pylori*. *Surg Endosc* 23(11): 2531–2534.
67. Printen, K.J., Scott, D., Mason, E.E. (1980). Stomal ulcers after gastric bypass. *Arch Surg* 115(4): 525–527.
68. Patel, J.A., Patel, N.A, Piper, G.L. *et al.* (2009). Perioperative management of cholelithiasis in patients presenting for laparoscopic Roux-en-Y gastric bypass: have we reached a consensus? *Am Surg* 75(6): 470–476.
69. Lopes, T.L., Clements, R.H., Wilcox, C.M. (2009). Laparoscopy-assisted ERCP: experience of a high-volume bariatric surgery center (with video). *Gastrointest Endosc* 70(6): 1254–1259 (Epub 2009 Oct 28).
70. Dapri, G., Himpens, J., Buset, M. *et al.* (2009). Laparoscopic transgastric access to the common bile duct after Roux-en-Y gastric bypass. *Surg Endosc* 23(7): 1646–1648.
71. Moreels, T.G., Hubens, G.J., Ysebaert, D.K. *et al.* (2009). Diagnostic and therapeutic double-balloon enteroscopy after small bowel Roux-en-Y reconstructive surgery. *Digestion* 80(3): 141–147.

72. Andersen, L.P., Klein, M., Gogenur, I. *et al.* (2008). Incisional hernia after open versus laparoscopic sigmoid resection. *Surg Endosc* 22(9): 2026–2029.
73. Champion, J.K., Williams, M. (2003). Small bowel obstruction and internal hernias after laparoscopic Roux-en-Y gastric bypass. *Obes Surg* 13(4): 596–600.
74. Ahmed, A.R., Rickards, G., Husain, S. *et al.* (2007). Trends in internal hernia incidence after laparoscopic Roux-en-Y gastric bypass. *Obes Surg* 17(12): 1563–1566.
75. Paroz, A., Calmes, J.M., Giusti, V. *et al.* (2006). Internal hernia after laparoscopic Roux-en-Y gastric bypass for morbid obesity: a continuous challenge in bariatric surgery. *Obes Surg* 16(11): 1482–1487.
76. Higa, K.D., Ho, T., Boone, K.B. (2003). Internal hernias after laparoscopic Roux-en-Y gastric bypass: incidence, treatment and prevention. *Obes Surg* 13(3): 350–354.
77. Iannelli, A., Buratii, M.S, Novellas, S. *et al.* (2007). Internal hernia as a complication of laparoscopic Roux-en-Y gastric bypass. *Obes Surg* 17(10): 1283–1286.
78. Clancy, T.E., Moore, F.D.J., Zinner, M.J. (2006). Post-gastric bypass hyperinsulinism with nesidioblastosis: subtotal or total pancreatectomy may be needed to prevent recurrent hypoglycaemia. *J Gastrointest Surg* 10(8): 1116–1119.
79. Kellogg, T.A., Bantle, J.P., Leslie, D.B. *et al.* (2008). Postgastric bypass hyperinsulinemic hypoglycaemia syndrome: characterization and response to a modified diet. *Surg Obes Relat Dis* 4(4): 492–499.
80. Z'graggen, K., Guweidhi, A., Steffen, R. *et al.* (2008). Severe recurrent hypoglycaemia after gastric bypass surgery. *Obes Surg* 18(8): 981–988.
81. Rivera, J., Ochoa-Martinez, C.I., Hermosillo-Sandoval, J.M. *et al.* (2007). Dumping syndrome in patients submitted to gastric resection. *Cir Cir* 75(6): 429–434.
82. Arts, J., Caenepeel, P., Bisschops, R. *et al.* (2009). Efficacy of the long-acting repeatable formulation of the somatostatin analogue octreotide in postoperative dumping. *Clin Gastroenterol Hepatol* 7(4): 432–437.
83. Ledoux, S., Msika, S., Moussa, F. *et al.* (2006). Comparison of nutritional consequences of conventional therapy of obesity, adjustable gastric banding, and gastric bypass. *Obes Surg* 16(8): 1041–1049.

84. Love, A.L. Billett, H.H. (2008). Obesity, bariatric surgery, and iron deficiency: true, true, true and related. *Am J Hematol* 83(5): 403–409.
85. Brolin, R.E., Gorman, J.H., Gorman, R.C. *et al.* (1998). Prophylactic iron supplementation after Roux-en-Y gastric bypass: a prospective, double-blind, randomized study. *Arch Surg* 133(7): 740–744.
86. Dalcanale, L., Oliveira, C.P., Faintuch, J. *et al.* (2009). Long-term nutritional outcome after gastric bypass. *Obes Surg* 20(2): 181–187 (Epub 2009 Aug 25).
87. Hamoui, N., Anthone, G., Crookes, P.F. (2004). Calcium metabolism in the morbidly obese. *Obes Surg* 14(1): 9–12.
88. DiGiorgi, M., Daud, A., Inabnet, W.B. *et al.* (2008). Markers of bone and calcium metabolism following gastric bypass and laparoscopic adjustable gastric banding. *Obes Surg* 18(9): 1144–1148.
89. Johnson, J.M., Maher, J.W., DeMaria, E.J. *et al.* (2006). The long-term effects of gastric bypass on vitamin D metabolism. *Ann Surg* 243(5): 701–704.
90. Ybarra, J., Sanchez-Hernandez, J., Gich, I. *et al.* (2005). Unchanged hypovitaminosis D and secondary hyperparathyroidism in morbid obesity after bariatric surgery. *Obes Surg* 15(3): 330–335.
91. Youssef, Y., Richards, W.O., Sekhar, N. *et al.* (2007). Risk of secondary hyperparathyroidism after laparoscopic gastric bypass surgery in obese women. *Surg Endosc* 21(8): 1393–1396.
92. De Prisco, C., Levine, S.N. (2005). Metabolic bone disease after gastric bypass surgery for obesity. *Am J Med Sci* 329(2): 57–61.
93. Clements, R.H., Yellumahanthi, K., Wesley, M. *et al.* (2008). Hyperparathyroidism and vitamin D deficiency after laparoscopic gastric bypass. *Am Surg* 74(6): 469–474.
94. Perugini, R.A., Mason, R., Czerniach, D.R. *et al.* (2003). Predictors of complication and suboptimal weight loss after laparoscopic Roux-en-Y gastric bypass: a series of 188 patients. *Arch Surg* 138(5): 541–545; discussion 545–546.
95. Schauer, P., Ikramuddin, S., Hamad, G. *et al.* (2003). The learning curve for laparoscopic Roux-en-Y gastric bypass is 100 cases. *Surg Endosc* 17(2): 212–215.
96. Sjostrom, L., Lindroos, A.K., Peltonen, M. *et al.* (2004). Lifestyle, diabetes, and cardiovascular risk factors 10 years after bariatric surgery. *N Engl J Med* 351(26): 2683–2693.

97. Fobi, M.A., Lee, H., Felahy, B. *et al.* (2005). Choosing an operation for weight control, and the transected banded gastric bypass. *Obes Surg* 15(1): 114–121.
98. Magro, D.O., Geloneze, B., Delfini, R. *et al.* (2008). Long-term weight regain after gastric bypass: a 5-year prospective study. *Obes Surg* 18(6): 648–651.
99. Brolin, R.E., Kenler, H.A., Gorman, J.H. *et al.* (1992). Long-limb gastric bypass in the superobese. A prospective randomized study. *Ann Surg* 215(4): 387–395.
100. Capella, J.F., Capella, R.F. (1996). The weight reduction operation of choice: vertical banded gastroplasty or gastric bypass? *Am J Surg* 171(1): 74–79.
101. MacLean, L.D., Rhode, B.M., Nohr, C.W. (2000). Late outcome of isolated gastric bypass. *Ann Surg* 231(4): 524–528.
102. Bessler, M., Daud, A., Digiorgi, M.F. *et al.* (2009). Adjustable gastric banding as revisional bariatric procedure after failed gastric bypass-intermediate results. *Surg Obes Relat Dis* 6(1): 31–35
103. Bessler, M., Daud, A., DiGiorgi, M.F. *et al.* (2005). Adjustable gastric banding as a revisional bariatric procedure after failed gastric bypass. *Obes Surg* 15(10): 1443–1448.
104. Dapri, G., Cadière, G.B., Himpens, J. (2009). Laparoscopic placement of non-adjustable silicone ring for weight regain after Roux-en-Y gastric bypass. *Obes Surg* 19(5): 650–654.
105. Sugerman, H.J., Wolfe, L.G., Sica, D.A. *et al.* (2003). Diabetes and hypertension in severe obesity and effects of gastric bypass-induced weight loss. *Ann Surg* 237(6): 751–756; discussion 757–758.
106. Mathus-Vliegen, E.M., de Weerd, S., de Wit, L.T. (2004). Health-related quality-of-life in patients with morbid obesity after gastric banding for surgically induced weight loss. *Surgery* 135(5): 489–497.
107. Guisado, J.A., Vaz, F.J. (2003). Personality profiles of the morbidly obese after vertical banded gastroplasty. *Obes Surg* 13(3): 394–398.
108. Tolonen, P., Victorzon, M. (2003). Quality of life following laparoscopic adjustable gastric banding — the Swedish band and the Moorehead-Ardelt questionnaire. *Obes Surg* 13(3): 424–426.
109. Boan, J., Kolotkin, R.L., Westman, E.C. *et al.* (2004). Binge eating, quality of life and physical activity improve after Roux-en-Y gastric bypass for morbid obesity. *Obes Surg* 14(3): 341–348.

110. Freys, S.M., Tigges, H., Heimbucher, J. *et al.* (2001). Quality of life following laparoscopic gastric banding in patients with morbid obesity. *J Gastrointest Surg* 5(4): 401–407.
111. Shai, I., Henkin, Y., Weitzman, S. *et al.* (2003). Determinants of long-term satisfaction after vertical banded gastroplasty. *Obes Surg* 13(2): 269–274.
112. Sabbioni, M.E., Dickson, M.H., Eychmuller, S. *et al.* (2002). Intermediate results of health related quality of life after vertical banded gastroplasty. *Int J Obes Relat Metab Disord* 26(2): 277–280.
113. Dymek, M.P., Le Grange, D., Neven, K. *et al.* (2002). Quality of life after gastric bypass surgery: a cross-sectional study. *Obes Res* 10(11): 1135–1142.
114. Choban, P.S., Onyejekwe, J., Burge, J.C. *et al.* (1999). A health status assessment of the impact of weight loss following Roux-en-Y gastric bypass for clinically severe obesity. *J Am Coll Surg* 188(5): 491–497.
115. Wadden, T.A., Sarwer, D.B., Womble, L.G. *et al.* (2001). Psychosocial aspects of obesity and obesity surgery. *Surg Clin North Am* 81(5): 1001–1024.
116. Kinzl, J.F., Traweger, C., Trefalt, E. *et al.* (2003). Psychosocial consequences of weight loss following gastric banding for morbid obesity. *Obes Surg* 13(1): 105–110.
117. Buddeberg-Fischer, B., Klaghofer, R., Sigrist, S. *et al.* (2004). Impact of psychosocial stress and symptoms on indication for bariatric surgery and outcome in morbidly obese patients. *Obes Surg* 14(3): 361–369.
118. Sannen, I., Himpens, J., Leman, G. (2001). Causes of dissatisfaction in some patients after adjustable gastric banding. *Obes Surg* 11(5): 605–608.
119. Kriwanek, S., Blauensteiner, W., Lebisch, E. *et al.* (2000). Dietary changes after vertical banded gastroplasty. *Obes Surg* 10(1): 37–40.
120. Foster, G.D., Wadden, T.A., Vogt, R.A. *et al.* (1997). What is a reasonable weight loss? Patients' expectations and evaluations of obesity treatment outcomes. *J Consult Clin Psychol* 65(1): 79–85.
121. Oria, H.E., Moorehead, M.K. (1998). Bariatric analysis and reporting outcome system (BAROS). *Obes Surg* 8(5): 487–499.
122. Hell, E., Miller, K.A., Moorehead, M.K. *et al.* (2000). Evaluation of health status and quality of life after bariatric surgery: comparison of standard Roux-en-Y gastric bypass, vertical banded gastroplasty and laparoscopic adjustable silicone gastric banding. *Obes Surg* 10(3): 214–219.
123. Adams, T.D., Gress, R.E., Smith, S.C. *et al.* (2007). Long-term mortality after gastric bypass surgery. *N Engl J Med* 357(8): 753–761.

Chapter 8

New Technologies in Bariatric Surgery

Matthias Lannoo and Andre D'Hoore

Introduction

In this chapter on new technologies in bariatric surgery two main subjects are addressed: sleeve gastrectomy and the new minimally invasive approaches of single incision laparoscopic surgery (SILS) and natural orifice transluminal endoscopic surgery (NOTES). There is increasing interest in primary sleeve gastrectomy either as a primary procedure to reduce morbidity related with duodenal switch procedures or as a 'stand alone' restrictive procedure. Furthermore, sleeve gastrectomy is a model for NOTES and SILS, both recent developments to further reduce the extent of access trauma by using a single port access. In NOTES a natural orifice is used to gain access to perform surgery and merges laparoscopic and endoscopic techniques. Reducing the surgical trauma is of utmost importance in the group of high-risk morbidly obese patients. Both methods however need to be validated.

Sleeve Gastrectomy

Introduction

Bariatric surgical procedures reduce caloric intake by modifying the anatomy of the gastrointestinal tract. These operations are classified as either restrictive or malabsorptive. Restrictive procedures limit intake by creating a small gastric reservoir with a narrow outlet to delay emptying and induce early satiety. Such procedures include the vertical banded gastroplasty (Mason) and the adjustable gastric banding.[1] A vertical restrictive sleeve gastrectomy (SG) is categorized as a restrictive operation: the volume of the stomach is reduced by 90 per cent and only the non-compliant smaller curvature part of the stomach is retained. The remainder of the stomach loses its capability to extend during eating,[2] and in contrast to former restrictive procedures where the outlet is created using a permanent ring, the outlet of the gastric sleeve is regulated by the pylorus.

After Gagner noticed the good results of the Mill and Magenstrasse procedure invented by Johnston *et al.*, he developed the SG as a first step procedure in biliopancreatic diversion (BPD) to reduce mortality and morbidity in super-obese patients.[3,4] Results showed an excess body weight reduction in the range of 45 per cent and amazingly not all patients regained weight despite the absence of a outlet calibration. These findings led to the strategy to propose SG as a primary procedure. Midterm follow-up outcome data in primary GS resections indicate that it could indeed be an effective procedure for a subgroup of morbidly obese patients. These positive results of SG challenge the 'mechanistic concept' that a calibrated outlet is the key to success for a restrictive procedure. Outcome after SG could be the result of neuro-humoral alterations influencing appetite control, early satiety and beneficial taste change. As a consequence SG could be an interesting model to study metabolic changes in an attempt to impact type II diabetes in the future.

History

SG was originally the restrictive part of a malabsorptive operation: the biliopancreatic diversion–duodenal switch (BPD–DS). Hess performed the first DS operation in March 1988[5,6] and Marceau *et al.* published the first paper.[7] In September 1999 Rabkin did the first hand-assisted laparoscopic DS (LDS),[8] and Gagner *et al.* performed the first totally laparoscopic DS (LDS).[9] Gagner's group published the concept of a two stage approach with a laparoscopic SG (LSG) as the first stage of the LDS in super-obese patients.[4]

LSG has been proposed as the first step in the treatment of super-obese patients, or in patients with high operative risk, to induce significant weight reduction and to reduce morbidity linked with the biliopancreatic diversion procedure. This would precede more complicated procedures such as laparoscopic BPD–DS or laparoscopic Roux-en-Y gastric bypass (LRYGBP).[10]

Definition

Sleeve gastrectomy is a term for partial gastrectomy that results in removal of most of the stomach, with the remainder resembling a 'banana' or 'half moon' (Fig. 1). The other names for this procedure are 'partial gastrectomy', 'longitudinal gastrectomy' and 'vertical gastrectomy'. The pylorus as natural outlet is the most important feature of this operation.

Technique

SG involves a longitudinal resection of the greater curvature of the stomach from the antrum, starting opposite to the nerve of Latarjet, up to the angle of His.[11] This longitudinal gastrectomy 'sleeves' the stomach to reduce it to a narrow tube and eliminates the gastric fundus, the dilating

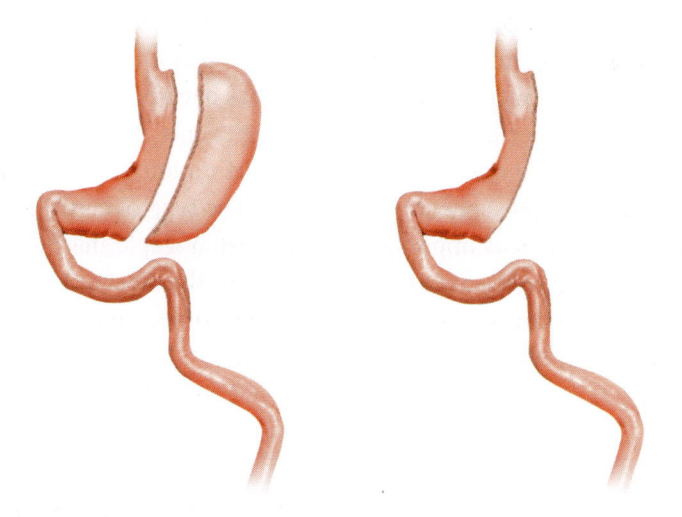

Figure 1. Sleeve gastrectomy, the greater curvature of the stomach is resected.

part of the stomach. A naso-gastric tube (bougie) is used to obtain a precise calibration and to avoid stenosis of the gastroplasty. There are multiple technical variations. There is variation in the size of bougie that calibrates the diameter of the sleeve. The size of the bougie used does not seem to ultimately influence weight loss. Large bougies (50 Fr and more) have been associated with ischemia and gastric fistula and small bougie on the other hand could herald a risk of stenosis. Dissection at the angle of His is critical to avoid the dreadful complication of iatrogenic stapling on the oesophagus.

There seems some agreement now over the use of a 32–36 Fr tube, which should be positioned along the smaller curvature. Stapling that is too wide (incorporating part of the fundus) will ultimately result in sleeve dilation on the long term. In addition, the distance to the pylorus where stapling on the greater curvature starts is variable. It looks more attractive to leave the antrum to regulate gastric emptying and to diminish the risk of narrowing the sleeve at the incisura angularis. Dissection close to the pylorus could eventually change antral motor activity and cross-stapling could be hazardous due to tissue thickness.[12] Leakage is most frequent at the upper and middle part of the stomach as a result of oesophageal trauma and/or high intraluminal pressure in this part of the sleeve due to narrowing more distally. Air insufflation and/or methylene blue instillation has been proposed to control staple line integrity during surgery. A gastrografin swallow in the early postoperative phase is highly advisable. Staple line reinforcement using Seamgard® has been proposed; this seems to significantly reduce postoperative bleeding events at the staple line and only to have a limited effect on the risk for perforation.[13,14] The data to use this reinforcement consequently are lacking. The type of cartridge used to perform the sleeve is of importance and indeed a staple that is too small could induce leaks certainly at the distal part of the sleeve. There are not enough data to advise a suturing over the staple line, which could have a detrimental effect on tissue healing.

Results

Discussion of the results of SG is not easy due to the small numbers of patients in most studies and the lack of standardization of procedures.

The main distinction we have to take into account is the possible difference in size of the sleeve: larger when it is part of the two-stage concept of a BPD–DS operation and smaller when it is a primary procedure.

Weight loss

It seems controversial to state that a procedure such as SG can induce a long-term sustainable weight loss, as there is no outlet restriction. On the other hand there has been no procedure until now where such an extensive part of the stomach is resected reducing the capacity by almost 100 per cent and virtually eliminating the production of the orexigenic hormone, ghrelin. Some data on a recent series of primary SG procedures with a follow-up of at least one year are presented in Table 1.

Ten studies have been selected. Most are observational cohort data except for the studies of Himpens and Vidal, which are prospective, randomized studies comparing the outcome of SG with LAGB and RYGB. At one year a significant loss of >50 per cent in weight or BMI is observed in most studies. No mortality was reported and major complications were around 5 per cent. Although these are data on primary procedures, patients' demographics are still different from the series of patients that undergo gastric bypass or gastric banding: higher preoperative BMI, older patients and higher portion of males. The results of these excellent results clearly favour the SG procedure.

It is important to mention a few studies separately as they specifically look at SG as a primary procedure. Meneakos has a series of 261 patients. At one year follow-up a median percentage EWL of 65.7 (range 33.8–102.3) is noted. The median BMI for the patients who had completed at least one year of follow-up is 30.5 kg/m^2 (range 21.2–42.7). The overall success rate after the first year for more than 50 per cent EWL is 74.3 per cent and even reaches 81.7 per cent with a BMI <35 as a cut-off.[25] The study of Jacobs and colleagues is most interesting as they have a total of 40 patients with a follow-up at two years and 157 patients eligible for follow-up at one year. Mean percentage EWL, for patients at one and two years are 78 per cent and 75 per cent respectively. There is no significant difference between the use of 46 Fr, 40 Fr

Table 1. Sleeve gastrectomy complications and results.

Author	Patients (n)	Sex	Mean age	Initial BMI (kg/m^2)	Complications	Deaths	EBL 1 year (%)	EWL 1 year (%)
Himpens[15]	40	9M, 31F	40 (22–65)	39 (30–53)	*Perioperative:* 1 bleeding (2.5%); 1 sleeve ischemia (2.5%) *Postoperative:* 2 gastric pain (5%); 1 frequent vomiting (2.5%); 2 mineral deficit (5%); 7 de novo GORD (21.8%)	None	Not Addressed (N/A)	57.7 (0–125.5)
Karamanakos[16]	16	1M, 15F	30.6 (19–50)	45.1 (37–51)	None	None	N/A	69.7 ± 14.6
Nocca[17]	163	57M, 111F	41.57	45.9	*Perioperative:* 9 staple line leaks (5.52%); 1 stapling of gastric tube (0.61%); 1 liver bleeding (0.61%) *Postoperative:* 6 gastric fistula (3.66%); 2 gastric stenosis (1.22%); 1 bleeding (0.66%) GORD 11.8%	None	N/A	49.45

(Continued)

Table 1. (Continued)

Author	Patients (n)	Sex	Mean age	Initial BMI (kg/m^2)	Complications	Deaths	EBL 1 year (%)	EWL 1 year (%)
Ou Yang[18]	138	49M, 89F	NA	50.6 (33–82)	*Perioperative overall*: (1.4%); 2 leakage (1.5%); 3 bleeding (2.2%); 1 pancreatitis (0.7%); 1 stricture 0.7%)	None	N/A	54.5 ± 22.32
Fuks[19]	135	22M, 113F	40 (18–65)	48.8 (37–72)	*Perioperative*: 10 bleeding (7.4%) 3 staple line leaks (2.2%) *Postoperative*: 7 gastric fistula (5.1%)	None	49.4	NA
Uglioni[20]	70	16M, 54F	43 (21–65)	46 (35–61)	5% major 7% minor	None	65 (9–127)	NA
Rubin[21]	120	22M, 98F	38 ± 11.8	43 (30–63)	None	None	53 ± 24	NA
Vida[22]	39	16M, 23F	50 ± 1.5	51.9 ± 1.2	NA	None	63 ± 2.89	NA
Lee[23]	216	43M, 173F	43 ± 11	49 ± 11	2.3% readmissions 2.8% reoperations 4.6% major 7.4% total complications	None	N/A	59 ± 17
Melissas[24]	23	7M, 16F	38.9 ± 11.9	47.2 ± 4.8	5.8% staple line leaks 15.3% haemorrhage 0% reoperations	None	72.5	NA

and 36 Fr bougie and no difference between the use of a 7 cm versus a 4 cm antral pouch.[26]

At the IFSO (International Federation for the Surgery of Obesity and Metabolic Disorders) congress of 2009, Angrisani et al. reported on 698 patients with more than half of them receiving an SG as a primary operation. The resulting percentage EWL at one, two and three years are 56 per cent, 43 per cent and 31 per cent respectively. These results are comparable to those seen after RYGBP. Vidal et al. prospectively compared SG with RYGB and found that 12 months after surgery, subjects undergoing SG and RYGB lose a similar amount of weight (percentage EBL: SG: 63.00 ± 2.89 per cent, RYGB: 66.06 ± 2.34 per cent).[22]

The report of the Spanish register on 540 patients by Carlos-Sanchez et al. shows they conclude with a mean follow-up of 16.5 ± 10.6 months (with a range of 1–73 months) and that LSG provides a mean percentage EWL at 12 months of 63.83 (n = 281), at 24 months of 68.5 (n = 120), and at 36 months of 67.12 (n = 30). They also decided after subanalysis for bougie size, initial BMI and age (cut-off of 50 years) that better results are obtained in younger patients with lowest BMI. Thinner bougies only give better weight loss the first six months. Cut-off of 38 Fr for bougie size analysis is perhaps a rather low to prove that dilatation over time is inevitable with larger bougie size as used in the early sleeve gastrectomies of 52–60 Fr. Sixty-eight per cent of the patients had a bougie of 32–34 Fr.[27]

When we look at the German registry at the results of their 144 SGs, we see that although a bougie of 32 Fr is used there was only a reduction of ten BMI points in comparison with the RYGBP patients who lost 16 BMI points. Mean preoperative BMI is of course significantly higher.[28]

In conclusion we can state that the weight loss after primary SG is almost in the same range as after gastric bypass when care is taken to resect the entire fundus of the stomach.[16,29] A smaller bougie size is probably more suitable in achieving this goal. The weight loss will probably be insufficient for super-obese patients and a second stage operation will be necessary for this subpopulation. The possible mechanisms that account for the limited weight loss or weight regain after SG include the spontaneous dilation of the gastric tube over time or the switch to a high caloric, soft, liquid diet.[11] It is also important to mention the excellent food tolerance in contrast with the other restrictive procedures.[27]

Of course, long term data are needed to evaluate the potential danger of weight regain, as no calibration outlet is present in this restrictive procedure. In this context it is important to mention the five year follow-up data of Johnston *et al.* who invented and validated the Mill and Magenstrasse operation. This procedure consists of a similar gastric tube as used in an SG without an outlet besides the pylorus, with the difference that the greater curvature is not resected. This procedure achieves a percentage EWL of 61 long term.[3,23]

Co-morbidities

It appears that SG catalogued as a restrictive procedure, could have more potential than expected. Resolution of co-morbidities is on first sight is as high as after gastric bypass procedures and higher than after the purely restrictive procedures. Preliminary data suggest that it could also have a very fast effect and so possibly partly independent of the weight loss.

Two large studies looked at the effect of SG on co-morbidities. Cottam *et al.* describe resolution of type II diabetes in 81 per cent and improvement in an additional 11 per cent of patients. Sleep apnoea is improved or resolved in 87 per cent, hypertension in 85 per cent of the patients. Remarkable too is a 70 per cent resolution of GORD after SG in this large series.[30]

The series of Moon Han *et al.* are even more impressive with an almost complete response of type II diabetes and sleep apnoea in sleeve patients. Of course, the metabolic syndromes of Korean and Indian populations are very different from that of Caucasians.[31,32]

Rosenthal did a retrospective review of a prospectively maintained database to investigate the effect of SG on type II diabetes patients. His conclusion is that the effect of this procedure is fast, as 27 per cent of the patients are already free of diabetes after two months and 63 per cent after six months. The longer the disease exists and the lower the percentage EWL after surgery means that the chances of total recovery will be lower.[33]

Most interesting is the prospective randomized study done by Vidal *et al.* on Type II diabetes mellitus and the metabolic syndrome following sleeve gastrectomy in severely obese subjects between SG and RYGBP regarding the effect on diabetes. They conclude that at 12 months after surgery, SG is as effective as GBP in inducing remission of type II diabetes mellitus.

Recently Peterli *et al.* looked more into the standard meal induced changes of the glucose metabolism. The almost comparable results showing beneficial changes in glucose metabolism between gastric bypass patients and SG patients at the earliest time point (one week postoperatively) suggests that SG may possibly have an effect independent of weight loss.[34]

SG has more therapeutic potential than other restrictive procedures and probably the same as an RYGBP. In the future SG will possibly be part of the new procedures to treat the metabolic syndrome even in leaner patients.

Complications

Short term

General complications such as pulmonary, cardiovascular and wound problems are also possible after SG as in other operative procedures in obese patients. The possible advantage of this procedure is a reduction in these complications due to a shorter operating time. The absence of an anastomosis can influence the leakage rate positively. The long stapler line can, on the other hand, neutralize this advantage.

Overall, the complication rate of SG published in the literature is equivalent to Roux-en-Y gastric bypass for the greater part of a high-risk population (see Table 1). Akkary *et al.* have been synthesising the literature and found that the incidence of complications among the selected publications, including 646 patients who underwent SG were:

- reoperation (4.5 per cent);
- leak (0.9 per cent);
- strictures (0.7 per cent);
- postoperative bleeding (0.3 per cent);
- pulmonary embolism (0.3 per cent);
- delayed gastric emptying (0.3 per cent);
- intra-abdominal abscess (0.1 per cent);

- wound infection (0.1 per cent);
- splenic injury (0.1 per cent);
- trocar site hernia (0.1 per cent).

Four mortalities were reported (0.6 per cent).[35] Brethuaer *et al.* selected the studies on primary SG separately and found a mortality rate in this series of only 0.17 per cent comparable to laparoscopic gastric banding.[36]

It has been suggested that SG might have an adverse effect on the function of the lower oesophageal sphincter due to gastric resection at the angle of His, predisposing the patient to postoperative reflux symptoms. Himpens *et al.* showed GORD incidence of 21.8 per cent at one year follow-up with subjective improvement of the symptoms (3.1 per cent) at three years.[15] Melissas *et al.* showed that gastric emptying was accelerated after SG a physiological change that might play a beneficial role in improving GORD symptoms gradually over time.[24] We have to take into account that one third of the patients might need treatment with proton pump inhibitors in the first year after the operation.

The German registry data analysed by Stroh show us another important issue about SG. In this report there is a rather high leakage rate of 7 per cent and a mortality rate of 1.2 per cent. SG was performed at 17 different hospitals, and the volume of surgeries performed at each ranged from one to 67 operations. Only three hospitals carried out more than ten operations per year. In contrast the leakage and mortality rate of the Spanish registry is much lower: 2 per cent and 0.36 per cent respectively. This can probably be explained by the fact that the same number of hospitals treated four times as many patients.[27] In this respect, it is important to stress that an SG is probably technically more demanding than it looks. Sillechia *et al.* published their learning curve: for the first 40 cases, the incidence of major complications was 9/40 (22.5 per cent), higher than in the last 45 cases, which had a complication rate of 5/47 (10.6 per cent).[37] In addition the patients have the same high-risk profile as those patients subjected to other bariatric operations. Adequate training and an experienced team are obligatory and will provide better results with SG in the future. There is still nothing proven about the necessity to use stapler line reinforcement or to place sutures to prevent leaks and/or bleeding. The studies concerning this topic are missing power or randomization.[27,38]

Long term

In the long term SG will probably have a benefit over RYGB: it does not involve any digestive anastomosis, no mesenteric defects are created (eliminating the risk of internal hernia), no foreign material is used as in the case of gastric banding and the whole digestive tract remains accessible to endoscopy. It is not associated with dumping syndrome, the risk of peptic ulcer is low and the absorption of nutrients, vitamins, minerals and drugs is less altered.[11]

Concerning vitamin deficiencies it is important to stress that around 15 per cent of the morbidly obese patients already have deficiencies before surgery. Theoretically patients are prone to develop vitamin B12 and iron deficiency after SG. In one study mean ferritin levels decreased significantly but stayed well within the normal range, without any patient developing deficiency after one year.[39] In another, development of iron deficiency was 4.9 per cent and insignificant compared to the higher rate after RYGBP.[40]

Longer term follow-up data are of course essential to detect complications. The most important topic will be weight regain or insufficient weight loss.

Mechanisms of action

Weight loss

As mentioned before the weight loss cannot be explained by a purely restrictive mechanism because of the lack of a restrictive outlet of the small gastric sleeve. Nevertheless the resected part of the stomach, due to the massive compliance of the fundus, is more than 90 per cent of the total stomach capacity;[2] see Fig. 2 (a) and (b).

We propose two possible mechanisms that individually or synergistically act on the process of losing weight by reducing the feeling of hunger and inducing early satiety:

1. the consistent acute deprivation of ghrelin;
2. a rapid emptying of the SG induces a possible RYGBP effect in the proximal jejunum through an increase of GLP-1 and PYY levels postprandial. These hormonal alterations decrease hunger and induce

New Technologies in Bariatric Surgery 211

(a)

(b)

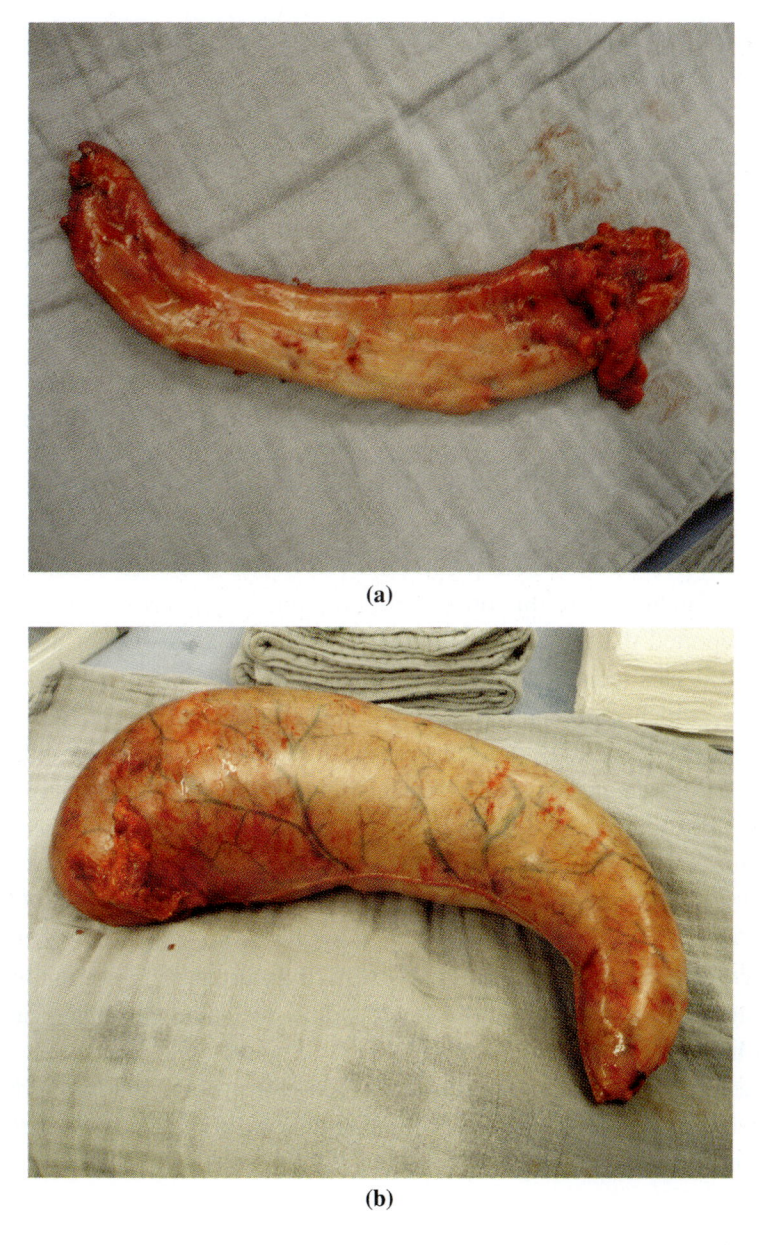

Figure 2. (a) Resected part of the stomach. (b) Resected part after injection of 2000 cc of saline.

early satiety. This mechanism may exert an additional positive effect on glucose homeastasis.[24,41]

The hormonal modifications induced by SG differ from those found after a purely restrictive procedure like laparoscopic adjustable gastric banding. Ghrelin, a peptide hormone mainly produced in the fundus of the stomach, is involved in the mechanisms regulating hunger. It is secreted by the endocrine cells of the stomach (X/A-like cells), which reside in the oxyntic glands of the gastric fundus. The gastric fundus contains 10–20 times more ghrelin per gram of tissue than the duodenum, with diminishing concentrations being found in the jejunum and ileum. Ghrelin regulates the secretion of growth hormone release and is a potent appetite-stimulating peptide. This last effect is mediated by the activation of ghrelin receptors in the hypothalamus/pituitary area.[42]

A decrease of circulating ghrelin levels occurs due to resection of the gastric fundus where this orexigenic hormone is primarily secreted.[43] It was reported that ghrelin is significantly reduced after SG but not after LAGB.[44] This reduction remains stable at follow-up six months postoperatively, which may contribute to the superior weight-loss of SG when compared with LAGB. A recent prospective randomized double-blinded study by Karamanakos et al. compared the postoperative hormonal levels in RYGB to SG: the reduction in the fasting ghrelin levels and increase in peptide YY are greater in the SG group.[16] Weight loss and the loss of feelings of hunger after one and three years are better after SG than LAGB.[15]

Another possible mechanism of weight loss after SG is accelerated gastric emptying. Bergmann et al. showed a correlation between echographic gastric emptying and appetite, where the antral expansion causes less hunger, an anatomical change achieved by the SG.[45] This rapid emptying for food and solids was confirmed on gastric emptying scintigraphy but discordant with the data of Rosenthal et al. who evaluated the patients pre- and postoperatively.[46,47]

Diabetes

The effect of exclusion of the duodenum in RYGBP could be mimicked by the rapid emptying of food into the proximal intestine. This could explain the good early results of SG on type II diabetes.[33] The rapid and profound effect on glucose metabolism, very similar to that seen after gastric bypass, could also be due to an increase of circulating GLP-1 and PYY. This has been confirmed recently by Peterli *et al.* who showed a similar increase in meal-stimulated GLP-1 immediately after SG and RYGBP in a randomized comparative study.[34]

Indications

SG as part of a two-step approach in super-obese patient (BMI > 55)

Although in some very experienced hands there is no difference in co-morbidity and mortality between super-obese patient and the morbidly obese patient, it is overall safer to perform first a sleeve gastrectomy.[48] When after one year significant weight loss is established, a second step procedure (RYGBP or BPD-DS) is performed in case of insufficient weight loss and/or insufficient controlled co-morbidities.[18]

SG as a primary bariatric operation

There is hesitancy in confirming this in the literature. The main reason is probably that cataloguing SG as a bariatric procedure in itself is premature due to the lack of sufficient long term follow-up data (< 4 years of follow-up). In consequence SG can be proposed to a patient but fully informed consent and understanding about the probability of a second operation in case of insufficient weight loss or eventual weight regain is mandatory. This should in fact be required for every bariatric procedure. On the other hand the short term weight loss data, which are similar to RYGBP, and the excellent metabolic control after SG are confirmed and likely to be sufficient confirmation.

SG is the best option in certain specific clinical situations

When the patient has had extensive abdominal surgery in the lower abdomen SG is the safest option.

In patients with Crohn's disease and colitis ulcerosa, compromising the small intestine is avoided when performing an SG.

In cases of persistent *Helicobacter pylori* (HP) infection after multiple eradication schemes or in populations at high risk for stomach cancer, SG is the only option. There are observations that pylorus-preserving surgery might even lead to HP eradication.[49]

SG is a good alternative in the young patient because of the preserved duodenal calcium absorption necessary to complete the bone formation that continues until the age of 25. Dumping syndromes can cause many problems in the hectic life style of adolescents. The elderly benefit more from a short operation with a low mortality that controls co-morbidities. Long term results are less important and quality of life is of primary importance. Laparoscopic banding is known to have bad results in these two subpopulations of patients.

Given the shorter operating time it can be beneficial to perform an SG in patients with ASA IV. There is always the possibility of performing a second stage operation later when the ASA score has improved.

It is clear that a BPD–DS operation is potentially hazardous in patients non-compliant towards eating habits and/or follow-up. On the other hand it is probably true that a subpopulation of morbidly obese patients are not sufficiently treated with a gastric bypass, for example the super-obese, sweet eaters and grazers. In these patients it is advisable first to perform an SG and then to check that the postoperative diet contains sufficient proteins and that there is no snacking. Given a good follow-up, a BPD–DS can safely be performed in this patient. SG is an ideal tool for patient tailoring.

More and more patients are being introduced to bariatric surgery before or after transplant procedures, and SG has several advantages in this setting. In the case of liver transplantation specifically, stable immunosuppressive medication trough levels and access to the biliary tract are attractive advantages. In dialysis patients, SG is more likely to preserve a good peritoneal dialysis and adequate immunosuppressant state after kidney transplantation.

New Minimally Invasive Techniques in Bariatric Surgery

Natural orifice transluminal endoscopic surgery

Natural Orifice Transluminal Endoscopic Surgery (NOTES) is the term that covers all conventional surgical procedures that are performed after gaining access to the peritoneum or retroperitoneum via natural body openings such as the mouth, anus, vagina and bladder. The motivating factor for NOTES is that elimination of abdominal scars will further reduce the invasiveness of surgery resulting in less pain, shortened convalescence, improved cosmesis and absence of abdominal wound infections and hernias. Although this hypothesis is largely unproven and many significant hurdles exist for application of natural orifice surgery, since the first report on NOTES by Kalloo *et al.* in 2004, there has been great enthusiasm with regard to different diagnostic and therapeutic interventions and much financial and research effort has been undertaken. The NOTES concept has been triggering many technological innovations broadly applicable to minimally invasive diagnostic and therapeutic strategies.

In recent years multiple feasibility and safety studies in animals (mainly pigs) have been reported. To date, the first NOTEStm case reports and small series reported on humans have mainly used cholecystectomy as an educational and research model. This study acts as a bridge between the classic field of laparoscopic surgery and conventional endoscopic procedures to facilitate the progress of NOTES[tm]. Most issues addressed in the 2006 White Paper by Rattner *et al.* have been dealt with, such as access to the peritoneal cavity, intestinal closure, prevention of infection and management of complications and physiologic events, such as intraperitoneal pressure measurements.

In animal models multiple groups are performing NOTES or hybrid NOTES, with the use of additional trocars. An SG in a porcine model using vaginal route visualization and additional 12 mm portal for the stapler and 2 2mm portals for traction purposes has been reported.[50] Others used the rectum as the port of entry to the peritoneal cavity, and the stomach was manipulated endoluminally using a gastroscope, the gastric remnant being removed through the rectal incision. Successful operations on five pigs were reported.[51]

One group stated that as a gastrotomy is part of the procedure anyway, RYGB might be a procedure that is suited for NOTES through the oral route. They performed a combined transvaginal and transgastric gastric bypass (TVTG-GBP) in a human cadaver.[52]

Recently it has become more and more apparent that transvaginal NOTES represents the safest and most applicable natural orifice route. It is relatively independent of advanced technological development, with a potential benefit of easy decontamination, controllable access and easy closure under direct vision. The safety of the transvaginal route also has been well documented for numerous gynaecologic procedures. In addition, the transvaginal route seems logical for most upper abdominal procedures. Male patients clearly cannot be operated upon in this way. The largest series consisting of two successful cases were submucosal tumours which were resected in a full NOTES procedure.[53]

It is too early to highlight any advantage of NOTES in bariatric surgery. It will be imperative to gain more than only a cosmetic benefit when implementing difficult and potentially more dangerous procedures in a subject as difficult as a morbidly obese patient. On the other hand it is an outstanding platform for the development of new materials and new metabolic and bariatric procedures.

Single incision laparoscopic surgery

Single incision laparoscopic surgery (SILS), also known as laparoendoscopic single-site surgery or single-port access surgery, is an area of active investigation for abdominal surgery with more immediate applicability in the clinics on first sight. Although the advantages that have been proposed include cosmetics (scarless abdominal surgery performed through an umbilical incision), less incisional pain and the ability to convert to standard multiport laparoscopic surgery if needed, these are less convincing in a bariatric surgery setting.

Single-access laparoscopy involves the introduction of special multichannel access devices that allow laparoscopic surgery to be performed through one incision. Ideally this is done with special instruments and endoscopes that are currently being developed. Several access devices are available to insert two or three instruments and a scope into the abdomen through an umbilical incision in an airtight fashion. The potential advantages of this approach are related to limiting the port incisions to one site, in addition to the advantages of traditional minimally invasive surgery. Positioning the single access within the umbilicus results in better cosmetics and avoids muscle penetration, which minimizes incision pain.

Single incision cholecystectomy was described by Piskun *et al.* as early as 1999, with the insertion of two trocars through the umbilical incision and additional stay sutures to stabilize the gallbladder.[54] Today almost all common laparoscopic procedures are performed with SILS technology.[55]

The first bariatric operation through a single incision was a gastric banding. In this case the whole operation was performed through a single supra-umbilical incision, necessary to place the port and to introduce the band.[51,56] The SG is of course a better procedure to be performed scarless using the SILS technology, because of the absence of any foreign body material that has to be introduced. The groups of Nguyen *et al.* and Reavis *et al.* describe the first successful procedure through an 2.5 cm supra-umbilical incision and one year later, without any visible scar, through an incision in the umbilicus, the latest natural orifice to be used.[57,58] The largest series describes a total of seven successful single-incision transumbilical laparoscopic SGs. Two patients required lysis for adhesions, one patient underwent an umbilical hernia repair during the procedure and one patient required the insertion of an additional trocar. The mean operating time was 143 minutes. There were no mortalities or postoperative complications noted during the mean follow-up period of 1.5 months.[59] One possible complication related to the technique is an umbilical hernia; the follow-up data in the published studies are too short to exclude this.

Many new instruments, trocars and flexible laparoscopes have been developed in recent years and will now become commercially available. In consequence the SILS technology will be available for every bariatric surgeon. Nevertheless it is very important to realize that there will be an important learning curve, which may result in possibly devastating complications in a morbidly obese patient. The necessary technology to perform full NOTES procedures and the validation of standard techniques are not yet available, so it is only performed in research settings and mainly in animal models.

References

1. DeMaria, E.J. (2007). Bariatric surgery for morbid obesity. *N Engl J Med* 356(21): 2176–2183.

2. Yehoshua, R.T., Eidelman, L.A., Stein, M. *et al.* (2008). Laparoscopic sleeve gastrectomy-volume and pressure assessment. *Obes Surg* 18(9): 1083–1088.
3. Johnston, D., Dachtler, J., Sue-Ling, H.M. *et al.* (2003). The Magenstrasse and Mill operation for morbid obesity. *Obes Surg* 13(1): 10–16.
4. Regan, J.P., Inabnet, W.B., Gagner, M. *et al.* (2003). Early experience with two-stage laparoscopic Roux-en-Y gastric bypass as an alternative in the super-super obese patient. *Obes Surg* 13(6): 861–864.
5. Hess, D.S., Hess, D.W. (1998). Biliopancreatic diversion with a duodenal switch. *Obes Surg* 8(3): 267–282.
6. Hess, D.S., Hess, D.W., Oakley, R.S. (2005). The biliopancreatic diversion with the duodenal switch: results beyond 10 years. *Obes Surg* 15(3): 408–416.
7. Marceau, P., Biron, S., Bourque, R.A. *et al.* (1993). Biliopancreatic diversion with a new type of gastrectomy. *Obes Surg* 3(1): 29–35.
8. Rabkin, R.A., Rabkin, J.M., Metcalf, B. *et al.* (2003). Laparoscopic technique for performing duodenal switch with gastric reduction. *Obes Surg* 13(2): 263–268.
9. Ren, C.J., Patterson, E., Gagner, M. (2000). Early results of laparoscopic biliopancreatic diversion with duodenal switch: a case series of 40 consecutive patients. *Obes Surg* 10(6): 514–523; discussion 524.
10. Langer, F.B., Bohdjalian, A., Felberbauer, F.X. *et al.* (2006). Does gastric dilatation limit the success of sleeve gastrectomy as a sole operation for morbid obesity? *Obes Surg* 16(2): 166–171.
11. Iannelli, A., Dainese, R., Piche, T. *et al.* (2008). Laparoscopic sleeve gastrectomy for morbid obesity. *World J Gastroenterol* 14(6): 821–827.
12. Deitel, M., Crosby, R.D., Gagner, M. (2008). The first international consensus summit for sleeve gastrectomy (SG), New York City, October 25–27, 2007. *Obes Surg* 18(5): 487–496.
13. Chen, B., Kiriakopoulos, A., Tsakayannis, D. *et al.* (2009). Reinforcement does not necessarily reduce the rate of staple line leaks after sleeve gastrectomy. A review of the literature and clinical experiences. *Obes Surg* 19(2): 166–172.
14. Consten, E.C., Gagner, M., Pomp, A. *et al.* (2004). Decreased bleeding after laparoscopic sleeve gastrectomy with or without duodenal switch for morbid obesity using a stapled buttressed absorbable polymer membrane. *Obes Surg* 14(10): 1360–1366.
15. Himpens, J., Dapri, G., Cadière, G.B. (2006). A prospective randomized study between laparoscopic gastric banding and laparoscopic isolated sleeve gastrectomy: results after 1 and 3 years. *Obes Surg* 16(11): 1450–1456.

16. Karamanakos, S.N., Vagenas, K., Kalfarentzos, F. *et al.* (2008). Weight loss, appetite suppression, and changes in fasting and postprandial ghrelin and peptide-YY levels after Roux-en-Y gastric bypass and sleeve gastrectomy: a prospective, double blind study. *Ann Surg* 247(3): 401–407.
17. Nocca, D., Krawczykowsky, D., Bomans, B. *et al.* (2008). A prospective multicenter study of 163 sleeve gastrectomies: results at 1 and 2 years. *Obes Surg* 18(5): 560–565.
18. Ou Yang, O., Loi K., Liew, V. *et al.* (2008). Staged laparoscopic sleeve gastrectomy followed by Roux-en-Y gastric bypass for morbidly obese patients: a risk reduction strategy. *Obes Surg* 18(12): 1575–1580.
19. Fuks, D., Verhaeghe, P., Brehant, O. *et al.* (2009). Results of laparoscopic sleeve gastrectomy: a prospective study in 135 patients with morbid obesity. *Surgery* 145(1): 106–113.
20. Uglioni, B., Wolnerhanssen, B., Peters, T. *et al.* (2009). Midterm results of primary vs. secondary laparoscopic sleeve gastrectomy (LSG) as an isolated operation. *Obes Surg* 19(4): 401–406.
21. Rubin, M., Yehoshua, R.T., Stein, M. *et al.* (2008). Laparoscopic sleeve gastrectomy with minimal morbidity early results in 120 morbidly obese patients. *Obes Surg* 18: 1567–1570.
22. Vidal, J., Ibarzabal, A., Romero, F. *et al.* (2008). Type II diabetes mellitus and the metabolic syndrome following sleeve gastrectomy in severely obese subjects. *Obes Surg* 18(9): 1077–1082.
23. Lee, C.M., Cirangle, P.T., Jossart, G.H. (2007). Vertical gastrectomy for morbid obesity in 216 patients: report of two-year results. *Surg Endosc* 21(10): 1810–1816.
24. Melissas, J., Koukouraki, S., Askoxylakis, J. *et al.* (2007). Sleeve gastrectomy: a restrictive procedure? *Obes Surg* 17(1): 57–62.
25. Menenakos, E.M., Stamou, K., Albanopoulos, K. *et al.* (2010). Laparoscopic sleeve gastrectomy performed with intent to treat morbid obesity: a prospective single-center study of 261 patients with a median follow-up of 1 year. *Obes Surg* 20(3): 276–282.
26. Jacobs, M., Bisland, W., Gomez, E. *et al.* (2010). Laparoscopic sleeve gastrectomy: a retrospective review of 1- and 2-year results. *Surg Endosc* 24(4): 781–785.
27. Sanchez-Santos, R., Masdevall, C., Baltasar, A. *et al.* (2009). Short- and midterm outcomes of sleeve gastrectomy for morbid obesity: the experience of the Spanish national registry. *Obes Surg* 19(9): 1203–1210.

28. Stroh, C., Birk, D., Flade-Kuthe, R. et al. (2009). Results of sleeve gastrectomy data from a nationwide survey on bariatric surgery in Germany. *Obes Surg* 9(5): 632–640
29. Colquitt, J.L., Picot, J., Loveman, E. (2009). Surgery for obesity. *Cochrane Database Syst Rev* 2: CD003641.
30. Cottam, D., Qureshi, F.G., Mattar, S.G. et al. (2006). Laparoscopic sleeve gastrectomy as an initial weight-loss procedure for high-risk patients with morbid obesity. *Surg Endosc* 20(6): 859–863.
31. Moon Han, S., Kim, W.W., Oh, J.H. (2005). Results of laparoscopic sleeve gastrectomy (LSG) at 1 year in morbidly obese Korean patients. *Obes Surg* 15(10): 1469–1475.
32. Shah, P.S., Todkar, J.S., Shah, S.S. (2010). Effectiveness of laparoscopic sleeve gastrectomy on glycemic control in obese Indians with type II diabetes mellitus. *Surg Obes Relat Dis* 6(2): 138–141.
33. Rosenthal, R., Li, X., Samuel, S. et al. (2009). Effect of sleeve gastrectomy on patients with diabetes mellitus. *Surg Obes Relat Dis* 5(4): 429–434.
34. Peterli, R., Wolnerhanssen, B., Peters, T. et al. (2009). Improvement in glucose metabolism after bariatric surgery: comparison of laparoscopic Roux-en-Y gastric bypass and laparoscopic sleeve gastrectomy: a prospective randomized trial. *Ann Surg* 250(2): 234–241.
35. Akkary, E., Duffy, A., Bell, R. (2008). Deciphering the sleeve: technique, indications, efficacy, and safety of sleeve gastrectomy. *Obes Surg* 18(10): 1323–1329.
36. Brethauer, S.A., Hammel, J.P., Schauer, P.R. (2009). Systematic review of sleeve gastrectomy as staging and primary bariatric procedure. *Surg Obes Relat Dis* 5(4): 469–475.
37. Silecchia, G., Rizzello, M., Casella, G. et al. (2009). Two-stage laparoscopic biliopancreatic diversion with duodenal switch as treatment of high-risk super-obese patients: analysis of complications. *Surg Endosc* 23(5): 1032–1037.
38. Assalia, A., Ueda, K., Matteotti, R. et al. (2007). Staple-line reinforcement with bovine pericardium in laparoscopic sleeve gastrectomy: experimental comparative study in pigs. *Obes Surg* 17(2): 222–228.
39. Toh, S.Y., Zarshenas, N., Jorgensen, J. (2009). Prevalence of nutrient deficiencies in bariatric patients. *Nutrition* 25(11–12): 1150–1156
40. Hakeam, H.A., O'Regan, P.J., Salem, A.M. et al. (2009). Impact of laparoscopic sleeve gastrectomy on iron indices: 1 year follow-up. *Obes Surg* 19(11): 1491–1496

41. Wang, Y., Liu, J. (2009). Plasma ghrelin modulation in gastric band operation and sleeve gastrectomy. *Obes Surg* 19(3): 357–362.
42. Kojima, M., Hosoda, H., Date, Y. *et al.* (1999). Ghrelin is a growth-hormone-releasing acylated peptide from stomach. *Nature* 402(6762): 656–660.
43. Cummings, D.E., Weigle, D.S., Frayo, R.S. *et al.* (2002). Plasma ghrelin levels after diet-induced weight loss or gastric bypass surgery. *N Engl J Med* 346(21): 1623–1630.
44. Langer, F.B., Reza, Hoda, M.A. *et al.* (2005). Sleeve gastrectomy and gastric banding: effects on plasma ghrelin levels. *Obes Surg* 15(7): 1024–1029.
45. Bergmann, J.F., Chassany, O., Petit, A. *et al.* (1992). Correlation between echographic gastric emptying and appetite: influence of psyllium. *Gut* 33(8): 1042–1043.
46. Bernstine, H., Tzioni-Yehoshua, R., Groshar, D. *et al.* (2009). Gastric emptying is not affected by sleeve gastrectomy-scintigraphic evaluation of gastric emptying after sleeve gastrectomy without removal of the gastric antrum. *Obes Surg* 19(3): 293–298.
47. Braghetto, I., Davanzo, C., Korn, O. *et al.* (2009). Scintigraphic evaluation of gastric emptying in obese patients submitted to sleeve gastrectomy compared to normal subjects. *Obes Surg* 19(11): 1515–1521.
48. Suter, M., Calmes, J.M., Paroz, A. *et al.* (2009). Results of Roux-en-Y gastric bypass in morbidly obese vs superobese patients: similar body weight loss, correction of comorbidities, and improvement of quality of life. *Arch Surg* 144(4): 312–318.
49. Keren, D., Matter, I., Rainis, T. *et al.* (2009). Sleeve gastrectomy leads to *Helicobacter pylori* eradication. *Obes Surg* 19(6): 751–756.
50. Marchesini, J.C., Cardoso, A.R., Nora, M. *et al.* (2008). Laparoscopic sleeve gastrectomy with NOTES visualization — a step toward NOTES procedures. *Surg Obes Relat Dis* 4(6): 773–776.
51. Mintz, Y., Horgan, S., Savu, M.K. *et al.* (2008). Hybrid natural orifice translumenal surgery (NOTES) sleeve gastrectomy: a feasibility study using an animal model. *Surg Endosc* 22(8): 1798–1802.
52. Madan, A.K., Tichansky, D.S., Khan, K.A. (2008). Natural orifice transluminal endoscopic gastric bypass performed in a cadaver. *Obes Surg* 18(9): 1192–1199.
53. Nakajima, K., Nishida, T., Takahashi, T. *et al.* (2009). Partial gastrectomy using natural orifice translumenal endoscopic surgery (NOTES) for gastric

submucosal tumors: early experience in humans. *Surg Endosc* 23(12): 2650–2655.
54. Piskun, G., Rajpal, S. (1999). Transumbilical laparoscopic cholecystectomy utilizes no incisions outside the umbilicus. *J Laparoendosc Adv Surg Tech A* 9(4): 361–364.
55. Merchant, A.M., Cook, M.W., White, B.C. et al. (2009). Transumbilical Gelport access technique for performing single incision laparoscopic surgery (SILS). *J Gastrointest Surg* 13(1): 159–162.
56. Nguyen, N.T., Hinojosa, M.W., Smith, B.R. et al. (2008). Single laparoscopic incision transabdominal (SLIT) surgery-adjustable gastric banding: a novel minimally invasive surgical approach. *Obes Surg* 18(12): 1628–1631.
57. Nguyen, N.T., Reavis, K.M., Hinojosa, M.W. et al. (2009). Laparoscopic transumbilical sleeve gastrectomy without visible abdominal scars. *Surg Obes Relat Dis* 5(2): 275–277.
58. Reavis, K.M., Hinojosa, M.W., Smith, B.R. et al. (2008). Single-laparoscopic incision transabdominal surgery sleeve gastrectomy. *Obes Surg* 18(11): 1492–1494.
59. Saber, A.A., El-Ghazaly, T.H. et al. (2009). Single-incision transumbilical laparoscopic sleeve gastrectomy. *J Laparoendosc Adv Surg Tech* 9(6): 755–759.

Chapter 9

Imaging of Complications After Bariatric Surgery

Jose C. Varghese and Shuvro H. Roy-Choudhury

Introduction

Weight reduction (bariatric) surgery can be of the malabsorptive, restrictive or mixed types, depending on the anatomical and physiological alterations surgically brought about to effect weight loss. The earlier purely malabsorptive surgeries have latterly given way to the more restrictive and mixed types because of improved patient tolerance and safety.[1-3] Currently, the most popular type of bariatric surgery in Europe is the laparoscopic adjustable gastric banding (LAGB), and that in the United States is the Roux-en-Y gastric bypass (RYGB).[4]

Complications after bariatric surgery can be broadly categorized as enteric or nonenteric in origin. The enteric complications — such as obstruction, perforation and herniation — often require reoperation for treatment. In contrast, the nonenteric complications — such as pulmonary embolism, myocardial infarction and infection — are treated medically. The remainder of the chapter will deal with the diagnosis and management of enteric complications that are often specific to bariatric surgery.

Imaging plays a vital role in the diagnosis and management of complications after bariatric surgery.[5-8] The upper gastrointestinal (UGI) series and computed tomography (CT) are by far the two most commonly used modalities in this regard. The UGI provides endoluminal and functional information related to the gastrointestinal tract itself, whilst CT provides a more comprehensive tomographic visualization of the extra-luminal structures. In addition, ultrasonography, nuclear scintigraphy and interventional radiology all have their limited but specific uses.

Laparoscopic Adjustable Gastric Banding

Laparoscopic adjustable gastric banding (LAGB) is the most commonly performed weight reduction surgery in Europe, with over 300,000 procedures having been performed worldwide to date.[9] It is a purely restrictive type of surgery that is designed to reduce receptive gastric volume, leading to early satiety and weight loss. The procedure involves the wrapping of a silicone band — with an attached inner lining balloon — around the upper stomach, to segment a small proximal portion of the stomach (the 'pouch') from the remainder of the distal stomach. The band is held in position by its circular wrapping effect, its positioning above the lesser omentum (using a pars flaccida technique), and the burying of the anterior portion of the band in a seromuscular tunnel (Fig. 1a) formed by gastro-gastric over sewing of the anterior gastric wall. The luminal constriction produced by the band is called the 'stoma', and its size is adjusted by inflation or deflation of the inner lining balloon using fluid injected through a subcutaneous port (Fig. 1b).

This combined restriction brought about by a small gastric pouch (< 15 ml in volume) and narrow stoma (2–4 mm in diameter) results in the feeling of early satiety after eating of small quantities of food, leading to weight loss. With appropriate patient selection, this technique can lead to a steady and sustained excess weight loss of around 62 per cent at three years.[10] However, complications can be frequent with a yearly major complication rate of 3–4 per cent,[11] and reoperation rate of 0.8–21 per cent.[11,12] Therefore, LAGB patients require close scrutiny in the days and months following surgery, and radiology plays an important part in this process.

The main imaging modality used to investigate patients after LAGB is the UGI series. The three main indications for performing UGI are to:

1. document baseline anatomy;
2. diagnose post-surgical complications;
3. guide port access/band adjustment.

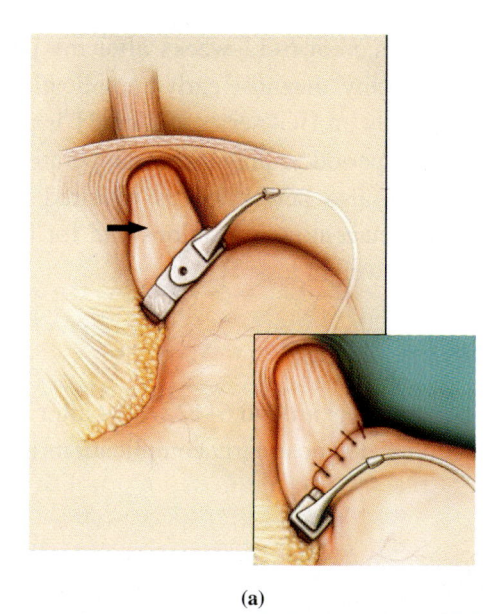

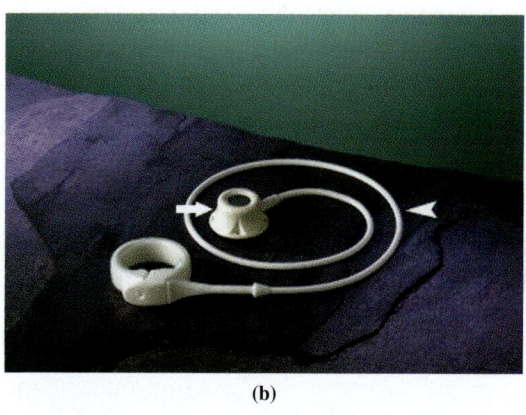

Figure 1. Laparoscopic adjustable gastric band. **(a)** Schematic diagram of a laparoscopic adjustable gastric band placed across the proximal stomach — above the insertion of the lesser omentum (suprabursal placement) — to create a 'neostomach' or pouch (arrow). This suprabursal placement reduces the risk of slippage. Slippage is further reduced by fixation of anterior band using seromuscular gastro-gastric sutures (inset). (Images by courtesy of BioEnterics Corp, MA, USA, and reprinted with permission from Dr. Shuvro H. Roy-Choudhury and Elsevier.[8] **(b)** Photograph of a laparoscopic adjustable band showing a port (arrow) connected to the band through a connecting tube (arrowhead). This port can be accessed externally like other similar devices. Filling the port fills an inflatable circumferential reservoir (not shown) around the inside of the band, which can tighten the stoma.

An UGI is usually performed at 6–12 weeks after the initial surgery to evaluate the baseline anatomy, diagnose early complications and assist in band inflation. Occasionally an UGI series and/or CT is performed in the immediate post-operative period to diagnose postoperative leak or cause of acute dysphagia. It is also performed as required in symptomatic patients to diagnose intercurrent complications and for band adjustment when there is a plateau in weight loss.

Early post-operative evaluation

An UGI is usually performed at around 6–12 weeks after initial surgery to evaluate baseline anatomy, diagnose early complications and guide stomal adjustment.

Imaging technique

A control film is taken to evaluate the position and orientation of the band, tubing and port (Fig. 2a). Following this, a semi erect barium swallow in the frontal and lateral projections is performed to evaluate oesophageal transit and any evidence of obstruction (Fig. 2b). If the initial study is normal, the procedure can be continued with the use of thick barium for stomal adjustment as described below.

Baseline anatomy

Some of the baseline imaging characteristics of a normal LAGB is as follows:

- the silicone band should lie approximately 1–2 cm below the gastro-oesophageal junction;
- the band should lie 30–45° inclined to the horizontal plane in the AP projection;
- the pouch should measure less than 15 ml in volume;
- the stoma should be large enough to allow passage of contrast medium without obstruction and, yet, tight enough to cause restriction (2–4 mm).

A normal early UGI after LAGB is shown in Fig. 2.

Imaging of Complications After Bariatric Surgery 227

(a)

(b)

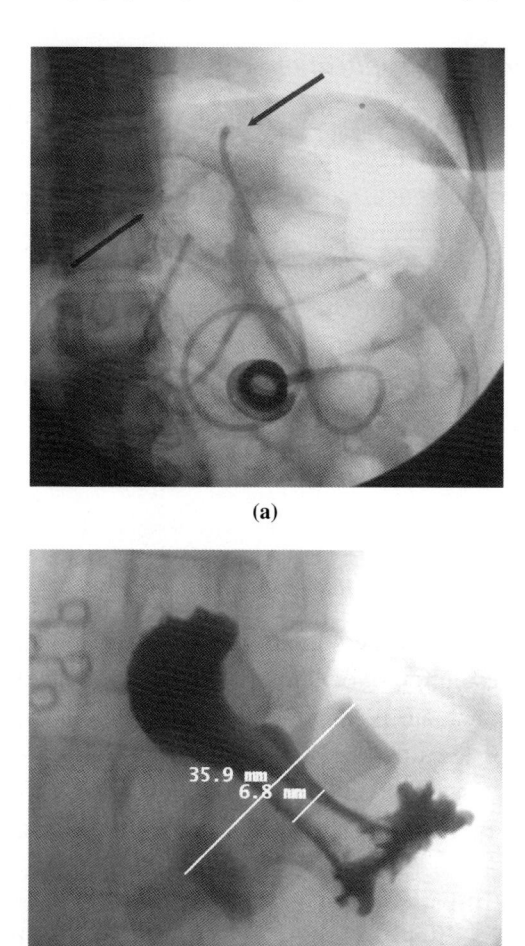

Figure 2. Normal postoperative appearance at barium swallow performed eight weeks following surgery. **(a)** Control film showing band faintly seen (between two arrows), but normally angled (30–45°) to the horizontal. The port is seen connected to the band through a connecting tube without any kink. **(b)** An initial contrast swallow in the anteroposterior (AP) projection shows unobstructed passage of contrast through the band with a wide stoma. Stomal size may be calculated by calibrating with the known diameter of the band. A lateral/oblique swallow examination should also be performed (not shown) to ensure the band is around the stomach. Reprinted with permission of Dr. Shuvro H. Roy-Choudhury and Elsevier.[8]

Early postoperative complications

Possible early post-operative complications would include obstruction, perforation and haemorrhage. These complications are often technical in origin and their incidence varies according to the surgical technique used and operator experience. Complications of obstruction, band slippage and gastric herniation are fairly obvious at UGI and are further discussed below. Perforation may be obvious on the UGI series (Fig. 3a), but continued clinical concern for perforation or haemorrhage in the face of a normal UGI mandates a CT. The latter may show extraluminal gas (Fig. 3b) and intra-abdominal fluid collections (Fig. 3c) indicative of perforation, or intra-abdominal high-density fluid indicative of haemorrhage.

Port access and stomal adjustment

The LAGB balloon is not fully inflated at the time of surgery to allow time for healing and resolution of oedema. Despite this, some weight reduction ensues in the immediate post-operative period due to the baseline constrictive effect of the device. However, from around 6–12 weeks after surgery and periodically thereafter — based on rate of patient weight loss — graduated inflation of the balloon is required to promote sustained weight loss.

The process of balloon inflation with stomal tightening can be performed with[5,8,13] or without[14] fluoroscopic guidance. If fluoroscopic guidance is used, a modified UGI technique is recommended that includes the use of thick barium to fully distend the pouch, visualization of the stoma in anterior and lateral projections, and an imaging rate of at least two frames per second to accurately measure stomal size.[8,15] A left anterior oblique projection can be useful when the band is obscured after the initial swallows. The port is accessed using a sterile technique and a non-coring needle, similar to the techniques used with traditional chemotherapy ports. A C-arm device and appropriate angulation may be useful to view a tilted port end-on (Fig. 4a) to facilitate puncture.

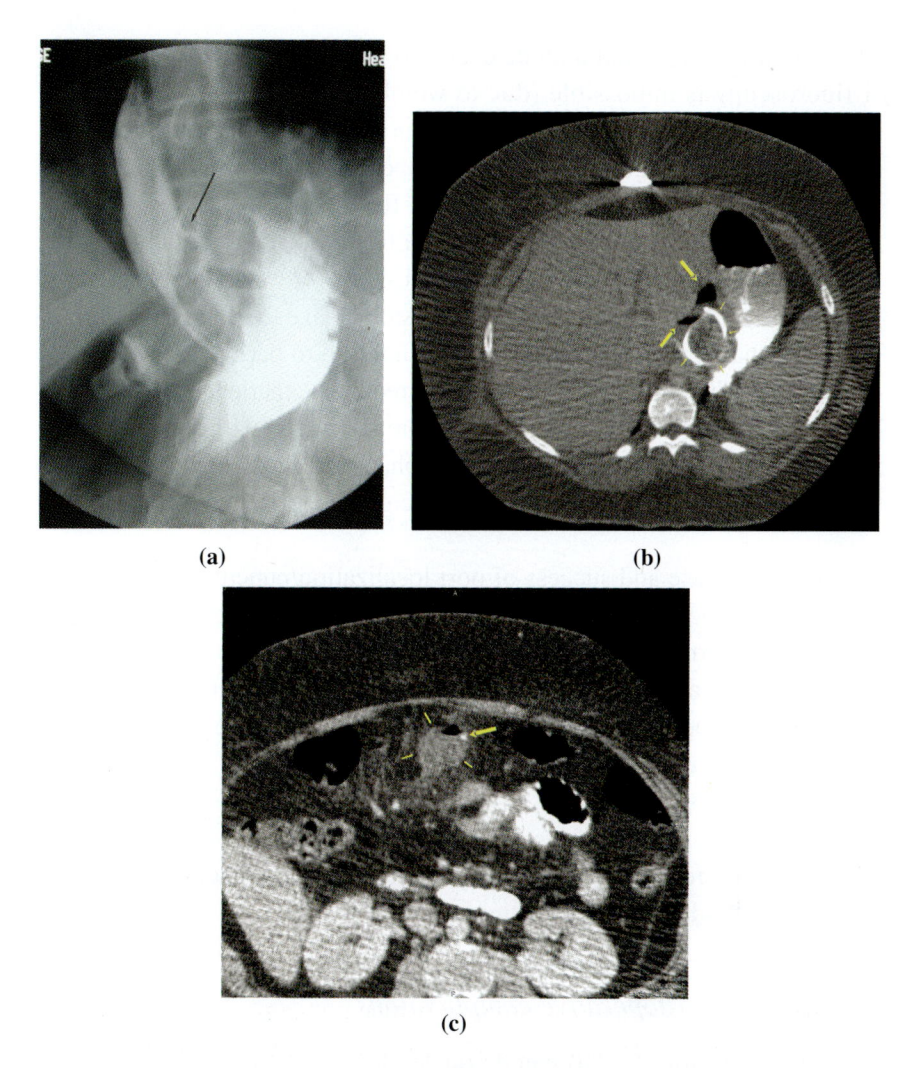

Imaging of Complications After Bariatric Surgery 229

Figure 3. Early perforation after laparoscopic gastric banding. (a) Water soluble contrast swallow performed 96 hours after surgery shows a leak from the distal oesophagus (arrow), just above the gastro-oesophageal junction. (b) Axial CT through upper abdomen after the contrast swallow shows free air (long arrows) adjacent to the band (small arrows) indicating perforation. (c) Axial CT just below (b) shows inflammation extending along the connecting tube (large arrow) with loculated fluid collection (small arrows).

Occasionally ultrasound may be useful to localize and puncture the port if fluoroscopy is impossible (due to weight limit of tables) or difficult.

Several generations of bands have been used over the last ten years and an accurate knowledge of their normal appearances and reservoir capacity is critical to optimally inflate the band. Reservoir capacity varies from 4–14 ml, with the later generation of larger bands having a greater capacity. Based on the band used, 1–8 ml of normal saline (or water soluble contrast medium, see below) is injected to adjust stomal size to around 2–4 mm in diameter, that is sufficient to cause mild hold-up to barium without causing total obstruction.[5,8,13] This assessment requires experience, but a rule of thumb is that the barium should clear from the pouch within two or three peristalsis without persistent gastro-oesophageal reflux (Figs 4b, 4c).

The advantages of using fluoroscopic guidance are the following:

1. increased ease and success of port localization/puncture;
2. increased accuracy of stomal size adjustments (patient sensation of hold-up correlates poorly with optimal stomal size, particularly with the older bands where as little as 0.5 ml of injectate may make a difference between optimal tightening and over-tightening);
3. the opportunity to diagnose occult complications related to the stomach or the prosthesis.

One group has reported the use of dynamic radioisotope scintigraphy as a superior method for band adjustment.[16]

Diagnosis of postoperative complications

Complications after LAGB can be related to:

1. the stomach (e.g. gastro-oesophageal reflux, pouch dilatation, obstruction, herniation);
2. the prosthesis used (silicone band, balloon, connecting tubing, subcutaneous port);
3. surgery in general (e.g. pulmonary embolism, wound infection). These complications can occur in the early (< 30 days), or the late post-operative period (> 30 days).

Imaging of Complications After Bariatric Surgery 231

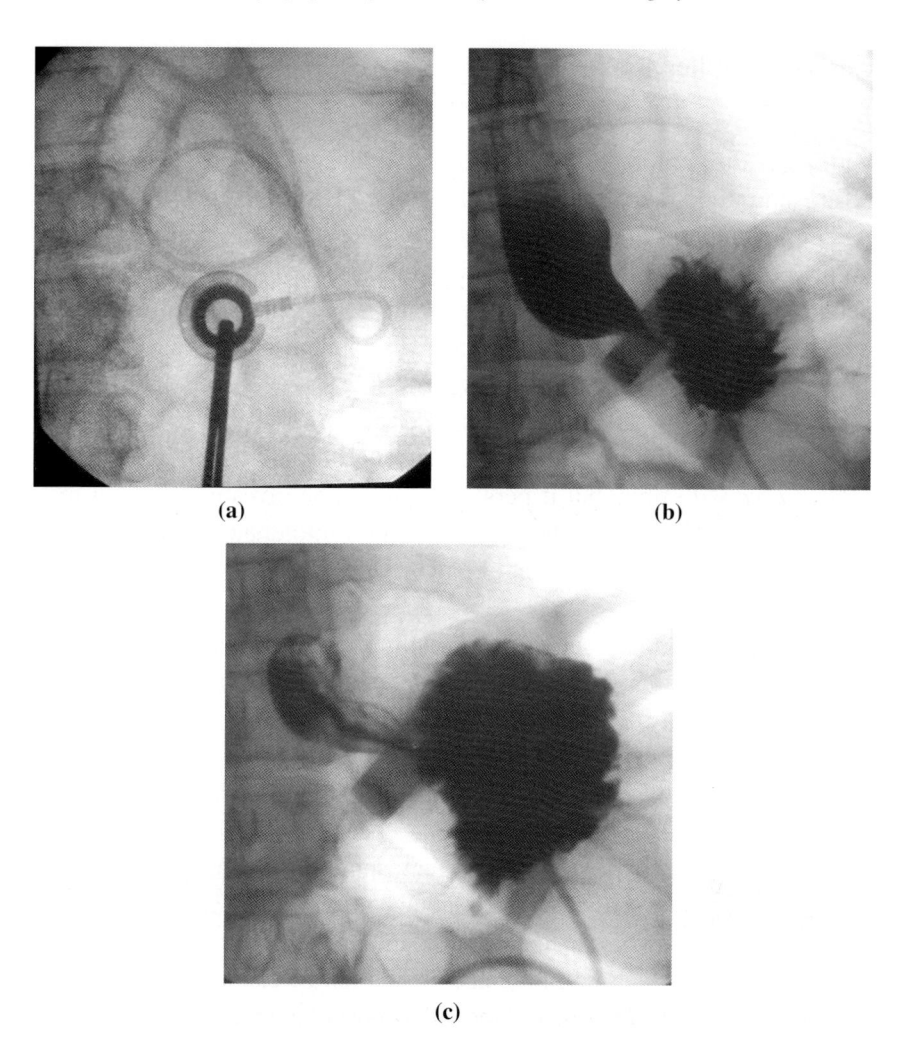

Figure 4. A typical radiological band adjustment sequence following normal assessment. (**a**) The port is localized; sometimes oblique screening may facilitate port puncture. (**b** and **c**) Dilute contrast solution is injected through the port in a graduated manner with intermittent check barium swallows. Optimal amount depends on the type of band and requires some experience. Radiological adjustment is often subjective with clearance after two or three peristaltic waves being about right. Adjustment should also take into account the specific patient's needs and the weight loss curve. With smaller bands, fine adjustment may be necessary with 0.5 ml making the critical difference.

Gastric complications

Pain and gastro-oesophageal reflux disease

Pain and discomfort due to gastro-oesophageal (pouch-oesophageal) reflux and food intolerance to solids after LAGB is not uncommon. Although studies have shown a reduction of preoperative reflux in up to 70 per cent of cases due to the constrictive effect of the band, reflux still persists in a significant minority of patients.[17,18] This is probably related to a high prevalence of undiagnosed gastro-oesophageal reflux disease prior to surgery in this patient group. Appropriate eating habits and dietetic advice is critical in this setting. Pain and discomfort can also be due to a high band or too tight stoma. In the majority of patients these symptoms will resolve with time, but if persistent should be investigated, as it may be a sign of underlying pathology. Total food intolerance can develop in the long term in up to 8 per cent of patients, sometimes necessitating band removal.[12]

Another important issue is the problem of oesophageal dysmotility following band insertion. The presence of occult hiatal hernia and dysmotility prior to surgery may be aggravated by band surgery leading to a pseudoachalasia-like syndrome.[19] A band predisposes to progressive oesophageal dilatation — particularly if placed high at the gastro-oesophageal junction — with significant dilatation seen in up to 2.6 per cent of cases (Fig. 5). There is often pre-existing lower oesophageal sphincter deficiency and these patients are prone to show lack of compliance, poor satiety and tend to abuse their distal oesophagus as an extension of their pouch.[20] However, this entity is different from pouch dilatation and should not be classed as a complication unless it necessitates band removal, as occurs in around 0.6 per cent of cases. In severe cases, these can be dealt with by controlled radiological deflation, although band adjustments in these patients may be extremely difficult.[21] Some authors therefore advocate routine pre-operative screening for these features so that an alternative to band surgery such as RYGB can be offered to such patients right from the start.[22]

Pouch dilatation

Pouch dilatation occurs with a reported incidence of 5–18 per cent.[5,15] Depending on the underlying cause and chronicity, the pouch can dilate

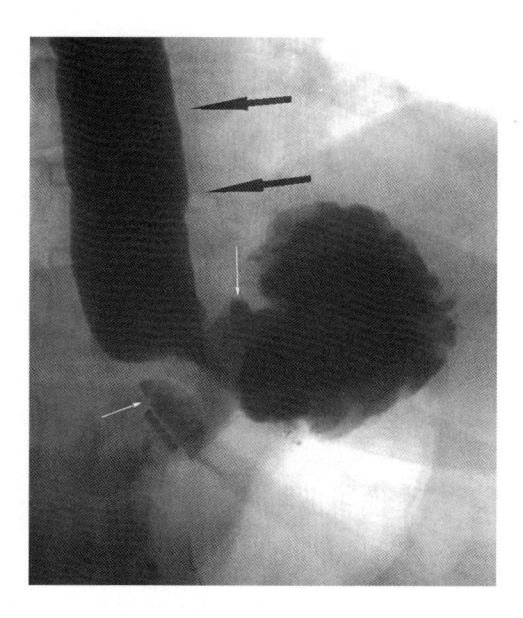

Figure 5. Oesophageal dilatation due to high band placement. Barium swallow examination showing marked dilatation of the oesophagus in spite of a patent and normal gastro-oesophageal junction. This is often associated with poor motility and can show tertiary contractions (arrows). This is particularly seen in bands placed too high with a small pouch and can be very difficult to adjust.

from less than 15 ml to over 500 ml in volume.[5] These patients can present with a constellation of symptoms including inappropriate weight loss, epigastric pain, gastro-oesophageal reflux and intractable vomiting.

Based on the underlying cause, pouch dilatation can be described as being: a) acute concentric; b) chronic concentric; or c) eccentric. Acute concentric pouch dilatation occurs in patients with stomal stenosis resulting from over-inflation of the balloon (Fig. 6). They present with dysphagia and painful swallowing soon after band inflation. UGI shows a dilated pouch with little or no passage of contrast material into the distal stomach. Immediate radiological deflation of the balloon followed by surgical referral is required for treatment.[23] If the stenosis is relatively recent, the stoma will reopen easily with immediate symptom relief. However, in chronic pouch stenosis, peri-stomal fibrosis may prevent reopening and device removal would be required for treatment.[15]

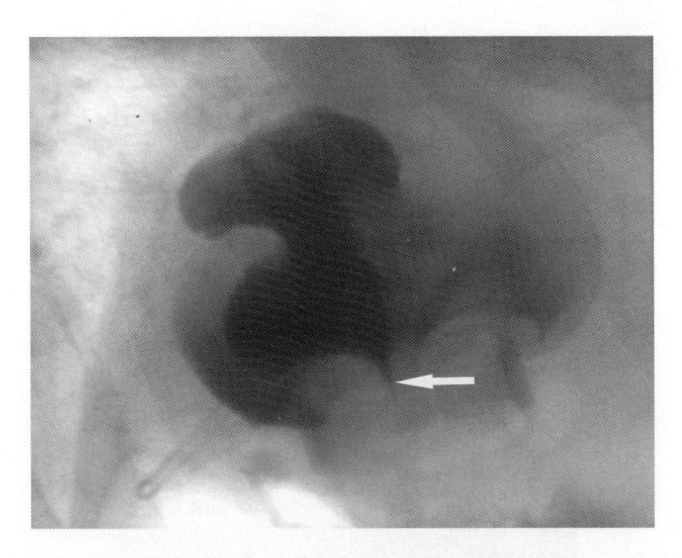

Figure 6. Acute concentric pouch dilatation following over-inflation of balloon. Dilute barium swallow shows narrow stoma (arrow) with very little contrast passing through. Note the moderately dilated proximal pouch, which is symmetrically dilated.

Chronic concentric dilatation results from chronic ingestion of large volumes of poorly masticated food. The stoma is open and of normal size or slightly dilated, but there is overstretching of the gastric pouch from chronic retention of poorly digested solid foods. UGI series will show a markedly distended pouch with open stoma and passage of contrast material into the distal stomach. Associated oesophageal dilatation and gastro-oesophageal reflux are frequent findings. Treatment requires dietary modification and patient education before return of the pouch to normal size.[5]

Eccentric pouch dilatation occurs relatively commonly and is due to either posterior or anterior band slip. This occurs as part of the 'band slip–hernia–pouch dilatation' complex described below. Patients with this complex present with food intolerance, vomiting and rapid weight loss. During UGI assessment, the control film shows abnormal angulation of the gastric band with a more horizontal lie that is suspicious of slippage. On the frontal view, a pouch above and lateral to the band usually indicates an anterior slip (Fig. 7), whilst a pouch below the band indicates a posterior slip.[24] This can easily be confirmed by lateral fluoroscopy that is

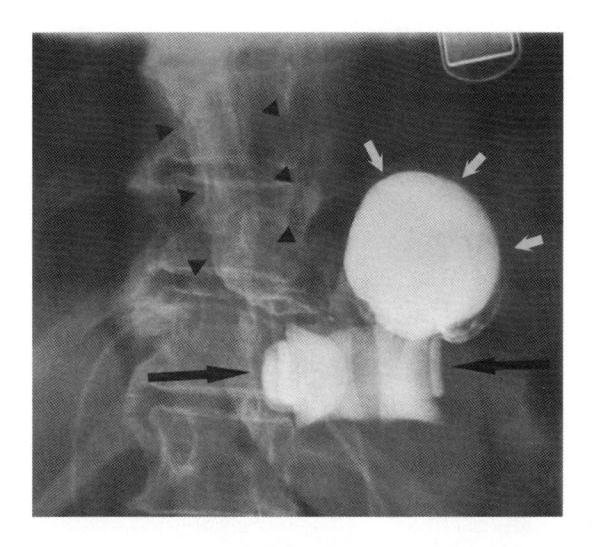

Figure 7. Eccentric pouch dilatation due to anterior band slippage. Dilute barium swallow shows posterior and lateral extension of pouch (white arrows) above the band typical of eccentric pouch dilatation due to anterior slippage of band. Note the horizontal orientation of the band (between black arrows), probably due to the gastro-gastric sutures giving way. There is very little of the administered contrast passing through the stoma, and the oesophagus is moderately dilated (arrowheads).

very helpful in the evaluation of patients with food intolerance where band slippage is suspected. Emptying of the pouch is usually poor. If a dilated pouch is seen, it is usual practice to immediately deflate the band before urgent surgical referral.

Occasionally, an excess of anterior fundus may be above the band, which may simulate a pouch (Fig. 8). The band angulation remains in excess of 20° and the pouch empties spontaneously. Band adjustments are difficult in these cases, but a policy of careful under-inflation with frequent follow-up may be adopted for these unusual patients (Mr H. Kumar, consultant surgeon, Birmingham, UK, *pers. comm.*).

Gastric herniation
Gastric herniation can be concentric or eccentric in nature. Concentric gastric herniation occurs with an incidence of 1.8–5 per cent[21,25] and results from cephalad migration of the stomach through the band due

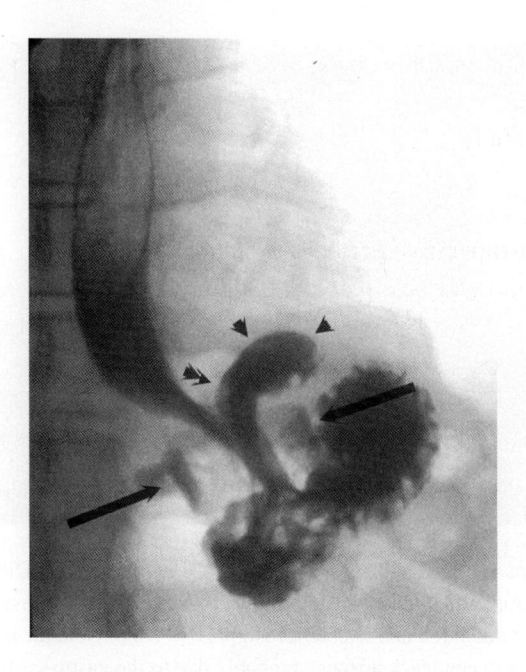

Figure 8. Excess anterior fundus above band simulating appearance of a pouch. Dilute barium swallow shows small redundant mucosa above the band due to gathering of anterior fundus above the band (small arrows). This should be differentiated from an eccentric pouch by the normal passage of barium through the band (between large arrows), and the relatively normal band angulation.

to high pouch pressures 'pulling' gastric tissue up from below the band. Eccentric gastric herniation usually occurs as part of the band slip–hernia–pouch dilatation complex.[24]

Patients with gastric herniation can present with severe upper abdominal pain, intractable vomiting and inability to swallow. On UGI series, a constellation of findings including malpositioning of the silicone band, eccentric pouch dilatation and partial or complete obstruction to outflow of contrast material may be seen. Occasionally slippage may be associated with a volvulus, where there is abnormal orientation of the stomach with transposition of the greater curvature above the lesser curvature in the organoaxial plane. Associated acute gastric obstruction is usual with complete non-passage of contrast material into the distal stomach. These findings constitute a surgical emergency that requires decompression of the balloon by the radiologist and urgent surgical referral. Band relocation with gastric reduction and surgical fixation is required for long-term symptomatic relief.[13]

Gastric obstruction

In the early postoperative period, oesophageal obstruction can occur due to inappropriate band size (e.g. small band in a super-obese patient) or postoperative oedema.[26,27] Passage of a nasogastric tube and conservative treatment usually leads to symptom resolution with the latter.

In the late postoperative period, gastric obstruction can be caused by a number of entities including over-tightening of the stoma and band slippage. Less common causes would include stomal obstruction from food bolus (Fig. 9) or bezoar,[28] and extrinsic compression from proximal axial gastric herniation.[13] In all these cases, UGI determination of band

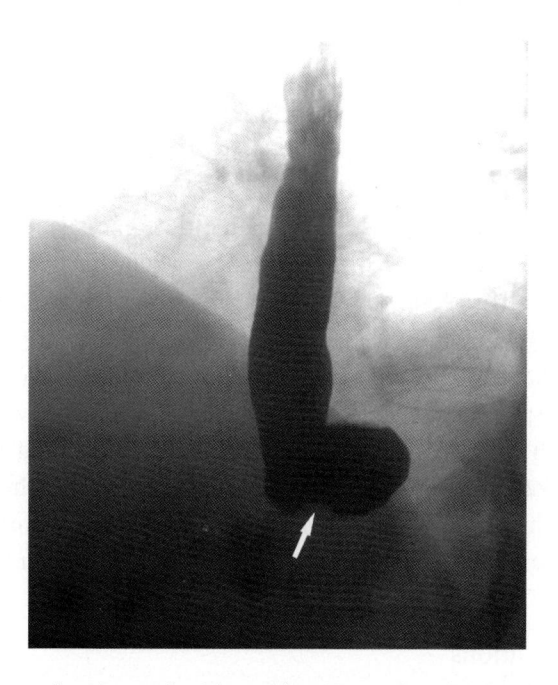

Figure 9. Obstruction due to food impaction 11 months after band insertion. Dilute barium swallow shows complete oesophageal obstruction at the level of the band in a patient with acute onset dysphagia. Note the indentation at the stoma (arrow) due to an obstructive food bolus. This was removed at endoscopy.

position, gastric orientation, pouch size, presence of any pouch filling defects and stomal patency helps in establishing the presence and cause of obstruction with a great deal of accuracy. CT with multiplanar reconstructions can also be useful in confirmation of the diagnosis.

Gastric perforation

Gastric perforation is an infrequent perioperative complication that occurs with an incidence of around 0.5 per cent, often related to deep suture bites being taken during gastric mobilization and imbrication of the silicone band.[12] The commonest cause of leak during the late postoperative period is from band erosion as described below. Finally, any cause of gastric ischemia — such as acute gastric dilatation or volvulus — can lead to necrosis and perforation. These are diagnosed by the finding of contrast extravasation during UGI, or extraluminal fluid and gas on CT (Fig. 3).

Intra-abdominal haemorrhage

Intra-abdominal haemorrhage can be intra- or extra-gastric in location. During the early postoperative period, extra-gastric haemorrhage results from bleeding of perigastric blood vessels damaged during gastric mobilization and prosthetic insertion.[29] The bleeding is usually self-limiting and asymptomatic. However, if the patient becomes haemodynamically unstable, a CT can be performed to show acute haematoma or active bleeding. Usually, blood transfusion and conservative measures are sufficient for treatment.

During the late post-operative period, intragastric bleeding can be related to the specific complication of gastric band erosion, where the band erodes through blood vessels in the gastric wall.[30] Depending on the degree and acuity of vascular injury, the presentation can vary from chronic anaemia to acute life threatening haematemesis. Emergency laparotomy with band removal with cautery of bleeding vessels may be required for treatment.

Band complications

Band erosion

This is a late complication resulting from pressure necrosis of the gastric wall leading to translocation of part or whole of the band into the gastric lumen. It is seen in up to 11 per cent of cases (mean, 3 per cent), with a time to presentation of 19–23 months.[22,31] Patients present with slowing of weight loss, or even weight gain. Even though the band has penetrated through the gastric wall, there is rarely free intraperitoneal leak due to the protracted nature of the process, allowing time for fibrosis and healing to take place. A very characteristic presentation of band erosion is that of port infection from tracking of infection along the tubing. In fact, protracted access port infection is often the first sign of band erosion.[30]

Band erosions can occasionally present with severe life threatening complications such as haematemesis,[32] or gastric outlet obstruction.[33,34] Yet it can also be completely asymptomatic and found incidentally at endoscopy or barium assessment.[30] The finding on UGI is pathognomonic with contrast outlining the band seen as a filling defect (Fig. 10) within the gastric lumen.[35] If intra-abdominal abscess is suspected, oral and

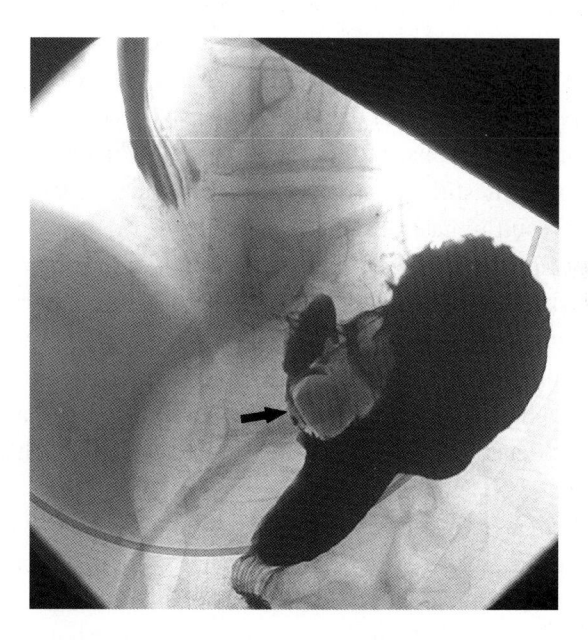

Figure 10. Intragastric erosion two years after band insertion. Water soluble contrast swallow shows a thin sliver of contrast outlining the outside edge of the band (arrow), signifying band erosion inside the stomach. Reprinted with permission of Dr. Shuvro H. Roy-Choudhury and Elsevier.[8]

intravenous contrast enhanced CT can show abnormal perigastric fluid collections and extraluminal gas that is useful in making this diagnosis.[30]

Band slippage

This band is held in position by its circular wrapping effect, positioning above the lesser omentum (using a *pars flaccida* technique), and suture fixation of the anterior band in an anterior gastric seromuscular tunnel. Band slippage has been associated with a number of factors including the surgical technique used, type of band employed and history of intractable vomiting. The band can slip anteriorly or posteriorly, of which the latter is more common due to anchoring of the band anteriorly to the stomach using sutures. Anterior or posterior slip can result in associated gastric herniation and eccentric pouch dilatation as part of the band slip–hernia–pouch dilatation complex (Fig. 7).

Patients with slipped band present with food intolerance, vomiting and rapid weight loss (see above). Posterior slippage used to happen very commonly with the older technique of transbursal band placement. However, the incidence of posterior slippage has reduced markedly from 30 per cent to less than 1–6 per cent since the use of the *pars flaccida* technique.[10,11] Band slip is also reduced with the use of newer larger sized bands,[36] although it still has a reported incidence of 0.3 per cent.[37] If severe, it can result in gastric volvulus and/or gastric obstruction.

Anterior slippage is usually due to disruption of the anterior seromuscular tunnel sutures, or the gathering of too much of the anterior fundus to form the pouch. If the fundus is redundant and emptying poorly, it will continue to enlarge and present as an enlarged pouch superior and lateral to the band. A high seromuscular suture to the diaphragmatic crus can reduce this incidence to 0.01 per cent (Mr Paul Super, consultant surgeon, Heart of England NHS Trust, *pers. comm.*).

During UGI assessment of patients with band slip, the control film shows abnormal angulation of the gastric band lying in a more horizontal plane than usual, suspicious for slippage. The anterior or posterior nature of the slippage can easily be diagnosed on lateral or oblique swallows. In a few patients, the band slippage can be intermittent in nature resulting in symptomatology only when the obstruction is present. In these patients, the examination may be normal when the band has fallen back to its native position. It may take several UGI examinations before the correct diagnosis is made.[5] The easiest way to make the diagnosis is to perform the UGI when the patient is acutely symptomatic.

Balloon complications

Balloon deflation

True balloon leakage occurs with an incidence of 4 per cent. Its cause is usually iatrogenic (inappropriate surgical handling with inadvertent puncture) if presenting early, and degenerative (tears in the balloon or breaks at the edge of the inner side of the balloon from fatigue) if presenting late. This leads to eventual patient weight gain due to increase in stomal size.[38] This complication can be diagnosed clinically by rapid loss of effect of inflation or radiologically by port injection of radiopaque contrast material, which should leak out from the band (Fig. 11). Port injection

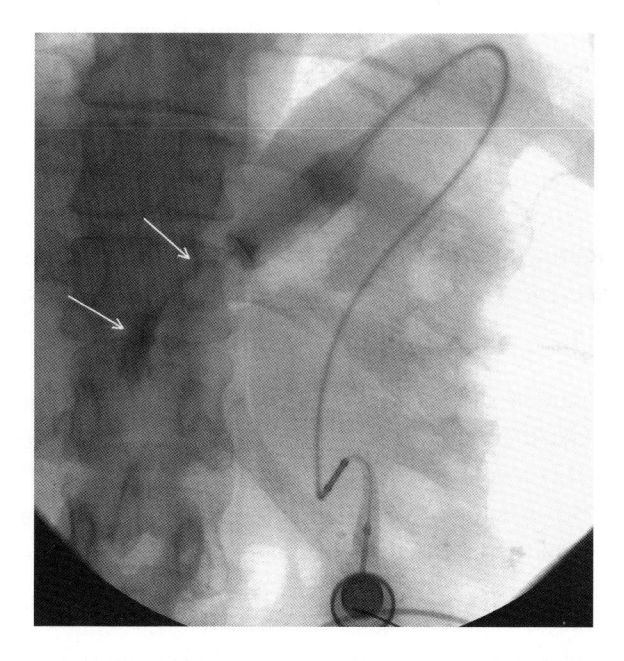

Figure 11. Band leakage in a patient with repeated loss of effect following band adjustments. Injection of water-soluble contrast material through the port confirms leakage from the band (arrows). Reprinted with permission of Dr. Shuvro H. Roy-Choudhury and Elsevier.[8]

using Tc99-colloid and scintigraphy detection of leak has also been described as a more accurate way to diagnose this complication.[38]

A more indolent cause for loss of balloon integrity has also been postulated. The balloon acts as a semi-permeable membrane and can slowly leak out normal saline over a prolonged period of time, resulting in balloon deflation and loss of restriction.[39] Use of contrast material diluted with water to make it iso-osmolar to plasma (150 mg/ml) for balloon inflation better maintains volume and leads to fewer such complications.[39] It is important to note that the use of hyperosmolar contrast material can have the opposite effect with absorption of water and over-inflation of the balloon.

Eccentric balloon herniation
Focal weakness with herniation of the balloon is a rare complication that occurred more frequently with the older bands. A localized weakness in the balloon can lead to focal eccentric herniation that is only seen in certain imaging projections.[5,8] Thus, if the stoma is not visualized with the herniation in profile, the size of the stoma can be overestimated during band inflation. This can lead to over-tightening of the stoma and eventually concentric pouch dilatation. Thus, it is vitally important to inject the balloon with water-soluble contrast material and view it in all projections to identify any focal eccentric band herniation in patients presenting with acute concentric pouch dilatation.[5,8]

Connecting tube and port complications

These are common and seen in 7–14 per cent of patients. In a series of 1,272 port related complications were seen in 91 patients who required 103 revisional procedures. These included 62 system leaks, 19 infections and 12 others.[40] Routine use of radiology and sterile techniques are the keys to reducing these complications.

Connecting tube complications
Connecting tube complications would include kinking (Fig. 12), twisting and detachment (Fig. 13) from its connection to the band or port. The latter is more common with Swedish bands and can be reduced by scrunching the connecting tube to the port attachment at the time of

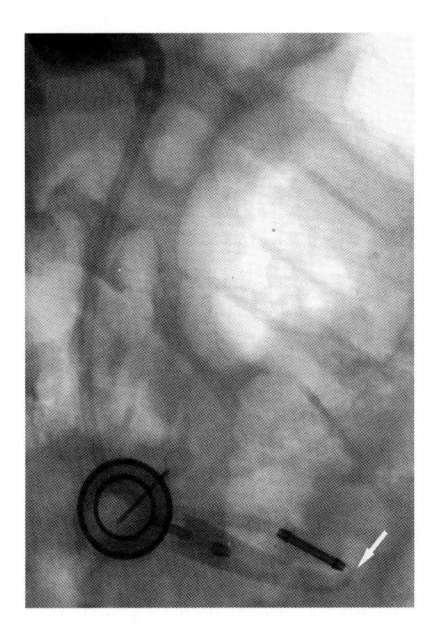

Imaging of Complications After Bariatric Surgery 243

Figure 12. Connecting tube kink. Scout film form a fluoroscopic study shows kink in the connecting tube (arrow) acting as a one-way valve, making aspiration more difficult than injection.

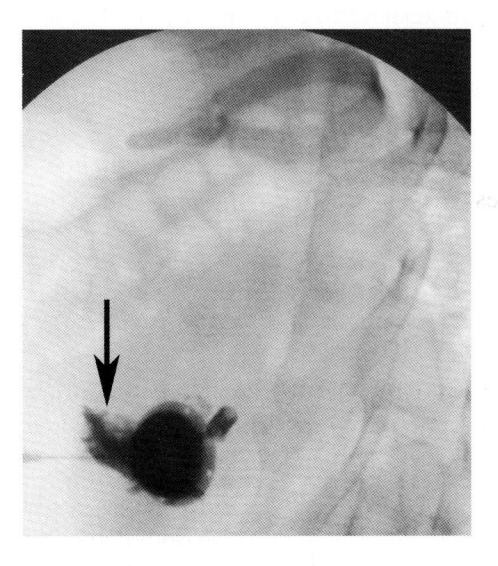

Figure 13. Disconnection of connecting tube from the port. Injection of water-soluble contrast medium through the port immediately results in leakage of contrast material around the port (arrow) indicative of disconnection of connecting tube at the port site.

insertion. Having a shorter loop of tube in the subcutaneous tissue can reduce tube kinkage (Mr Paul Super, *pers. comm.*). Similar to diagnosis of balloon integrity, a radiographic method involving water-soluble contrast material injection into the port under fluoroscopy, or a nuclear isotope injection (Technetium or Thallium) with gamma camera detection can be used for diagnosis of kinks and leaks.

Port complications
Port complications include port inversion and infection. Despite being attached to the anterior rectus sheath using sutures, the port can tilt, migrate or invert due to patient manipulation or spontaneous dislocation. The commonest port-related problem is tilting, which makes clinical and radiological access for puncture difficult. The use of C-arm fluoroscopy or ultrasound guidance may be required for successful access. Occasionally, the port is totally inverted such that it requires surgical revision. This problem can be reduced if the port is fixed at all four corners at the time of surgery close to the xiphisternum (Mr Paul Super, *pers. comm.*).

Port infection can be due to localized infection from dermal flora,[15,41,42] or deep-seated infection arising from band erosion.[30] In fact, port infection may be the first sign of band erosion and requires investigation to exclude this possibility. In deep-seated infections, surgical removal of the band and intravenous antibiotic therapy is needed for treatment. If in doubt, port infection can be diagnosed using radionuclide techniques such as Technetium- or Indium-labelled white blood cell studies.

Miscellaneous

Other rare complications reported include paragastric Richter's hernia,[43] small bowel obstruction resulting from the connecting tube,[44] and chronic unremitting cough cured by band deflation.[45]

In summary, in spite of the complications outlined, LAGB is a remarkably safe and well-tolerated procedure that is minimally invasive, totally reversible and adjustable to the patient's needs. Long term (>10 years) complication and failure rates are yet to be fully evaluated though. Overall mortality is very low (3/5,827 cases) with excess weight loss of 50–65 per cent, which can be maintained over time.[46] However, morbidity from complications does occur and can be related to the stomach, the prosthesis or surgery in general. They can occur in the early or late post-operative period. UGI series is invaluable in diagnosing these and a radiologist conversant with the expected findings should be an integral member of the multidisciplinary team. The routine use of UGI is not always necessary but recommended for port access and stomal size adjustment as it provides a more objective assessment of the anatomy. CT is complementary in the diagnosis of complications.

Roux-en-Y Gastric Bypass (RYGB)

The Roux-en-Y gastric bypass (RYGB) is a 'mixed-type' of surgery that uses a combination of restriction (gastric partitioning) and malabsorption (proximal small bowel bypass) to effect weight loss.[47] It is the most commonly performed bariatric surgery in the United States and is performed using the laparoscopic technique in the majority of cases.[48]

The technique involves dividing the stomach into two completely separate compartments by placement of a staple line across the cardia. This creates a small proximal compartment called the 'pouch' in continuity with the oesophagus, which should measure between 15 and 30 ml in volume for effective restriction. The remaining distal stomach consisting of the fundus, body and antrum is called the 'remnant' and is excluded from the food stream by the staple line partition.

Drainage from the newly created gastric pouch is facilitated through the creation of a 'gastrojejunal' anastomosis. To do this, the proximal jejunum is divided approximately 30–50 cm from the Ligament of Treitz to form two separate small bowel limbs. The proximal limb that is in continuity with the duodenum is called the 'biliopancreatic limb', and the distal limb that is in continuity with the remainder of the distal small bowel is called the 'Roux-en-Y' limb (or Roux limb for short). The cut end of the Roux limb is over sawn and brought up in front of the transverse colon (ante colic) and stomach (ante gastric), to be anastomosed in an end-to-side fashion with the gastric pouch to form the gastrojejunal anastomosis. Ideally, this opening should measure around 10–12 mm in diameter so as to provide adequate resistance to emptying without causing obstruction. The oversawn end of the Roux limb forms a short blind ending 'stump' at the gastrojejunostomy that should not be confused with a diverticulum or ulcer.[48]

The biliopancreatic limb free end is oversawn and anastomosed side-to-side with the Roux limb — approximately 75–150 cm downstream from the gastrojejunal anastomosis — to form the 'jejunojejunal' or 'Roux-en-Y' anastomosis. Downstream from this anastomosis, food coming from the Roux limb mixes with bile and pancreatic juices draining from the biliopancreatic limb as it passes distally through the remainder of the small bowel. In summary, this surgery creates two gastric compartments (pouch and remnant), two small bowel limbs (biliopancreatic and Roux), and two anastomosis (gastrojejunal and jejunojejunal) that work in concert to restrict and divert food to bring about weight loss. A schematic diagram of Roux-en-Y reconstruction is shown in Fig. 14.

As with any major surgery, there are complications associated with this procedure.[50] Complications occur in 3–20 per cent of morbidly obese

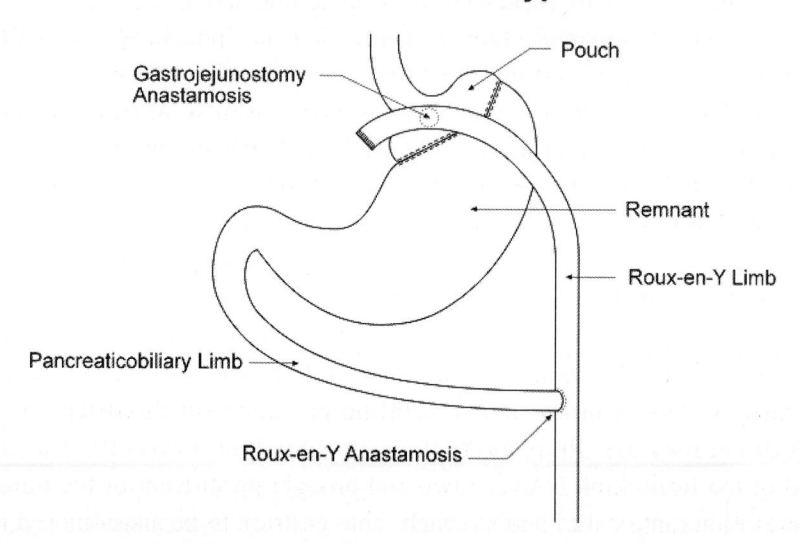

Figure 14. Diagram showing normal Roux-en-Y surgical anatomy. Reprinted, with permission, from Farraye F.A. and Forse R.A. (eds).[49]

patients after RYGB. A recent study[51] of 38,501 patients undergoing RYGB over a period of 19 years found a 30-day operative mortality of 0.24 per cent (93/38,501). The commonest causes of death were pulmonary embolism in 32 per cent (30/93), gastrointestinal leaks in 15 per cent (14/93) and bowel obstruction in 9 per cent (8/93). The enteric complications after RYGB can be divided into early (<30 days) and late (>30 days) postoperative complications. The most commonly encountered early complications are leaks, anastomotic obstruction and bleed. The most commonly encountered late complications are marginal ulceration, staple line failure (also known as gastrogastric fistula) and bowel obstruction.

The use of radiological investigations is crucial in the early and accurate diagnosis of complications after bariatric surgery.[47] In general, UGI and CT are the two most commonly used radiological tests in this regard. A UGI performed during the first or second postoperative day, before commencing oral intake, has been found to be very useful in the detection of early complications such as leaks and obstruction.[7,52,53] It is also particularly useful in the diagnosis of delayed complications such as staple line failure and gastrojejunostomy stricture. A normal UGI after RYGB is shown in Fig. 15.

CT gives a more comprehensive evaluation of the extraluminal pathology within the abdominal cavity. It is able to detect free intraperitoneal gas, intra-abdominal fluid collections, mesenteric inflammatory changes and bowel dilatation. Therefore, it is particularly useful in the diagnosis of leaks, abscess and small bowel obstruction.[7] A normal CT after RYGB is shown in Fig. 16.

Early postoperative complications

Anastomotic leak

Gastric leak is the most serious enteric complication associated with RYGB surgery with an incidence of 1–6 per cent[52,54–62] (Fig. 17). If not recognized and treated early, it can be a potentially lethal with a reported mortality of 6 per cent resulting from peritonitis and ensuing sepsis.[47,60,61] Therefore, early detection of postoperative leak is critical for minimizing morbidity and preventing mortality.[59,63,64]

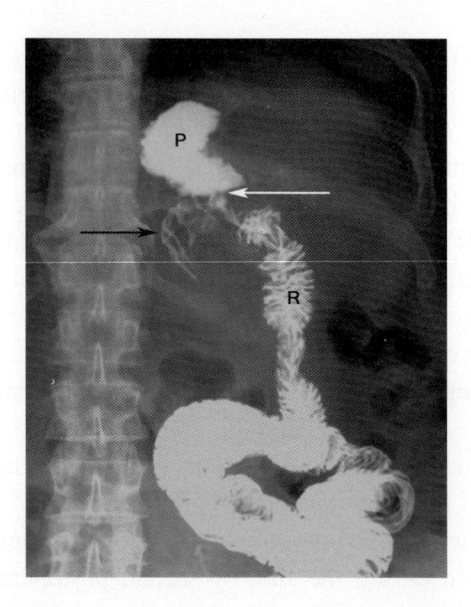

Figure 15. Normal post-operative anatomy on upper gastrointestinal series. A single contrast barium upper gastrointestinal series shows the gastric pouch, side-to-side gastrojejunostomy anastomosis (white arrow), blind ending Roux loop stump (black arrow), and the Roux limb. P = Pouch; R = Roux limb. Reprinted, with permission, from Farraye F.A. and Forse R.A. (eds).[49]

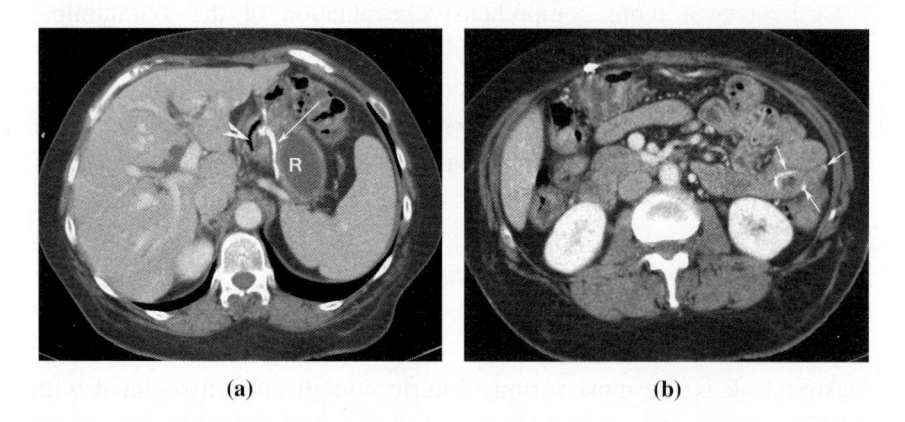

Figure 16. Normal post-operative anatomy on CT. An intravenous contrast enhanced axial CT without oral contrast at the level of the proximal anastomosis **(a)** shows the pouch (arrow head), fluid filled remnant and the dividing staple line (arrow). The same study through the lower anastomosis **(b)** shows the staples of the jejunojejunostomy (arrows), just anterior to the left mid kidney. R = Remnant.

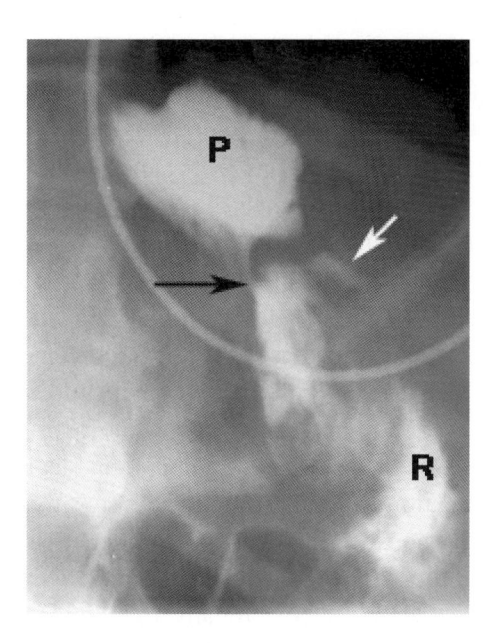

Figure 17. Anastomotic leak in the early post-operative period. Gastrografin upper gastrointestinal series in the immediate postoperative period showing a small localized leak (white arrow) arising from the gastrojejunostomy anastomosis. Note the site of the gastrojejunostomy anastomosis (black arrow). P = Pouch, R = Roux limb. Reprinted, with permission, from Farraye F.A. and Forse R.A. (eds).[49]

Leaks almost always occur in the early postoperative period (<30 days) and arise from the site of the gastrojejunal anastomosis in the vast majority of cases.[7] However, leaks can also arise less frequently from the gastric pouch, distal oesophagus, jejunal stump, staple line, bypassed gastric remnant and the jejunojejunal anastomosis. Leaks at the gastrojejunal anastomosis result from ischemic necrosis and focal perforation; excessive tension caused by drag from the Roux-en-Y limb, suboptimal surgical technique and dilatation of the Roux limb from distal obstruction are all presumed causative factors. Associated staple line dehiscence with gastrogastric fistula has been found in 31 per cent of patients with a leak.[61]

Most leaks extend to the left subphrenic and perisplenic areas.[7,61] This can cause hiccups, referred shoulder pain and left pleural effusion with associated passive lung atelectasis. Associated enteric findings would include ileus and/or small bowel obstruction (at the jejunojejunal anastomosis or gastrojejunal anastomosis).[61] There is an increased incidence of wound infection, chronic enterocutaneous fistula, deep venous thrombosis, pulmonary embolism and gastrointestinal bleed in patients with a leak.

Patients with leak often present with tachycardia, hypotension and acute respiratory distress (tachypnea, hypoxia), signs which raise concerns of pulmonary embolism. During the early stages of a leak, fever and peritonitis may be absent, leading to false reassurance for a primary abdominal abnormality.[7] Chest radiograph may show a left pleural effusion (due to sympathetic effusion from left subphrenic collection) that may further raise concern for pulmonary embolism. However, the rapid onset of increasing abdominal pain and leucocytosis should alert the clinician to the true diagnosis of an intra-abdominal leak.[61]

Clinical examination is often difficult and insensitive in the diagnosis of a leak due to the nonspecific signs (as mentioned above) and patient size. However, radiological evaluation has been shown to be of value in the early detection of leak.[7,55,63] Specifically, the routine use of UGI in the first or second post-operative day — before commencing oral intake — has been advocated for detection of leaks.[55,58,63,65,66] The finding of oral contrast extravasation that communicates with a peritoneal collection or surgical drain is diagnostic.[50] The use of this type of planned early UGI has been suggested to reduce morbidity.[65]

When performing UGI, a meticulous technique should be used to diagnose even the smallest leak. A control (scout) film should always be taken before contrast administration to distinguish small leaks from overlying artefacts. If a nasogastric tube is present, this should be pulled back into the gastric pouch to prevent obturation of any small potential leak sites.[53]

A single contrast study without oral gas administration is sufficient for diagnosis. The patient is placed in a supine position on the fluoroscopy table. While performing fluoroscopy, small volumes (20–30 ml) of water-soluble contrast medium are given orally or instilled down the nasogastric tube until there is adequate filling of the pouch. Observation is made for any evidence for oesophageal hold-up, hiatal hernia, reflux or leak, as these will modify the course of the examination.

After filling of the pouch, the patient should be rotated as much as possible to extreme lateral positions to maximize the detection of leak.

Turning the patient into a prone position is often not possible due to patient size, postoperative discomfort and restriction from attached lines/tubes. Continuous vigilance with intermittent fluoroscopic examination for contrast opacification of the left subdiaphragmatic space, perigastric region, abdominal peritoneal spaces and any surgical drains present should be performed to detect subtle leaks (Fig. 18).

If the initial water-soluble contrast examination is normal, it is prudent to repeat the examination using dilute barium to better detect subtle leaks. The examination is not completed until delayed imaging with overhead radiographs is obtained of the contrast reaching the distal small bowel to exclude possible obstruction and/or leak at the jejunojejunostomy anastomosis.

If CT is performed to detect anastomotic leak, the use of oral and intravenous contrast material is highly beneficial. CT has the added advantage that an initial CT pulmonary angiogram can be performed to exclude a potential pulmonary embolus before scanning through the abdomen. In patients with a leak, CT can show mesenteric stranding (indicative of

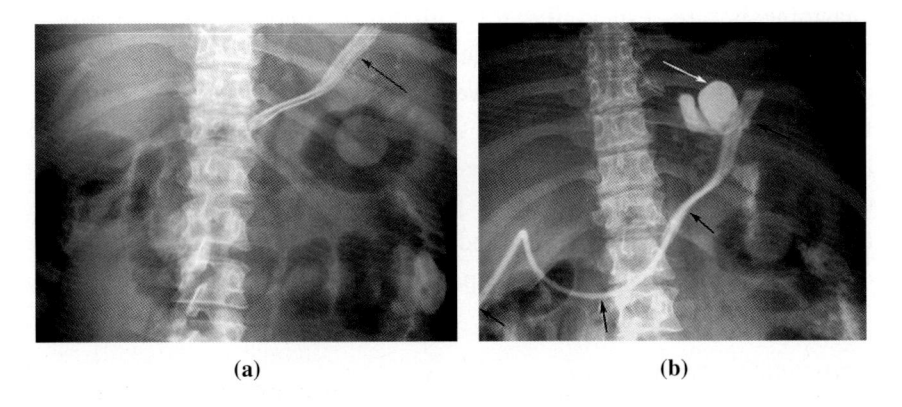

(a)   (b)

Figure 18. Early post-operative leak shown only by opacification of a surgical drain *in situ*. (a) The scout film taken before a Gastrografin upper gastrointestinal study shows the opaque portion of a Jackson–Pratt surgical drain in position (arrow). (b) After administration of Gastrografin, there is filling of the gastric pouch (white arrow) with subsequent contrast opacification of the length of the surgical drain (black arrows), indicative of a leak arising from the region of the gastrojejunostomy. A small amount of contrast is seen draining into the Roux loop situated at the left upper quadrant of the abdomen. Reprinted, with permission, from Farraye F.A. and Forse R.A. (eds).[49]

peritonitis), free intraperitoneal gas, and abnormal fluid collections that may also contain oral contrast.[6,67] However, the finding of free intraperitoneal gas *per se* should be interpreted with caution, as this can be a normal finding after recent operation.[61] Also, caution is required so that a distended but otherwise normal gastric fundus containing air/fluid levels — and possible oral contrast material — is not confused with a leak. Remember also that contrast can enter the gastric remnant by retrograde reflux through the jejunojejunal anastomosis. Careful confirmation of the fundus being in continuity with the gastric antrum will help to distinguish this normal variation from a pathological leak with collection.[67]

Whether to perform a CT or UGI as the initial study in the diagnosis of a leak depends on many factors including the patient condition, local expertise/experience and expediency. CT or UGI may individually be sufficient to make the diagnosis in many instances. However, when one test is negative or equivocal, performance of the other test is recommended as they can be complementary and increase the diagnostic yield. However, it must be emphasized that a negative CT, UGI, or both, does not necessarily exclude a life-threatening leak. Leaks from the jejunojejunal anastomosis are especially difficult to diagnose radiologically.[68] Therefore, a patient with high clinical suspicion for bowel leak should be assumed to have a leak until proven otherwise at surgery; waiting and watching can lead to sepsis, rapid multiorgan failure and death in these high-risk patients.[68,69] Percutaneous catheter drainage of gastric leak is only indicated in clinically stable patients with organized well-defined fluid collections that are easily and safely reached using a catheter. All others should undergo emergent laparotomy for diagnosis and treatment.

Anastomotic obstruction

Gastrojejunal anastomotic obstruction occurs in the early postoperative period with an incidence of 1.4 per cent.[52] This may be due to oedema, intraluminal lesion, fibrotic stenosis, or suboptimal surgical technique. There is an increased incidence of this complication in patients operated on by inexperienced surgeons during their early learning curve.[70-72] Patients present with epigastric pain, inability to swallow saliva, and dry retching; the diagnosis is usually clear at UGI or upper endoscopy.[69]

It is not unusual to find mild delay in pouch emptying in patients undergoing routine UGI studies after RYGB.[52,53] However, most of these patients have temporary hold-up at the gastrojejunal anastomosis due to post-operative oedema (Fig. 19). The challenge is to identify the small number of patients who have irreversible obstruction (fibrosis, iatrogenic closure) that would require surgical revision. Manoeuvres such as examining the patient in an erect position and using delayed films will help with this distinction. Even the slightest drainage of contrast from the pouch at any stage is a good prognostic sign and should warrant continued conservative management. With gradual resolution of oedema, there should be establishment of rapid pouch emptying with symptomatic relief and a good clinical outcome. However, if there is persistent hold-up of barium at the gastrojejunostomy, a nasogastric tube should be placed under fluoroscopy for decompression and the examination repeated a day or two later. In patients with non-oedematous obstruction, there is complete and persistent pouch obstruction. After endoscopic confirmation, these patients should be taken back to the operating room for take down and refashioning of the obstructed gastrojejunostomy.

Gastrojejunostomy obstruction in the early postoperative period due to intraluminal clot is a rare but well described finding (Fig. 20).[52] It is not unusual to find small clots in the stomach and jejunum of patients after bariatric surgery.[52] However, in the vast majority of patients these clots are too small to cause obstruction and resolve spontaneously. However, if they do result in obstruction, treatment with endoscopic removal or nasogastric tube lavage can be effective.

Obstruction at the jejunojejunal anastomosis is a rare complication and is more common after laparoscopic compared to open RYGB surgery.[73] In at least one study,[74] it was found to be the commonest cause of early small bowel obstruction. It occurs due to anastomotic oedema or iatrogenic occlusion of the jejunojejunal anastomosis.[69] Depending on the extent of involvement, it can lead to obstruction of the Roux limb, the biliopancreatic limb or both. Obstruction of the biliopancreatic limb is equivalent to a closed-loop obstruction that can lead to dilatation of the duodenum and gastric remnant with retained biliary and pancreatic secretions.[75] Developing tension can lead to staple line dehiscence and/or

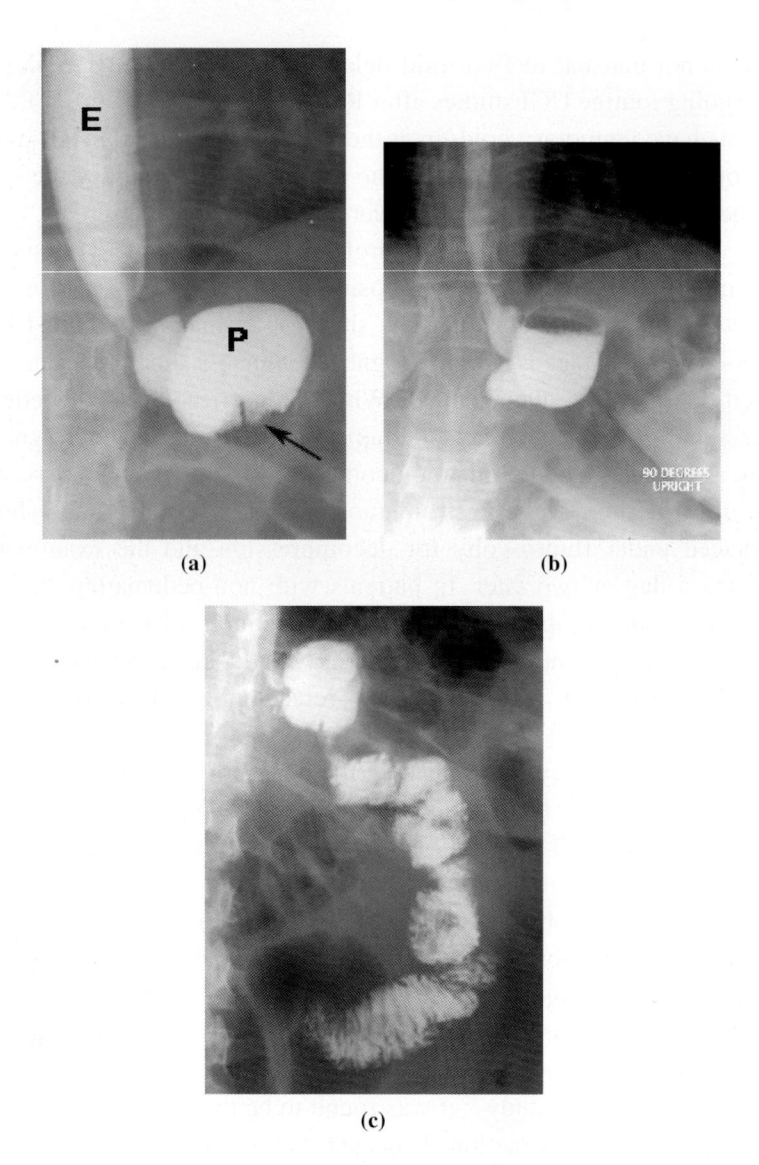

Figure 19. Temporary hold-up of contrast at the gastrojejunostomy due to oedema. Gastrografin upper gastrointestinal series shows: **(a)** opacification of the oesophagus and gastric pouch, with complete obstruction to flow of contrast at the gastrojejunostomy anastomosis (arrow); **(b)** even with placing the patient in a semi-erect position, there is no flow of contrast past the proximal anastomosis; **(c)** however, a supine film half an hour later shows normal drainage of contrast into the Roux limb suggestive of anastomotic oedema. E = Oesophagus, P = Pouch.

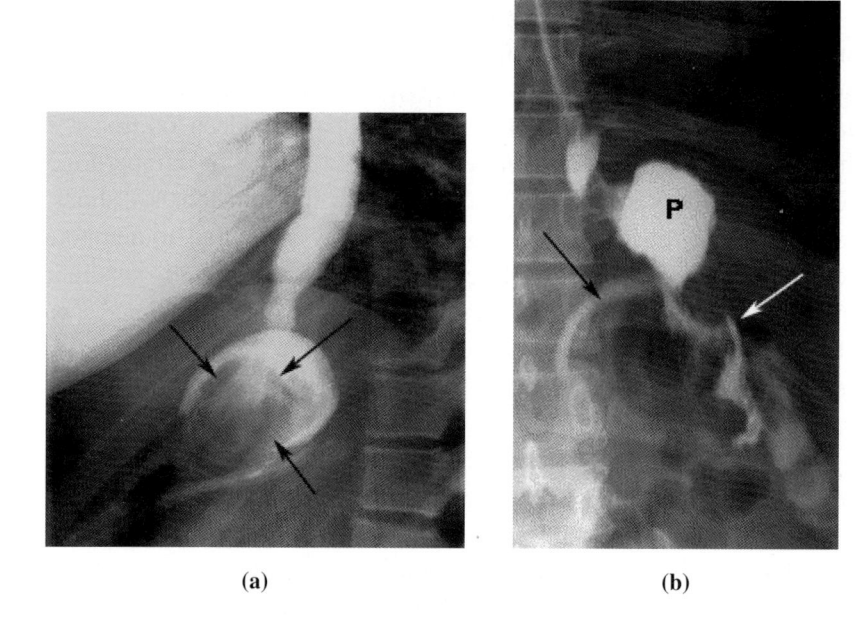

Figure 20. Gastrojejunostomy obstruction due to clot in the early post-operative period. Gastrografin upper gastrointestinal series showing: **(a)** large clot (arrows) within the gastric pouch causing complete obstruction to drainage of contrast from the stomach; **(b)** a repeat study 24 hours after saline lavage through a nasogastric tube shows resolution of clot with normal contrast opacification of the Roux limb (white arrow). Note the opaque portion of a Jackson–Pratt drain close to the gastrojejunostomy site (black arrow). P = Pouch.

gastrojejunostomy leak.[53] Because of its closed loop nature, this complication can be difficult to diagnose using UGI or upper endoscopy. CT is the modality of choice for investigation of patients with abdominal bloating and hiccups, suspicious for this diagnosis.[53,74]

Haemorrhage

Haemorrhage is a relatively uncommon complication after RYBG with an incidence of 0.5–5 per cent. However, many of these patients are on prophylactic anti-thrombotic medication for prevention of venous thromboembolic disease or co-morbid cardiac conditions that can aggravate these bleeding complications.[76]

Haemorrhage in the early postoperative period can originate from many sites including fresh staple lines (gastric partition, gastrojejunostomy anastomosis, jejunojejunostomy), cut edges of the mesentery, damaged blood vessels (short gastrics), damaged spleen or trocar site injury. The site of bleeding can be intraluminal, mural or intraperitoneal, depending on the cause. Patients can present with haematemesis, shock or gastrointestinal obstruction. Larger clots may give rise to temporary bowel obstruction (Fig. 20). More often than not, bleeding is subclinical and self-limiting. Most of the time these patients can be managed with blood transfusion and supportive care. Bleeding in the late postoperative period occurs most often due to marginal ulceration[77] and is described in more detail below.

The best test for the investigation of bleeding is the upper GI endoscopy as it can visualize the bleeding site and treat the cause. If endoscopy is normal, occult intra-abdominal haemorrhage should be suspected and a CT of the abdomen performed. CT will show free fluid or, more probably, a localized haematoma of varying appearance and density, depending on age. Occasionally, associated gastric wall thickening will also be found due to a mural haematoma. UGI is relatively insensitive in the diagnosis of marginal ulcers unless they are large and deep. Occasionally, selective mesenteric angiography may be required for diagnosis and treatment of intractable bleeding.

Bleeding arising from the bypassed stomach and duodenum should be considered when no other site is identified at endoscopy or standard radiological imaging. As the bypassed biliopancreatic limb is a relatively 'blind' area that is not readily accessible to a scope or contrast from an UGI study, this poses a difficult and interesting challenge for imaging. In such patients, confirmation of bleeding from the biliopancreatic limb can be attempted using Tc-red cell labelled radionuclide studies.

Late postoperative complications

Marginal ulcer

This is a complication of the late postoperative period with an incidence of around 0.5–15 per cent.[6,47,78] Classically, marginal ulcers are shallow ulcers occurring at the jejunal side of the gastrojejunal anastomosis (Fig. 21). However, these can occur anywhere around the gastrojejunostomy margin and some can be very large. They can lead to complications with haemorrhage[77] and perforation.[79,80]

The aetiology of marginal ulcer remains unclear but has been postulated to be due to use of non-steroidal anti-inflammatory drugs, ischemia at the anastomotic site and infection with *Helicobacter pylori*. There is also an increased incidence of marginal ulcers with staple line failure, presumably due to exposure of this site to gastric acid from reflux through the gastrogastric fistula (Fig. 22).

Presentation of marginal ulcers includes severe dyspepsia, epigastric pain, vomiting and/or bleeding. As mentioned above, radiological investigations are relatively insensitive in their diagnosis as the ulcers are often small and shallow.[81] Larger ulcers can be diagnosed as elsewhere in the gastrointestinal system by the findings of an excavated mucosal defect associated with persistent barium pooling and radiating folds. Upper endoscopy is by far the most useful test for the diagnosis of marginal ulcers.

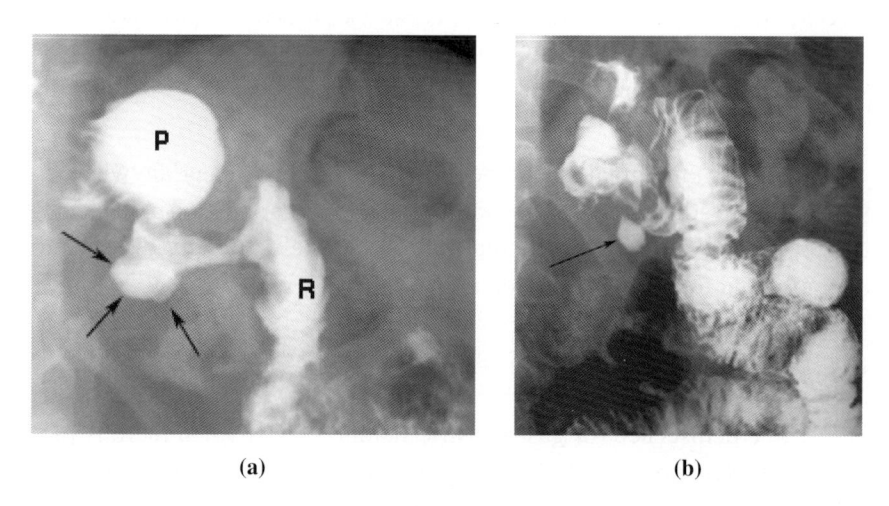

(a)   (b)

Figure 21. Marginal ulcer. Single contrast barium upper gastrointestinal series shows: **(a)** contrast filling of a large ulcer crater (arrows) situated at the jejunal side of the gastrojejunostomy; **(b)** persistent pooling of contrast (arrow) on delayed images indicative of an acute ulcer. P = Pouch, R = Roux limb. Reprinted, with permission, from Farraye F.A. and Forse R.A. (eds).[49]

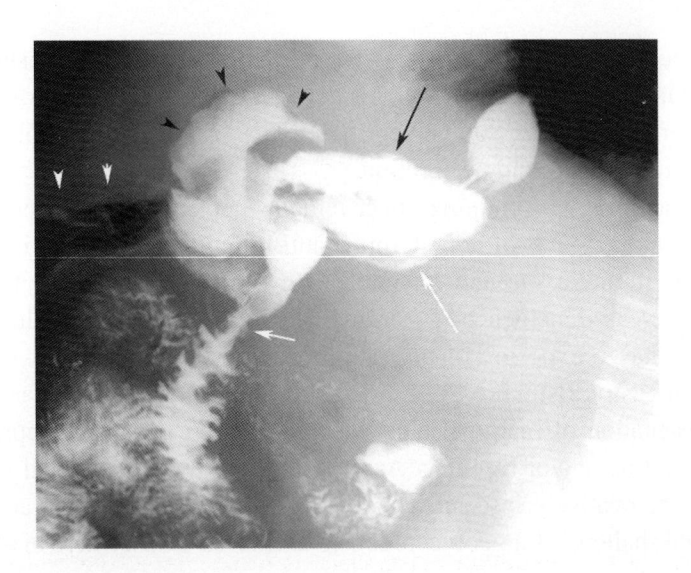

Figure 22. Giant marginal ulcer associated with gastrogastric fistula. Single contrast barium upper gastrointestinal series showing barium from gastric pouch (black arrow) communicating with gastric fundus (long white arrow), and coating an air filled antrum (white arrow heads) due to staple line dehiscence. There is drainage of barium from the pouch to the Roux limb (short white arrow) despite the presence of a giant ulcer (black arrow heads) arising from the gastrojejunostomy site. Reprinted, with permission, from Farraye F.A. and Forse R.A. (eds).[49]

Apart from marginal ulcers, peptic ulcers can also occur anywhere in the gastrointestinal tract, as in non-bariatric patients. Duodenal ulceration occurring in the biliopancreatic limb can be extremely difficult to diagnose and treat,[82] as discussed above.

Staple line dehiscence

Staple line dehiscence (or gastrogastric fistula) occurs when there is partial or complete breakdown of the partition between the gastric pouch and remnant, due to a tear or the staples coming away (Fig. 23). This usually occurs during the early postoperative period with an incidence of around 20 per cent. The aetiology is thought to be due to excessive strain being placed on the staple line from eating large volumes of poorly digested food with resultant chronic gastric pouch distention.[66] This breakdown of

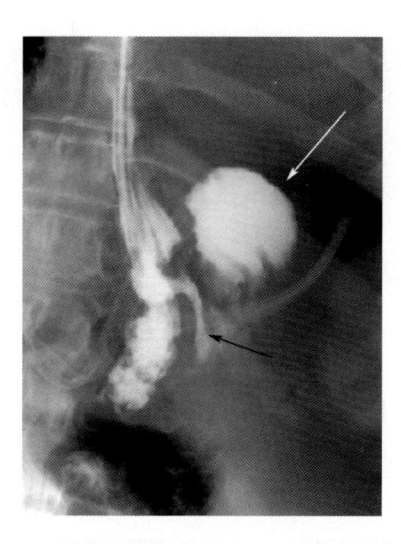

Figure 23. Staple line dehiscence. Gastrografin upper gastrointestinal series in the immediate post operative period shows contrast leak from the pouch (black arrow) filling the gastric remnant (white arrow), indicative of a gastrogastric fistula. Reprinted, with permission, from Farraye F.A. and Forse R.A. (eds).[49]

the staple line results in loss of the restrictive and bypass effects of the surgery leading to stabilization or regaining of weight, prompting further investigations.

UGI is by far the best test for diagnosis of gastrogastric fistula.[53] Endoscopy will show large defects, but UGI will reveal even the smallest gastrogastric fistula. It will show extravasation of contrast from the pouch with progressive opacification of the gastric remnant (Fig. 24). In the normal post-operative situation, there should be absolutely no contrast material seen entering the remnant, with all contrast exiting the pouch through the gastrojejunostomy. However, care must be taken not to confuse the occasional contrast opacification of the remnant resulting from retrograde filling through the jejunojejunostomy. In a true leak, there will be early and progressive contrast opacification of the remnant, well before there is contrast reaching the jejunojejunal anastomosis where reflux could occur.

In patients with staple failure, CT can also be diagnostic if performed with administration of oral contrast. In patients with a fistula, there is

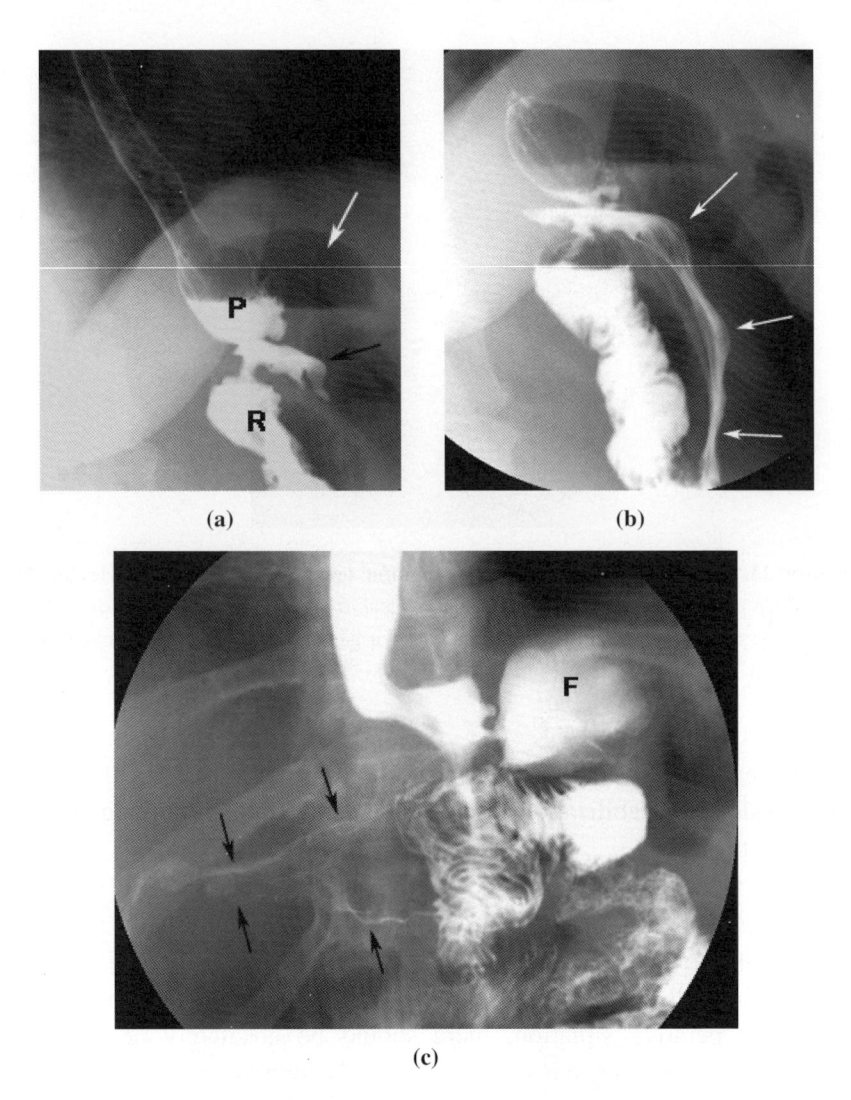

Figure 24. Staple line dehiscence. Gastrografin upper gastrointestinal series in the early post operative period shows: **(a)** contrast leak from the gastrojejunostomy (black arrow). Note an air/fluid level in the unopacified gastric fundus (white arrow); **(b)** a subsequent film shows progressive contrast coating of the gastric body (white arrows); **(c)** a delayed film shows progressive contrast filling of the gastric remnant with pooling of contrast within the fundus and coating of the gastric antrum (black arrows). P = Pouch, R = Roux limb, F = Fundus.

contrast opacification of the gastric body and antrum that is normally of fluid density (Fig. 25). With the advent of helical CT, many in the radiology community are now questioning the need for routine administration of positive oral contrast material in patients undergoing abdominal CT. Irrespective of the outcome of this debate, a history of RYGB should be an indication for routine administration of positive oral contrast material in order not to miss staple line dehiscence in both symptomatic and asymptomatic patients.

Bowel obstruction

Small bowel obstruction is usually a late complication of bariatric surgery with an incidence of 1–5 per cent.[6,47,62,73,74,83,84] They are most commonly caused by adhesion, stricture and internal herniation. Rare causes would include intussusception and bezoar related obstruction.[85,86]

UGI and CT are the most frequently used imaging tests in patients with suspected bowel obstruction, although CT has been shown to be

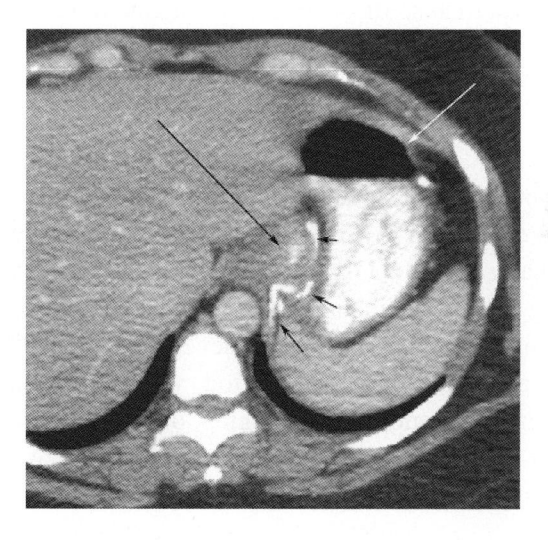

Figure 25. Staple line dehiscence. Oral contrast enhanced axial CT through the upper abdomen shows contrast material in the gastric pouch (long black arrow) as would be expected, but contrast material also in the gastric remnant (white arrow) that is abnormal and indicative of a gastrogastric fistula. Note portions of the dividing staple line (small black arrows). Reprinted, with permission, from Farraye F.A. and Forse R.A. (eds).[49]

superior to UGI in making this diagnosis.[74] Not only does CT enable the diagnosis of obstruction to be made, but it may also identify the underlying cause and exclude associated complications such as perforation and/or abscess. If the CT is normal or equivocal (and there is no obvious perforation) progressing to an UGI may identify functional or mucosal lesions that may explain patient symptomatology. Although these tests are complementary, CT is generally recommended before a UGI in the investigation of suspected bowel obstruction. Irrespective of the cause, the radiological hallmark of obstruction is the same: a change in bowel calibre (transition point) associated with proximally dilated and distally collapsed bowel loops. As obstructions tend to be proximal in the post-RYGB patient, characteristic findings at imaging includes dilatation of the oesophagus, gastric pouch dilatation, wide opening of the gastrojejunostomy and dilatation of the Roux limb (Fig. 26). CT also helps with the identification of the actual cause of obstruction in many patients, particularly when there are characteristic radiological findings such as that of intussusception. However, in a few patients, the exact cause of obstruction remains obscure until surgical exploration.

Adhesions

This is a leading cause of small bowel obstruction, particularly in patients undergoing RYGB using the open surgical technique.[73] However, with the advent of laparoscopic RYGB, the incidence has much decreased. The aetiology is related to organizing inflammatory peritoneal bands leading to extrinsic bowel compression. It can develop rapidly and usually presents in the early postoperative period with symptoms of colicky abdominal pain and vomiting. On imaging, dilated proximal small bowel with a sharp transition point is often identified (Fig. 27). Surgical exploration with release of adhesion is both diagnostic and therapeutic.

Anastomotic stricture

Anastomotic structure can occur at the gastrojejunal or the jejunojejunal anastomosis. Gastrojejunostomy stricture occurs with an incidence of

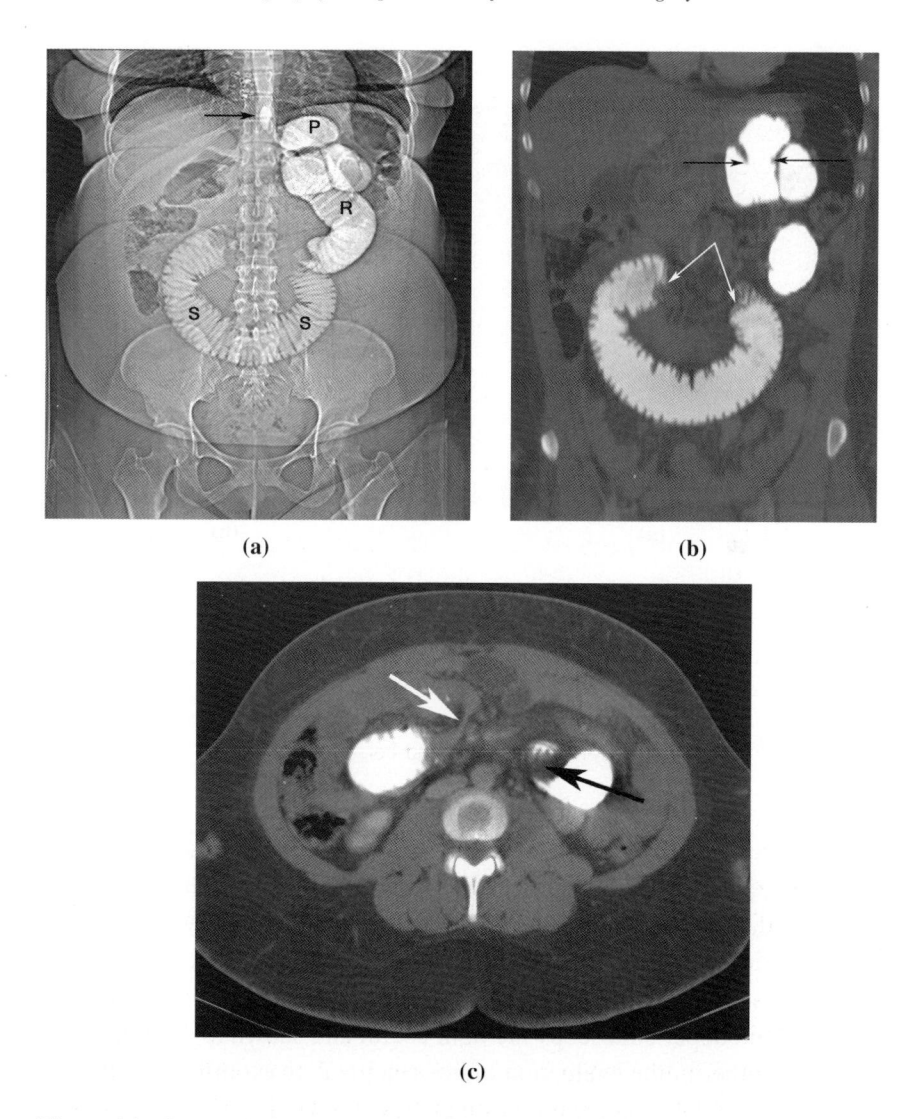

Figure 26. Petersen's hernia. Oral contrast material enhanced CT of the abdomen: **(a)** scout film from the study showing hold-up of oral contrast material in the oesophagus (black arrow), contrast filled dilated pouch, Roux limb and portion of the closed-loop obstructed herniated small bowel; **(b)** a coronal CT image shows dilated gastrojejunostomy anastomosis (black arrows) and sites of closed loop obstruction (white arrows); **(c)** an axial CT image shows the 'mushroom' sign where the herniated bowel together with its mesentery and blood vessels are pinched into a waist (arrows), as they pass through the hernial defect. P = Pouch, R = Roux limb, S = Small bowel.

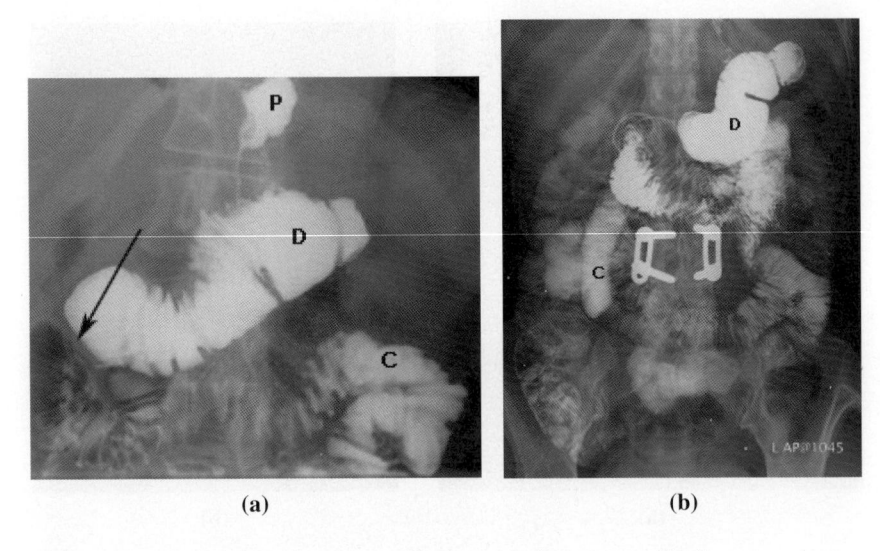

Figure 27. Bowel obstruction due to adhesion proved at surgery. Single contrast barium upper gastrointestinal series shows: **(a)** abnormal dilatation of the Roux limb, relatively collapsed distal bowel and a transition point (black arrow); **(b)** a delayed film shows persistently dilated contrast filled Roux limb and a relatively collapsed partially contrast filled distal small bowel. P = Pouch, D = Dilated Roux limb, C = collapsed distal small bowel. Reprinted, with permission, from Farraye F.A. and Forse R.A. (eds).[49]

3–27 per cent.[6,47,48,56,78,83,84] Patients usually present with nausea, vomiting, regurgitation, dysphagia or epigastric pain[87,88] during the late postoperative period, with a mean of 48 days from surgery in one study.[87] The cause of the stricture is thought to be due to ischemia from tension and compromised blood supply.[78,89]

UGI and upper endoscopy are both useful and shown to correlate well with each other in the evaluation of gastrojejunal anastomotic structure.[90] The most useful radiological investigation is the UGI, which may show a number of findings including concentric dilatation of the pouch, pinhole sized ostomy, delayed pouch emptying, open gastro-oesophageal junction and a dilated lower oesophagus associated with reflux[87] (Fig. 28). When performing the UGI, lateral and/or steep oblique (>45°) imaging is recommended for full visualization of the anteriorly placed gastrojejunostomy and any strictures that may be hidden on the frontal projection alone.[7,87]

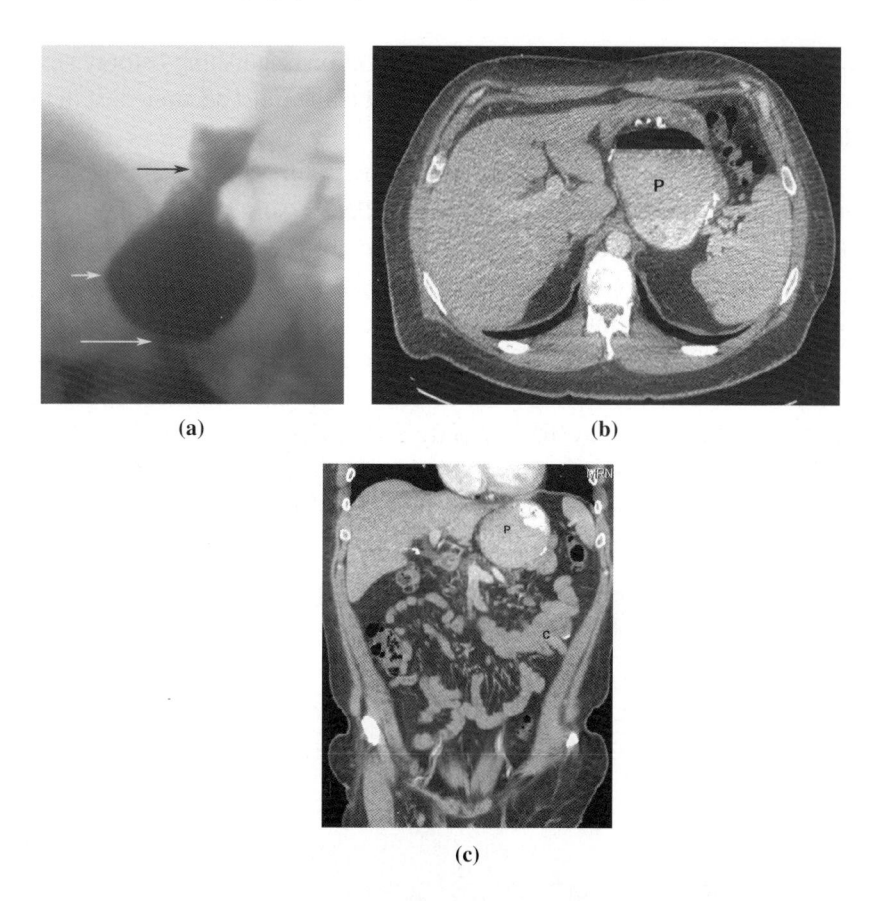

Figure 28. Gastrojejunostomy stricture. **(a)** A barium swallow study shows tight 'pinhole' stricture at the gastrojejunostomy (long white arrow), a concentrically dilated barium filled pouch (short white arrow) and barium hold-up in a dilated lower oesophagus associated with patulous gastro-oesophageal junction (black arrow). Reprinted, with permission, from Farraye F.A. and Forse R.A. (eds).[49] An oral and intravenous contrast material enhanced CT from another patient shows: **(b)** a markedly dilated fluid filled gastric pouch on axial imaging through the upper abdomen; **(c)** isolated dilatation of the gastric pouch with distally collapsed small bowel on a coronal reconstructions through the abdomen. P = Pouch, C = Collapsed distal small bowel.

Other rare causes of gastrojejunostomy obstruction include ostomy impaction from food or bezoar. Hiatal hernia, marginal ulceration and small bowel obstruction are among other conditions simulating gastrojejunostomy obstruction. When patients present with symptoms consistent with pouch obstruction, UGI can be useful in distinguishing ostomy stricture from many of these other conditions. It is the most accurate test in the diagnosis of hiatal hernia and reflux.

Stricture at the jejunojejunal anastomosis is a less frequent but, nevertheless, a serious complication after RYGB surgery (Fig. 29). The stricture at the jejunojejunostomy can cause obstruction of the Roux-en-Y limb alone, the biliopancreatic limb alone or both limbs simultaneously (with or without continuity between the two limbs). In most cases, an UGI will show a much dilated Roux-limb with obstruction at the anastomosis, except in the rare case of an isolated biliopancreatic limb obstruction. In the latter, the UGI may be perfectly normal with progress of barium through the distal small bowel. Thus a life-threatening closed loop obstruction (the biliopancreatic limb is closed off proximally by the

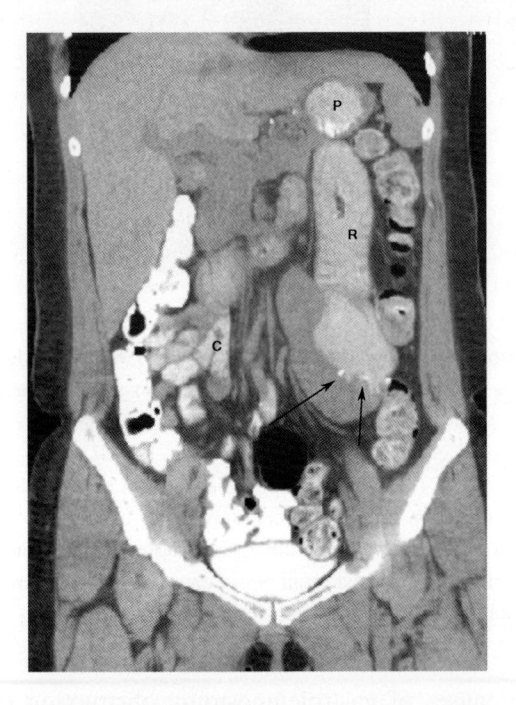

Figure 29. Jejunojejunostomy anastomosis stricture causing Roux limb obstruction. Oral contrast material enhanced coronal CT of abdomen showing fluid filled dilated pouch and Roux limb, with point of obstruction at the jejunojejunostomy where suture material is seen (arrows). P = Pouch, R = Roux limb, C = Collapsed distal small bowel.

gastric partitioning and closed off distally at the jejunojejunostomy) may be missed if UGI alone is performed. The closed off biliopancreatic limb distends markedly due to continuous filling with bile and pancreatic juice, leading to jaundice in severe cases. The diagnosis is solely and accurately made by CT, which will show a cystic fluid collection in the upper abdomen, posteromedial to the free margin of the liver.

Internal herniation

Internal herniation is the commonest cause of small bowel obstruction after RYGB surgery with a reported incidence of 0.2–5 per cent.[91–93] It is caused by herniation of small bowel through surgically created defects in the mesentery, resulting in a 'closed-loop' type of obstruction.[91,94] It may involve any portion or length of the small bowel, including variable portions of the Roux or biliopancreatic limbs. Although some have suggested increased incidence of internal hernias after laparoscopic as compared to open RYGB,[95] others have found no significant difference.[73]

There are three distinct types of internal hernias based on their anatomic sites of herniation: transmesenteric, transmesocolic and Petersen hernia. The transmesenteric herniation occurs through a defect in the small bowel mesentery near the jejunojejunal anastomosis (Fig. 30); the transmesocolic herniation occurs through a defect in the transverse mesocolon created for retrocolic passage of the Roux loop[88] (Figs. 31 and 32); and the Petersen herniation occurs through a mesenteric defect behind the Roux limb itself [91] (Fig. 26). Depending on the study, the transmesenteric,[96] transmesocolic[92,97] and Petersen[98] hernias have all been reported to occur with the most increased frequency. However the technique of bringing the Roux limb anterior to the transverse colon, (antecolic) rather than posteriorly through the transverse mesocolon, has considerably reduced the incidence of transmesocolic herniation. Many surgeons try to close any remaining mesenteric defects using nonabsorbable sutures at the time of the initial surgery to prevent the incidence of the other types of hernias also.

Internal hernias most commonly occur during the late postoperative period because mesenteric hernial defects enlarge with weight loss, making easier for herniation to take place. It is a potentially lethal

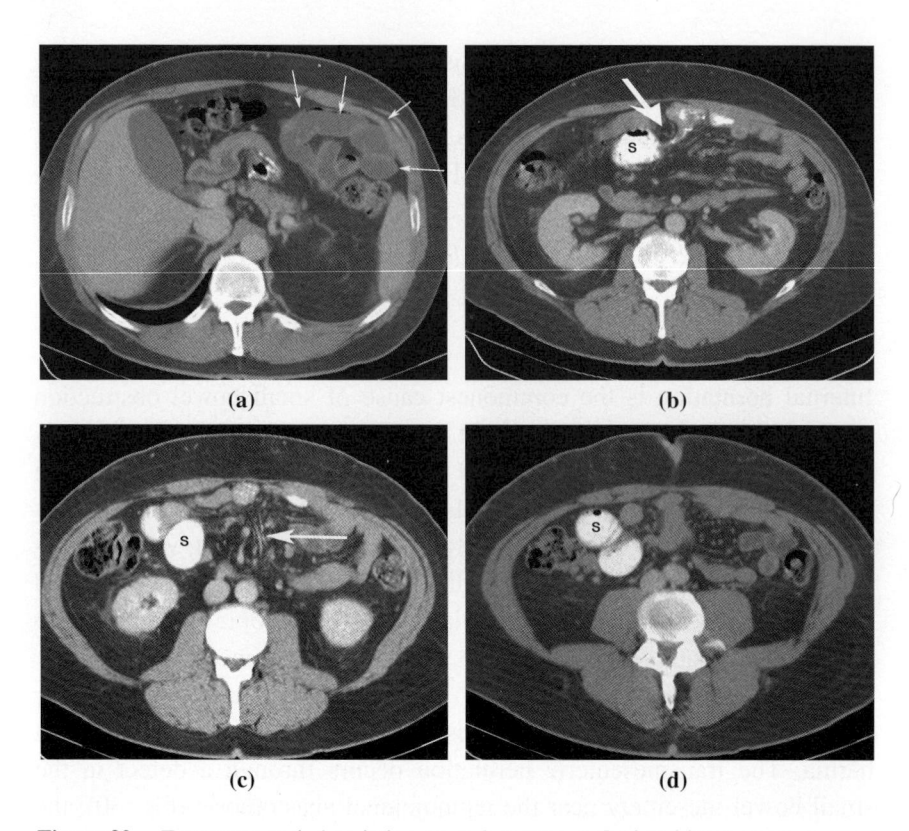

Figure 30. Transmesenteric herniation proved at surgery. Oral and intravenous contrast material enhanced axial CT shows: **(a)** dilated fluid-filled herniated small bowel loops at the left upper quadrant of abdomen (arrows); **(b)** the 'pinch sign' as the hernial defect indents on the side of the herniating bowel (arrow); **(c)** bunched-up blood vessels running in a unusual vertical orientation (arrow) in the root of the small bowel mesentery as it herniates; **(d)** dilated contrast-filled bowel proximal to the level of herniation. S = Small bowel dilated proximal to herniation.

complication with variable and nonspecific clinical presentation.[92,99,100] Patients typically present with intermittent postprandial colicky abdominal pain and nausea, with or without vomiting. If strangulation occurs, patients present with sudden onset of abdominal pain and peritonitis. However, in the majority of patients the herniation is intermittent and low-grade, with insidious symptoms and subtle imaging findings.[96]

Both UGI and CT have been used in the diagnosis of obstructed internal herniation.[6,7] On UGI, there is almost always the finding of dilated

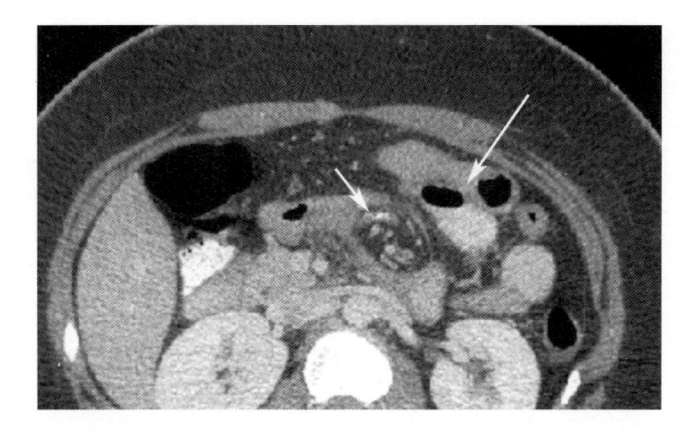

Figure 31. Transmesocolonic herniation proved at surgery. Oral and intravenous contrast material enhanced axial CT showing crowding and swirling of blood vessels through the mesenteric defect in the transverse mesocolon (small arrow), associated with dilatation of the herniated small bowel (large arrow).

contrast-filled oesophagus, gastric pouch and proximal Roux limb with a dilated gastrojejunal anastomosis.[6,7] In addition, the finding of fixed dilated loops of small bowel (the herniated bowel) at the left upper to mid abdomen is characteristic. If these fill with orally administered contrast material, they will show stasis and slow emptying. There is rarely adequate opacification of the collapsed distal small bowel. Despite these latter limitations, an UGI can be extremely helpful in confirming and delineating small bowel obstruction from internal herniation.

CT is the best diagnostic test for diagnosis of internal herniation. A recent study[98] looked at the usefulness of seven specific CT signs in the prediction of internal herniation:

1) the swirled appearance of mesenteric fat or vessels at the root of the mesentery (swirl-sign);
2) presence of small-bowel obstruction;
3) clustering of small bowel loops;
4) mushroom shape of the herniated mesenteric root with crowding and stretching of the mesenteric vessels;
5) tubular or round shape of distal mesenteric fat closely surrounded by bowel loops;

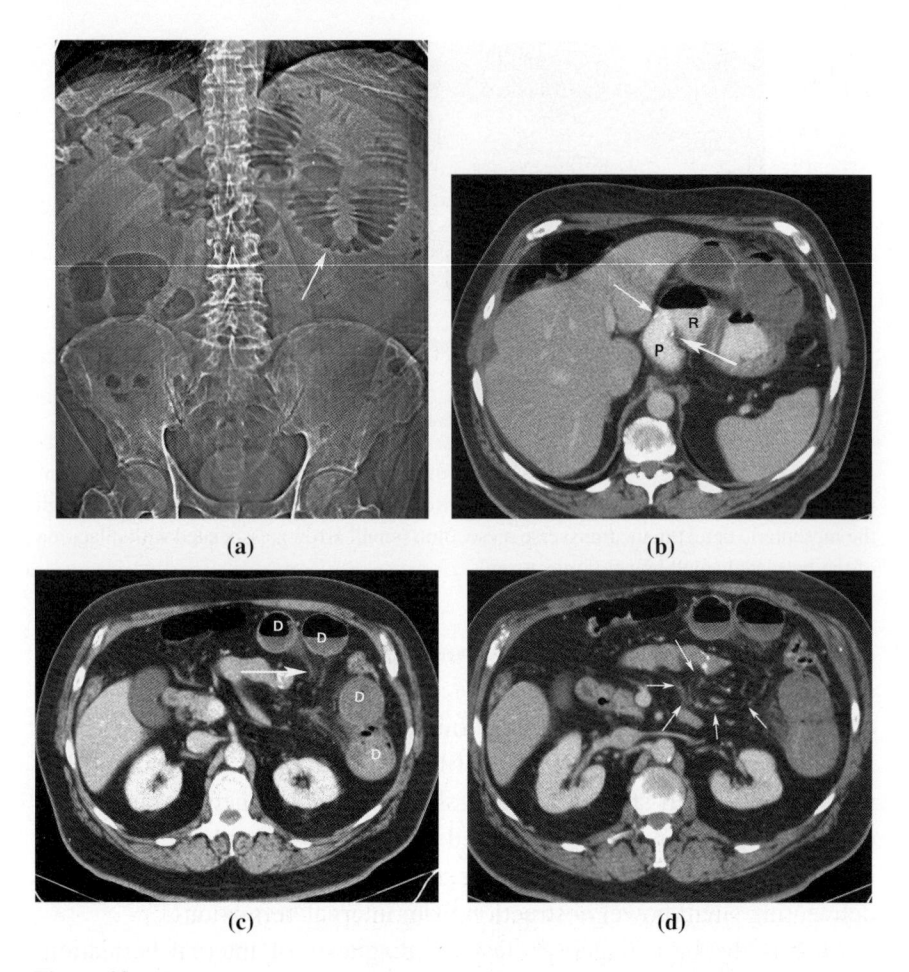

Figure 32. Transmesocolonic herniation proved at surgery. Oral and intravenous contrast material enhanced axial CT of the abdomen: (a) scout film from the study shows dilated loops of small bowel occupying the left upper quadrant of the abdomen (arrow); (b) an axial image through the upper abdomen shows dilated gastrojejunostomy anastomosis (arrows) due to obstruction; (c) engorged blood vessels (arrow) are seen in the mesentery of the herniated small bowel; (d) there is crowding and swirling of blood vessels in the root of the mesentery (arrows), at the site of herniation through the transverse mesocolon. P = Pouch, R = Roux limb, D = Dilated obstructed herniated small bowel.

6) small bowel other than duodenum passing posterior to the superior mesenteric artery;
7) right-sided location of distal jejunal anastomosis.

Of these, the 'swirl' sign was the most sensitive and single most useful sign in the diagnosis of internal herniation (Fig. 32). The addition of the 'mushroom' sign (Fig. 26) — the appearance of the herniated bowel mesentery and its vessels traversing the hernial defect — increased the sensitivity of the diagnosis. All the other signs were highly specific but poorly sensitive. Another specific but poorly sensitive indicator called the 'pinch sign' has also been described where the herniating bowel is pinched by the surrounding hernial defect (Fig. 30).[100]

The typical CT findings of small bowel obstruction due to internal herniation would include:

1) proximally situated fluid/contrast filled dilated oesophagus and pouch;
2) clustered fluid/contrast filled dilated loops of small bowel at the left upper to mid abdomen, corresponding to the internally herniated bowel undergoing closed loop obstruction;
3) distally collapsed poorly opacified small bowel loops situated predominantly at the right lower quadrant of abdomen/pelvis.

The findings of the 'swirl' and 'mushroom' signs would increase the diagnostic confidence. The presence of mesenteric congestion (increased fat attenuation) and peritoneal fluid will be determined by the grade and chronicity of obstruction. The finding of bowel wall pneumatosis and free intraperitoneal gas would be suggestive of bowel necrosis and perforation, respectively.

Specific CT features have been described to help with diagnosis of particular types of internal hernias. In cases of transmesocolic herniation, herniated small bowel is located posterior to the stomach and may exert a mass effect on its posterior wall.[7,94] In addition, the findings of a high riding jejunojejunal anastomosis may also point to this diagnosis.[100] With the transmesenteric hernia, clustered bowel is found pressed against the anterior abdominal wall with no overlying omental fat, causing central displacement of the colon. The Petersen hernia is difficult to diagnose because it has neither a confining sac nor a characteristic location, and its presence may be obvious only from the finding of engorgement and crowding of the mesenteric vessels and presence of small-bowel obstruction.[7,94]

Despite the above pointers, in actual practice it is difficult to distinguish between these various hernias with certainty, as the various hernial defects are very close to each other with little distinguishing features between them. Happily, excruciating efforts to make such fine distinction are not necessary, as it does not change clinical management. Once internal herniation is diagnosed, an experienced bariatric surgeon has to perform an exploratory laparotomy, 'run' the bowel, find which defect is causing the herniation, reduce the hernia and close the offending defect, as well as any other defects present.

When interpreting a CT in a RYGB patient with symptoms of small bowel obstruction, the primary concern of the radiologist is to determine whether a mechanical obstruction is present or not, and to diagnose any associated complications such as ischemia or perforation. Then, using the above-described imaging signs, the radiologist should be able to make a diagnosis of internal herniation with some degree of confidence. For the radiologist to obsess as to which of the three types of internal hernias is present is academically interesting but clinically unnecessary. In any centre where there is close cooperation between the surgeon and the radiologist, the surgeon should be able to reveal the exact diagnosis soon after surgery!

Intussusception

Intussusception after RYGB is an extremely rare complication and occurs almost exclusively at the jejunojejunal anastomosis.[101–105] It can be antegrade (isoperistaltic) or retrograde (antiperistaltic) in nature.[105] The aetiology remains unclear but is probably multifactorial involving a lead point (suture lines, adhesions, lymphoid hyperplasia)[103] motility disturbances,[101] and aberrant intestinal pacemakers.[106] It presents in the late postoperative period and so far has been only seen after open RYGB surgery.[105]

Patients can present with a range of symptomatology including nausea, retching vomiting, epigastric pain, intermittent diffuse abdominal pain, diarrhoea, and haematemesis. However, symptoms can be vague, physical examination nonspecific and patient condition stable with no toxicity.[105] Therefore, a high index of suspicion has to be maintained for early radiological evaluation and surgical intervention before severe complications of bowel necrosis and perforation occur.

CT is the first line imaging for the suspected diagnosis of intussusception.[106] It will show the characteristic target sign on transverse, and sausage-like appearance on the longitudinal sections taken along the centreline of the bowel. The finding of fat in the mesentery of the intussusceptum being dragged into the lumen of the intussuscipiens is diagnostic (Fig. 33). There is usually a fluid-filled dilation of the proximal Roux limb and pouch.

Bariatric surgery patients with intussusception invariably require reoperation to prevent life threatening complications. Therefore, the suspicion of intussusception on clinical or imaging grounds requires immediate consultation by an experienced bariatric surgeon. At exploratory laparotomy, the intussusception can be difficult to reduce and bowel infarction likely. The safest option might be en-bloc resection of the intussusception with reconstruction of the entire jejunojejunostomy.

Miscellaneous

Other complications after RYGB include incisional hernia, intra-abdominal abscesses unrelated to leak and liver/splenic infarctions.[53,62,67] The incidence of incisional hernia has decreased with the change from open to laparoscopic surgery, although this has brought its own complications with port-site hernias.[47] Intra-abdominal fluid collections and abscesses can occur unrelated to leaks in about 2 per cent of patients after RYGB.[6,69] Any suspicion of intra-abdominal sepsis should be investigated early using CT, as left undiagnosed can lead to multiorgan failure and death.[69]

Summary

Imaging is used in bariatric patients to evaluate the technical success of surgery, document baseline anatomy, and diagnose postoperative complications. The UGI series and CT are the most commonly used investigations for this purpose. Together they provide functional, dynamic and cross-sectional information that is sufficient to identify most postoperative complications. There should be a low threshold for performing

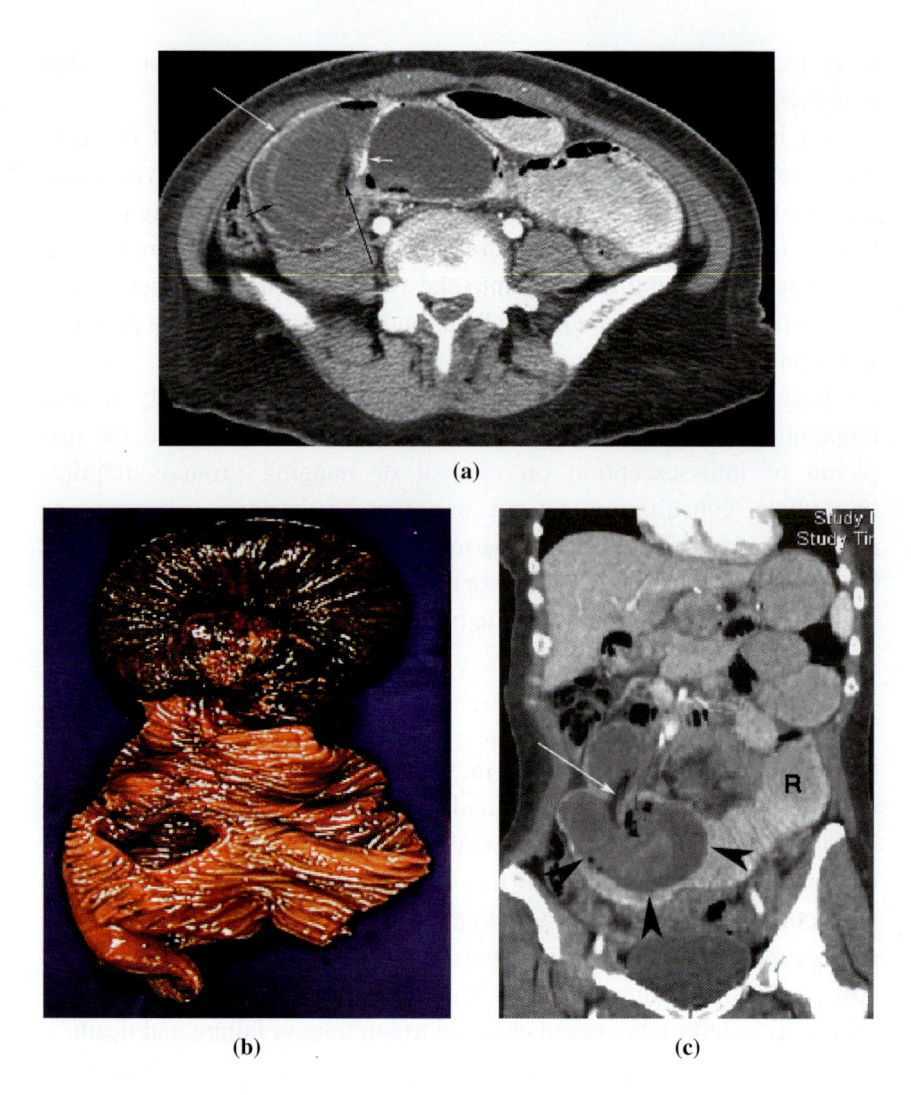

Figure 33. Retrograde intussusception at the Roux-en-Y anastomosis proved at surgery. Oral and intravenous contrast material enhanced CT abdomen: (**a**) axial CT through lower abdomen shows retrograde migration of distal jejunum (short black arrow) together with its mesentery (long black arrow) intussuscepting through the anastomosis (short white arrow) into the pancreaticobiliary limb (long white arrow); (**b**) coronal CT reconstruction shows the intussusceptum (arrow heads) and its mesenteric fat (arrow) more clearly. (**c**) Photograph of the en-bloc resection of the anastomosis shows the infarcted intussuscepted small bowel. R = Roux limb dilatation due to obstruction. Reprinted, with permission, from Farraye F.A. and Forse R.A. (eds).[49]

imaging in symptomatic patients, as early diagnosis can lead to lifesaving therapy.

Compared to the average subject, bariatric patients pose a greater diagnostic challenge to the radiologist due to their larger size. Therefore, robust imaging equipment[53] meticulous radiological technique and considerable interpreter expertise is required for diagnosis. Most importantly, any imaging finding should be interpreted in the light of the patient's clinical, laboratory and endoscopic findings in order to arrive at the most accurate diagnosis and the best management plan for the individual patient.

References

1. Schauer, P.R. (2003). Open and laparoscopic surgical modalities for the management of obesity. *J Gastrointest Surg* 7: 468–475.
2. Miller, K., Hell, E. (2003). Laparoscopic surgical concepts of morbid obesity. *Langenbecks Arch Surg* 388: 375–384.
3. Hocking, M.P., Davis, G.L., Franzini, D.A. *et al.* (1998). Long-term consequences after jejunoileal bypass for morbid obesity. *Dig Dis Sci* 43: 2493–2499.
4. Samuel, I., Mason, E.E., Renquist, K.E. *et al.* (2006). Bariatric surgery trends: an 18-year report from the International Bariatric Surgery Registry. *Am J Surg* 192: 657–662.
5. Wiesner, W., Schob, O., Hauser, R.S. *et al.* (2000). Adjustable laparoscopic banding in patients with morbid obesity: radiographic management, results and postoperative complications. *Radiology* 216: 389–394.
6. Blachar, A., Federle, M.P., Pealer, K.M. *et al.* (2002). Gastrointestinal complications of laparoscopic Roux-en-Y gastric bypass surgery: clinical and imaging findings. *Radiology* 223: 625–632.
7. Blachar, A., Federle, M.P. (2002). Gastrointestinal complications of laparoscopic Roux-en-Y gastric bypass surgery in patients who are morbidly obese: findings on radiography and CT. *AJR Am J Roentgenol* 179: 1437–1442.
8. Roy-Choudhury, S.H., Nelson, W.M., El Cast, J. *et al.* (2004). Technical aspects and complications of laparoscopic banding for morbid obesity — a radiological perspective. *Clin Radiol* 59: 227–236.

9. Parikh, M., Duncombe, J., Fielding, G.A. (2006). Laparoscopic adjustable gastric banding for patients with body mass index of < or = 35 kg/m^2. *Surg Obes Relat Dis* 2: 518–522.
10. Ponce, J., Paynter, S., Fromm, R. (2005). Laparoscopic adjustable gastric banding: 1,014 consecutive cases. *J Am Coll Surg* 201: 529–535.
11. Suter, M., Calmes, J.M., Paroz, A. et al. (2006). A 10-year experience with laparoscopic gastric banding for morbid obesity: high long-term complication and failure rates. *Obes Surg* 16: 829–835.
12. Belachew, M., Belva, P.H., Desaive, C. (2002). Long-term results of laparoscopic adjustable gastric banding for the treatment of morbid obesity. *Obes Surg* 12: 564–568.
13. Szucs, R.A., Turner, M.A., Kellum, J.M. et al. (1998). Adjustable gastric band for the treatment of morbid obesity: radiologic evaluation. *AJR Am J Roentgenol* 170: 993–996.
14. Fielding, G.A., Ren, C.J. (2005). Laparoscopic adjustable gastric band. *Surg Clin N Am* 85: 129–140.
15. Pretolesi, F., Camerini, G., Bonifacino, E. et al. (1998). Radiology of adjustable silicone gastric banding. *Br J Radiol* 71: 717–722.
16. Susmallian, S., Ezri, T., Charuzi, I. (2004). Dynamic radioisotope scintigraphy for gastric banding adjustment. *Obes Surg* 14: 520–523.
17. Dixon, J.B., O'Brien, P.E. (1999). Gastroesophageal reflux in obesity: the effect of lap-band placement. *Obes Surg* 9: 527–531.
18. Iovino, P., Angrisani, L., Tremolaterra, F. et al. (2002). Abnormal oesophageal acid exposure is common in morbidly obese patients and improves after a successful Lap-band system implantation. *Surg Endosc* 16: 1631–1635.
19. Klaus, A., Gruber, I., Westscher, G. et al. (2006). Prevalent oesophageal body motility disorders underlie aggravation of GERD symptoms in morbidly obese patients following adjustable gastric banding. *Arch Surg* 141: 247–251.
20. Wiesner, W., Hauser, M., Schob, O. et al. (2001). Pseudo-achalasia following laparoscopically placed adjustable gastric banding. *Obes Surg* 11: 513–518.
21. Dragnet, J. (2005). Oesophageal dilatation after laparoscopic adjustable gastric banding: definition and strategy. *Obes Surg* 15: 843–848.
22. Suter, M., Dorta, G., Giusti, V. et al. (2005). Gastric banding interferes with oesophageal motility and gastroesophageal reflux. *Arch Surg* 140: 639–643.

23. Angrisani, L., Lorenzo, M., Santoro, T. *et al.* (1999). Follow-up of Lap-Band complications. *Obes Surg* 9: 276–278.
24. Wiesner, W., Weber, M., Hayser, R.S. *et al.* (2001). Anterior versus posterior slippage: Two different types of eccentric pouch dilatation in patients with adjustable laparoscopic gastric banding. *Dig Surg* 8: 182–187.
25. Vertruyen, M. (2003). Repositioning the Lap-Band for proximal pouch dilatation. *Obes Surg* 13: 285–288.
26. Patel, S.M., Shapiro, K., Abdo, Z. *et al.* (2004). Obstructive symptoms associated with the Lap-Band in the first 24 hours. *Surg Endosc* 18: 51–55.
27. Bernante, P., Francini, F., Toniato, A. *et al.* (2005). Obstructive symptoms associated with the 9.75 cm Lap-Band in the first 24 hours using the pars flaccida approach. *Obes Surg* 15: 357–360.
28. Parameswaran, R., Ferrando, J., Sigurdsson, A. (2006). Gastric bezoar complicating laparoscopic adjustable gastric banding with band slippage. *Obes Surg* 16: 1683–1684.
29. Micheletto, G., Roviaro, G., Lattuada, E. *et al.* (2006). Adjustable gastric banding for morbid obesity. *Ann Ital Chir* 77: 397–400.
30. Hainaux, B., Agneessens, E., Rubesova, E. *et al.* (2005). Intragastric band erosion after laparoscopic adjustable gastric banding for morbid obesity: imaging characteristics of an underreported complication. *AJR Am J Roentgenol* 184: 109–112.
31. Abu–Abeid, S., Keidar, A., Gavert, N. *et al.* (2003). The clinical spectrum of band erosion following laparoscopic adjustable silicone gastric banding for morbid obesity. *Surg Endosc* 17: 861–863.
32. Rao, A.D., Ramalingham, G. (2006). Exsanguinating haemorrhage following gastric erosion after laparoscopic adjustable gastric banding. *Obes Surg* 16: 1675–1678.
33. Bueter, M., Thalheimer, A., Meyer, D. *et al.* (2006). Band erosion and passage, causing small bowel obstruction. *Obes Surg* 16: 1679–1682.
34. Pinsk, I., Dukhno, O., Levey, I. *et al.* (2004). Gastric outlet obstruction caused by total band erosion. *Obes Surg* 14: 1277–1279.
35. Pretolesi, F., Camerini, G., Gianetta, E. *et al.* (2001). Intraluminal penetration of the band in patients with adjustable silicone gastric banding: radiological findings. *Eur Radiol* 11: 412–416.

36. Wolnerhanssen, B., Kern, B., Peters, T. et al. (2005). Reduction in slippage with 11-cm Lap-Band and change of gastric banding technique. *Obes Surg* 15: 1050–1054.
37. Sherwinter, D.A., Powers, C.J., Geiss, A.C. et al. (2006). Posterior prolapse: an important entity even in the modern age of the pars flaccida approach to Lap-band placement. *Obes Surg* 16: 1312–1317.
38. Mittermair, R.P., Weiss, H.G., Nehoda, H. et al. (2003). Band leakage after laparoscopic adjustable gastric banding. *Obes Surg* 13: 913–917.
39. Wiesner, W., Hauser, M., Schob, O. et al. (2001). Spontaneous volume changes in gastric banding devices: complications of a semi permeable membrane. *Eur Radiol* 11: 417–421.
40. Keidar, A., Cameron, E., Szold, A. et al. (2005). Port complications following laparoscopic adjustable gastric banding for morbid obesity. *Obes Surg* 15: 361–365.
41. Favretti, F., Liberati, L., Curtolo, S. et al. (1997). Laparoscopic adjustable silicone gastric banding (LAP-BAND): how to avoid complications. *Obes Surg* 7: 352–358.
42. Chelala, E., Cadière, G.B., Favretti, F. et al. (1997). Conversions and complications in 185 laparoscopic adjustable silicone gastric banding cases. *Surg Endosc* 11: 268–271.
43. Srikanth, M.S., Oh, K.H., Keskey, T. et al. (2005). Critical extreme anterior slippage (paragastric Richter's hernia) of the stomach after laparoscopic adjustable gastric banding: early recognition and prevention of gastric strangulation. *Obes Surg* 15: 207–215.
44. Zappa, M.A., Lattuada, E., Mozzi, E. et al. (2006). An unusual complication of gastric banding: recurrent small bowel obstruction caused by the connecting tube. *Obes Surg* 16: 939–941.
45. Nemni, J. (2007). Severe chronic cough after Lap-Band gastric surgery. *Can Respir J.* 14: 171–172.
46. O'Brien, P.E., Dixon, J.B. (2002). Weight loss and early and late complications — the international experience. *Am J Surg* 184: 42–45.
47. Fobi, M.A.L., Hoil, L., Holness, R. et al. (1998). Gastric bypass operation for obesity. *World J Surg* 22: 925–935.
48. Schauer, P.R., Ikramuddin, S. (2001). Laparoscopic surgery for morbid obesity. *Surg Clin N Am* 81: 1145–1178.

49. Farraye, F.A. and Forse, R.A. (eds). (2006). *Bariatric Surgery: A Primer for Your Medical Practice*, Slack Incorporated, Thorofare, New Jersey, USA.
50. Scheirey, C.D., Scholz, F.J., Shah, P.C. et al. (2006). Radiology of the laparoscopic Roux-en-Y gastric bypass procedure: conceptualization and precise interpretation of results. *RadioGraphics* 26: 1355–1371.
51. Mason, E.E., Renquist, K.E., Huang, Y.H. et al. (2007). Causes of 30-day bariatric surgery mortality: with emphasis on bypass obstruction. *Obes Surg* 17: 9–14.
52. Raman, R., Raman, B., Raman, P. et al. (2007). Abnormal findings on routine upper GI series following laparoscopic Roux-en-Y gastric bypass. *Obes Surg* 17: 311–316.
53. Merkle, E.M., Hallowell, P.T., Crouse, C. et al. (2005). Roux-en-Y gastric bypass for clinically severe obesity: normal appearance and spectrum of complications at imaging. *Radiology* 234: 674–683.
54. Fisher, B.L., Schauer, P. (2002). Medical and surgical options in the treatment of severe obesity. *Am J Surg* 84: 9–16.
55. Ganci-Cerrud G., Herrera, M.G. (1999). Role of radiologic contrast studies in the early postoperative period after bariatric surgery. *Obes Surg* 9: 532–534.
56. Schauer, P.R., Ikramuddin, S., Gourash, W. et al. (2000). Outcomes after laparoscopic Roux-en-Y gastric bypass for morbid obesity. *Ann Surg* 232: 515–529.
57. Livingston, E.H., Ko, C.Y. (2002). Assessing the relative contribution of individual risk factors on surgical outcome for gastric bypass surgery: a baseline probability analysis. *J Surg Res* 105: 48–52.
58. DeMaria, E.J., Sugerman, H.J., Kellum, J.M. et al. (2002). Results of 281 consecutive total laparoscopic Roux–en–Y gastric bypasses to treat morbid obesity. *Ann Surg* 235: 640–645.
59. Buckwalter, J.A., Herbst, C.A. Jr (1980). Complications of gastric bypass for morbid obesity. *Am J Surg* 139: 55–60.
60. Buckwalter, J.A., Herbst, C.A. Jr (1988). Leaks occurring after gastric bariatric operations. *Surgery* 103: 156–160.
61. Carucci, L.R., Turner, M.A., Conklin, R.C. et al. (2006). Roux-en-Y gastric bypass surgery for morbid obesity: evaluation of postoperative extraluminal leaks with upper gastrointestinal series. *Radiology* 238: 119–127.

62. Flancbaum, L., Belsley, S. (2007). Factors affecting morbidity and mortality of Roux-en-Y gastric bypass for clinically severe obesity: an analysis of 1,000 consecutive open cases by a single surgeon. *J Gastrointest Surg* 11: 500–507.
63. Moffat, R.E., Peltier, G.L., Jewell, W.R. (1979). The radiological spectrum of gastric bypass complications. *Radiology* 132: 33–36.
64. Koehler, R.E., Halverson, J.D. (1982). Radiographic abnormalities after gastric bypass. *AJR Am J Roentgenol* 138: 267–270.
65. Serafini, F., Anderson, W., Ghassemi, P. et al. (2002). The utility of contrast studies and drains in the management of patients after Roux-en-Y gastric bypass. *Obes Surg* 12: 34–38.
66. Goodman, P., Halpert, R.D. (1991). Radiological evaluation of gastric stapling procedures for morbid obesity. *Crit Rev Diagn Imaging* 32: 37–67.
67. Yu, J., Turner, M.A., Cho, S.R. et al. (2004). Normal anatomy and complications after gastric bypass surgery: helical CT findings. *Radiology* 231: 753–760.
68. Marshall, J.S., Srivastava, A., Gupta, S.K. et al. (2003). Roux-en-Y gastric bypass leak complications. *Arch Surg* 138: 520–523.
69. Byrne, T.K. (2001). Complications of surgery for obesity. *Surg Clin North Am* 81: 1181–1193.
70. Lujan, J.A., Frutos, M.D., Hernandez, Q. et al. (2004). Laparoscopic versus open gastric bypass in the treatment of morbid obesity: a randomized prospective study. *Ann Surg* 239: 433–437.
71. Suter, M., Giusti, V., Heraief, E. et al. (2003). Laparoscopic Roux-en-Y gastric bypass: initial 2-year experience. *Surg Endosc* 17: 603–609.
72. Cottam, D., Lord, J., Dallal, R.M. et al. (2007). Medicolegal analysis of 100 malpractice claims against bariatric surgeons. *Surg Obes Relat Dis* 3: 60–66.
73. Nelson, L.G., Gonzalez, R., Haines, K. et al. (2006). Spectrum and treatment of small bowel obstruction after Roux-en-Y gastric bypass. *Surg Obes Relat Dis* 2: 377–383.
74. Schauer, M., Carrodeguas, L., Pinto, D. et al. (2006). Diagnosis and management of partial small bowel obstruction after laparoscopic antecolic antegastric Roux-en-Y gastric bypass for morbid obesity. *J Am Coll Surg* 202: 262–268.
75. Mason, E.E., Ito, C. (1967). Gastric bypass in obesity. *Surg Clin North Am* 47: 1345–1351.

76. Caruana, J.A., McCabe, M.N., Smith, A.D. et al. (2007). Risk of massive upper gastrointestinal bleeding in gastric bypass patients taking clopidogrel. *Surg Obes Relat Dis* 3: 443–445.
77. Madan, A.K., DeArmond, G., Ternovits, C.A. et al. (2006). Laparoscopic revision of the gastrojejunostomy for recurrent bleeding ulcers after past open revision gastric bypass. *Obes Surg* 16: 1662–1668.
78. Higa, K.D., Boone, K.B., Ho, T. (2000). Complications of Roux-en-Y gastric bypass: 1040 patients — what have we learned? *Obes Surg* 10: 509–513.
79. St Jean, M.R., Dunkle-Blatter, S.E., Petrick, A.T. (2006). Laparoscopic management of perforated marginal ulcer after laparoscopic Roux-en-Y gastric bypass. *Surg Obes Relat Dis* 2: 668.
80. Bramkamp, M., Muller, M.K., Wildi, S. et al. (2006). Perforated ulcer at the gastrojejunostomy: laparoscopic repair after Roux-en-Y gastric bypass. *Obes Surg* 16: 1545–1547.
81. Stellato, T.A., Crouse, C., Hallowell, P.T. (2003). Bariatric surgery: creating new challenges for the endoscopist. *Gastrointest Endosc* 57: 86–94.
82. Mittermair, R., Renz, O. (2007). An unusual complication of gastric bypass: perforated duodenal ulcer. *Obes Surg* 17: 701–703.
83. Higa, K.D., Boone, K.B., Ho, T. et al. (2000). Laparoscopic Roux–en–Y gastric bypass for morbid obesity: technique and preliminary results of our first 400 patients. *Arch Surg* 135: 1029–1033.
84. Matthews, B.D., Sing, R.F., DeLegge, M.H. et al. (2000). Initial results with a stapled gastrojejunostomy for the laparoscopic isolated Roux-en-Y gastric bypass. *Am J Surg* 179: 476–481.
85. Steele, K., Schweitzer, M., Lidoe, A. et al. (2006). Unusual case of gastric bezoar causing obstruction after Roux-en-Y gastric bypass. *Surg Obes Relat Dis* 2: 536–537.
86. Pinto, D., Carrodeguas, L., Soto, F. et al. (2006). Gastric bezoar after laparoscopic Roux-en-Y gastric bypass. *Obes Surg* 16: 365–368.
87. Jha, S., Levine, M.S., Rubesin, S.E. et al. (2006). Detection of strictures on upper gastrointestinal tract radiographic examinations after laparoscopic Roux-En-Y Gastric bypass surgery: importance of projection. *AJR Am J Roentgenol* 186: 1090–1093.
88. Ahmad, J., Martin, J., Ikramuddin, S. et al. (2003). Endoscopic balloon dilation of gastroenteric anastomotic stricture after laparoscopic gastric bypass. *Endoscopy* 35: 725–728.

89. Spaulding, L. (1977). The impact of small bowel resection on the incidence of stomal stenosis and marginal ulcer after gastric bypass. *Obes Surg* 7: 485–487.
90. Szomstein, S., Kaidar-Person, O., Naberezny, K. et al. (2006). Correlation of radiographic and endoscopic evaluation of gastrojejunal anastomosis after Roux-en-Y gastric bypass. *Surg Obes Relat Dis* 2: 617–621.
91. Cho, M., Pinto, D., Carrodeguas, L. et al. (2006). Frequency and management of internal hernias after laparoscopic antecolic antegastric Roux-en-Y gastric bypass without division of the small bowel mesentery or closure of mesenteric defects: review of 1400 consecutive cases. *Surg Obes Relat Dis* 2: 87–91.
92. Higa, K.D., Ho, T., Boone, K.B. (2003). Internal hernias after laparoscopic Roux en-Y gastric bypass: Incidence, treatment and prevention. *Obes Surg* 13: 350–354.
93. Onopchenko, A. (2005). Radiological diagnosis of internal hernia after Roux en- Y gastric bypass. *Obes Surg* 15: 606–611.
94. Blachar, A., Federle, M.P., Dodson, S.F. (2001). Internal hernia: clinical and imaging findings in 17 patients with emphasis on CT criteria. *Radiology* 218: 68–74.
95. Capella, R.F., Iannace, V.A., Capella, J.F. (2006). Bowel obstruction after open and laparoscopic gastric bypass surgery for morbid obesity. *J Am Coll Surg* 203: 328–335.
96. Paroz, A., Calmes, J.M., Giusti, V. et al. (2006). Internal hernia after laparoscopic Roux-en-Y gastric bypass for morbid obesity: a continuous challenge in bariatric surgery. *Obes Surg* 16: 1482–1487.
97. Garza, E. Jr, Kuhn, J., Arnold, D. et al. (2004). Internal hernias after laparoscopic Roux-en-Y gastric bypass. *Am J Surg* 188: 796–800.
98. Lockhart, M.E., Tessler, F.N., Canon, C.L. et al. (2007). Internal hernia after gastric bypass: sensitivity and specificity of seven CT signs with surgical correlation and controls. *AJR Am J Roentgenol* 188: 745–750.
99. Filip, J.E., Mattar, S.G., Bowers, S.P. et al. (2002). Internal hernia formation after laparoscopic Roux-en-Y gastric bypass for morbid obesity. *Am Surg* 68: 640–643.
100. Reddy, S.A., Yang, C., McGinnis, L.A. et al. (2007). Diagnosis of transmesocolic internal hernia as a complication of retrocolic gastric bypass: CT imaging criteria. *AJR Am J Roentgenol* 189: 52–55.

101. Hocking, M.P., McCoy, D.M., Vogel, S.B. *et al.* (1991). Antiperistaltic and isoperistaltic intussusception associated with abnormal motility after Roux-en-Y gastric bypass: a case report. *Surgery* 110: 109–112.
102. Goverman, J., Greenwald, M., Gellman, L. *et al.* (2004). Antiperistaltic (retrograde) intussusception after Roux-en-Y gastric bypass. *Am Surg* 70: 67–70.
103. Duane, T.M., Wohlgemuth, S., Ruffin, K. (2000). Intussusception after Roux-en-Y gastric bypass. *Am Surg* 66: 82–84.
104. Majeski, J., Fried, D. (2004). Retrograde intussusception after Roux-en-Y gastric bypass surgery. *J Am Coll Surg* 199: 988–989.
105. Edwards, M.A., Grinbaum, R., Ellsmere, J. *et al.* (2006). Intussusception after Roux-en-Y gastric bypass for morbid obesity: case report and literature review of rare complication. *Surg Obes Relat Dis* 2: 483–489.
106. Huang, B.Y., Warshauer, D.M. (2003). Adult intussusception: diagnosis and clinical relevance. *Radiol Clin North Am* 41: 1137–1151.

Chapter 10

Sequential Treatment of Obesity

*Maurizio De Luca, Luca Busetto,
Gianni Segato and Franco Favretti*

Introduction

The first laparoscopic procedure was undertaken in 1990, and this new approach was to influence the future of obesity surgery. Behind laparoscopy there is a new philosophy consisting in the evaluation of the risk/benefits ratio for each operation, related to the individual patient, and at the same time, a renewed respect for anatomy and physiology. So, the future of obesity is related to these concepts: laparoscopy, risk/benefits ratio, respect for anatomy and physiology. In a single phrase: quality of life.

Everybody knows that obesity is a global problem of epidemic proportions and morbid obesity can at present be treated only by surgery. There is now international agreement about the indications and contraindications for bariatric surgery. At the same time, despite knowledge of physiology and hundreds of international congresses, general disagreement about the choice of bariatric operation remains.

There is a grey zone in which the surgeon uses his experience, knowledge and the technology of his hospital to decide the best operation for a specific patient. So, day by day, it is becoming clear that obesity surgery is developing a philosophy.

Classification of Bariatric Operation

In the short history of bariatric surgery many tens of operations have been proposed, but most of them were not carried out because of the poor efficacy of the procedure, or due to concerns over serious co-morbidities.

At present, the most performed bariatric operations are:

(a) *Restrictive*: vertical banded gastroplasty Mason; vertical banded gastroplasty MacLean; sleeve gastrectomy; gastric banding.
(b) *Malabsorptive*: biliopancreatic diversion Scopinaro; duodenal switch sleeve gastrectomy;[1,2] duodenal switch with gastric restriction and preservation.[3]
(c) *Mixed*: gastric bypass.

All the above-mentioned operations can be performed by laparoscopy, and research and technology are opening up to surgeons the possibility of other laparoscopic and endoscopic procedures. These new approaches have still to be defined, and some of them need further clinical trials in order to clarify the best indications for their use. These approaches are:

(a) *Endoscopical*: intragastric balloon, endobarrier and POSE (Primary Obesity Surgery Endoluminal);[4]
(b) *Electrical stimulation*: gastric pacing,[5] vagal stimulation;[6]
(c) *Surgical*: LAP-BAND® + duodenal switch with ('Bandinaro'),[7] functional gastric bypass,[8] sleeve gastrectomy.[3,5]

Effectiveness/Invasiveness of Various Operations

The scientific community has accepted that the effectiveness of bariatric operations cannot be evaluated only in terms of weight lost. Other parameters should be considered. The Bariatric Analysis and Report Outcome System (BAROS),[9] for example, considers weight loss and the impact of weight loss on co-morbidities and quality of life. It is a complete and well standardized method.

Effectiveness is expressed in terms of percentage excess weight loss (EWL) because almost all results are expressed in this manner in the literature. Table 1 shows the effectiveness of various surgical techniques based on results in the literature in terms of percentage EWL.

Table 1. Effectiveness (percentage EWL) of the various surgical techniques currently available.

Risk of operation	% EWL
Intragastric Balloon (BIB)	25
Gastric Pacing	25
Lap-Band	50
Vertical Banded Gastroplasty (Mason)	55
Vertical Banded Gastroplasty (MacLean)	60
"Functional" Gastric Bypass	70
Duodenal Switch + Lap-Band (Bandinaro)	75
Gastric Bypass	75
Bilio Pancreatic Diversion	80
Duodenal Switch + Gastric Tubulisation	80

Then, evaluating the above-mentioned procedures laparoscopically (obviously only the intragastric balloon is performed by endoscopy) and evaluating the invasiveness of the operations, we indicate risk values according to the literature in Table 2.

Scoring from 0 to 4, the parameters considered in Table 2 are: general anaesthesia, incisions and/or suture of gastro-intestinal tract, anatomical and/or functional reversibility and morbidity.

Figure 1 evaluates both effectiveness (percentage EWL) and risk score of various operations.

'Operations with more effectiveness are operations with more risk'.

Undertreatment and Overtreatment

The literature illustrates the interesting similarities of any specific operation, when the general features of the patients (age, weight, BMI, weight loss, co-morbidities) are taken into account. In particular, operations with more effectiveness also have a higher risk.

Laparoscopic gastric banding, for example, has a huge diffusion worldwide (300,000 implantations) with percentage EWL of 45–55 and good results in 75–80 per cent of cases.

Evaluating these results in a different manner, we could say that the majority of patients has a good experience with LAP-BAND®, while

Table 2. Risk score of the various surgical techniques currently available.

Operation	General anesthesia	Invasiveness opening G.I. tract	Anatomical reversibility	Functional reversibility	Morb	Risk score
Intragastric Balloon (BIB)	0	0	0	—	0	0
Gastric Pacing	1	0	0	—	0	1
Lap-Band	1	0	0	—	1	2
Vertical Banded Gastroplasty (Mason)	1	1	—	1	2	5
Vertical Banded Gastroplasty (MacLean)	1	2	—	1	2	6
"Functional" Gastric Bypass	1	3	—	1	3	8
Duodenal Switch + Lap Band (Bandinaro)	1	3	—	1	3	8
Gastric Bypass	1	3	—	1	4	9
Bilio Pancreatic Diversion	1	4	—	1	4	10
Duodenal Switch + Gastric Tubulisation	1	4	—	1	4	10

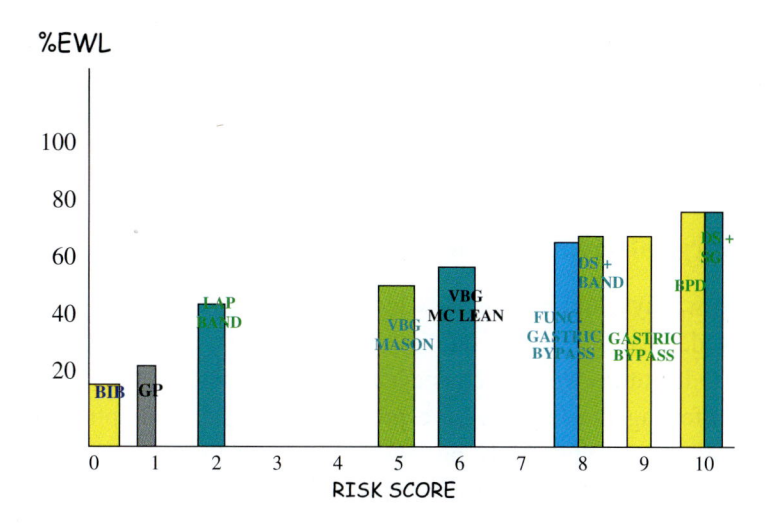

%EWL

[Bar chart showing effectiveness vs risk score]

BIB = Bioenterics Intragastric Balloon™
GP = Gastric Electrostimulation
LAP-BAND™ = Laparoscopic Gastric Banding
VBG MASON = Vertical Banded Gastroplasty (Mason)
VBG MACLEAN = Vertical Banded Gastroplasty (MacLean)
FUNC GASTRIC BYPASS: Functional Gastric Bypass
DS + BAND = Lap-Band + Duodenal Switch ("Bandinaro")
GASTRIC BYPASS = Gastric Bypass
BPD = Bilio Pancreatic Diversion
DS + SG= Duodenal Switch + Sleeve Gastrectomy

Figure 1. Effectiveness (percentage EWL) and risk score of the various surgical techniques currently available. BIB = BioEnterics® Intragastric Balloon BIB®; BPD = biliopancreatic diversion; DS + BAND = duodenal switch + LAP-BAND® ('Bandinaro'); DS + SG = duodenal switch + sleeve gastrectomy; FGB = functional gastric bypass; GB = gastric bypass; GP[QA2a] = gastric pacing; LAP-BAND® = laparoscopic gastric banding; VBG MACLEAN = vertical banded gastroplasty MacLean; VBG MASON = vertical banded gastroplasty Mason.

20–25 per cent of patients has a surgical undertreatment, but in both groups of patients, the risk score is very low (Table 2, risk score 2).

On the other hand, though, 60–70 per cent of obese patients undergoing gastric bypass (Table 2, risk score 9) or biliopancreatic diversion (Table 2, risk score 10) undergo useless overtreatment.

So, the surgeon has to decide if the patient can be treated with a minimally invasive procedure (e.g. LAP-BAND®) with a failure rate of

20–25 per cent, or with a more invasive procedure like gastric bypass and/or biliopancreatic diversion risking an overtreatment in 60–70 per cent of cases. For this reason the decision over which bariatric procedure to select becomes a philosophical judgment.

Surgical Treatment of Obesity

Nowadays, and increasingly in the future, the aim of obesity surgery will be defined in terms of quality of life.

In future we will consider the effectiveness of the approach, always preferring the less invasive procedure. Surgical complications in obese patients are absolutely be avoided because the management of them is more difficult than in a normal weight patient.

The literature, for example, shows that laparoscopic gastric bypass in patients with BMI > 60 results in about 50 per cent of peri- and post-operative surgical complications (M. Gagner, *pers. comm.*, 2001); in these patients it would be useful to reduce the BMI before the gastric bypass operation. Nowadays we can reduce the initial BMI with a less invasive procedure, such as the insertion of an intragastric balloon (BioEnterics® Intragastric Balloon or BIB® which is now called Orbera in our series), which is then followed by laparoscopic gastric banding.[4]

In a high rate of patients (78 per cent in our experience) this sequential treatment could be considered definitive and that a further, more invasive operation, such as gastric bypass or biliopancreatic diversion, is useless.

For patients with a low rate of percentage EWL and/or lack of compliance to the LAP-BAND® (22 per cent of patients in our experience), an operation with more effectiveness and more risk will be indicated and surely more justified. In this case the weight loss, even if modest, will be useful in order to reduce peri- and post-operative complications related to the higher BMI of the patient.

In our opinion the higher sensitivity to quality of life and risk/benefits concepts, two important parameters already applied in every other field of surgery, will be applied by bariatric surgeons to the sequential treatment of obesity.

We think that in the future we will use the surgical options that we already have today in different ways. So, at the beginning of a surgical

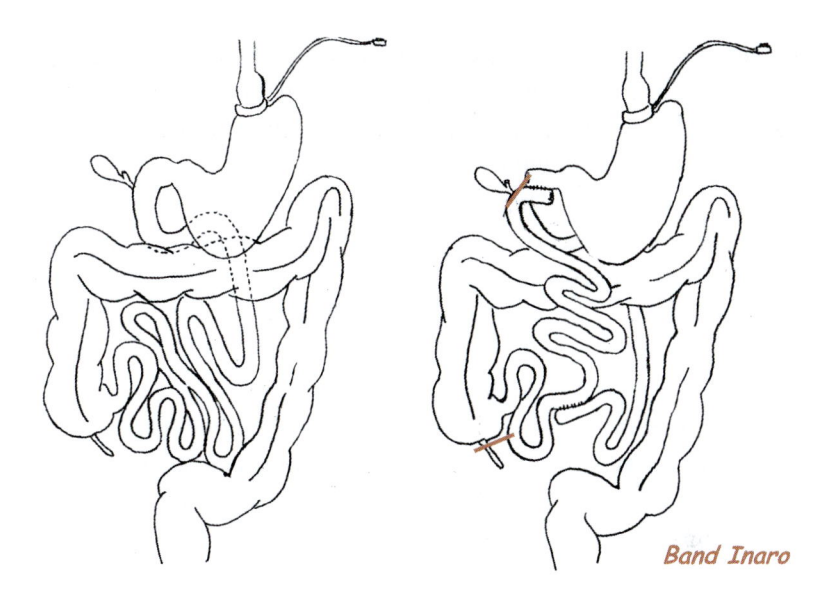

- Digestive loop = 200 cm.
- Common loop = 50 cm
- Bilio-pancreatic loop = remainder of small intestine

Figure 2. Bandinaro.

treatment, we usually perform the less invasive procedure with a good rate of effectiveness (2,245 LAP-BAND® patients in our series with 0 mortality), considering the second more invasive options (duodenal switch with gastric preservation or 'Bandinaro' in our series, Scopinaro procedure, gastric bypass or functional gastric bypass) only for patients for whom previous less invasive surgery has not given useful results. [9,10] Please see Fig. 2.

Conclusions

The future of bariatric surgery will be characterized by:

1. concepts of 'quality of life' and 'risk/benefits', which will influence the scientific community more and more;
2. the widespread use of a less invasive approach, such as laparoscopic gastric banding, due to the less invasive procedure;

3. some new techniques, already introduced, becoming more widespread (e.g. Bandinaro, functional gastric bypass, sleeve gastrectomy);
4. the intragastric balloon and gastric electrostimulation having a role in the sequential treatment of obesity;
5. consideration of the 'step by step' approach or 'sequential treatment of obesity', waiting for a sure indication that a specific operation is suitable for a specific patient.

References

1. Gagner, M., Rubino, F., Ren, C. (2000). Laparoscopic bilio-pancreatic diversion with duodenal switch: technical aspects. *Obes Surg* 10: 317–318.
2. Marceau, P., Hould, F.S., Simard, S. *et al.* (1998). Biliopancreatic diversion with duodenal switch. *World J Surg* 22 (9): 947–954.
3. Vassallo, C., Negri, L., Della Valle, A. *et al.* (1997). Bilio-pancreatic diversion with transitory gastroplasty preserving duodenal bulb: 3 yr experience. *Obes Surg* 7: 30–33.
4. Weiner, R., Gutberlet, L., Bockhorn, H. (1999). Preparation of extremely obese patients for laparoscopic gastric banding by gastric balloon therapy. *Obes Surg* 9(3): 261–264.
5. Shikora, S.A., Bessler, M., Fisher, B.L. *et al.* (2000). Laparoscopic insertion of the implantable gastric stimulator (IGS™): initial surgical experience. *Obes Surg* 10: 315.
6. De Luca, M., Segato, G., Busetto, L. (2004). Progress in implantable gastric stimulation. Summary of results of the European multicenter study. *Obes Surg* 14: S33–S39.
7. Cadière, G.B., Favretti, F., Himpens, J. *et al.* (2001). Anneau gastrique et derivation bilio-pancreatique par laparoscopie. *J Celio-Chir* 38: 33.
8. Furbetta, F., Gambinotti, G. (2002). Functional gastric bypass with an adjustable gastric band. *Obes Surg* 12: 876–880.
9. Favretti, F., Cadière, G.B., Segato, G. *et al.* (1998). Bariatric Analysis and Reporting Outcome System (BAROS) applied to laparoscopic gastric banding patients. *Obes Surg* 8: 500–504.
10. Favretti, F., Segato, G., Asthon, D. *et al.* (2007). Laparoscopic adjustable gastric banding in 1791 consecutive obese patients: 12-year results. *Obes Surg* 17: 168–175.

Chapter 11

Bariatric Surgery: When the Miracle is Not Enough

Melodie K. Moorehead

Introduction

For most patients, bariatric surgery is nothing short of an earthly miracle. Originally, bariatric surgery was intended for dangerously obese people. Currently, bariatric surgery also benefits non-obese people challenged with other metabolic issues, particularly diabetes. Most forms of bariatric or metabolic surgery impact the experience people have relating to food; as a result, it is the author's opinion that health-related psychological support is warranted for all people undergoing such surgery. This chapter, however, provides information that focuses on the role of psychology in a bariatric surgery programme for people suffering with severe obesity. The close of the chapter will highlight political actions that healthcare providers can take to help turn the tide of obesity throughout our world.

People who have been dangerously obese for years can shed hundreds of pounds after surgery; and often for the first time, these people feel welcomed by a society that had effectively shunned them all their lives.

Unfortunately, too often the weight-loss miracle alone is not enough. Bariatric surgery, although the nexus of successful treatment, is now recognized as foremost among other measures essential for effective, long-term treatment of morbid obesity.

New research provides compelling support for clinical and anecdotal evidence that, despite an initial dramatic weight loss, bariatric surgery is frequently challenged by the return of patients' former detrimental behaviour. Without a professionally managed long-term recovery programme predicated on pre- and post-operative mental health care, some patients suffer an undetected relapse, either by regaining weight or substituting hazardous coping behaviours, such as alcoholism, drug addiction, compulsive shopping or gambling. One key to widespread success after bariatric surgery is the effort made by the entire multi-disciplinary team of healthcare professionals. These are guided by a pathway of care intended for a long-term recovery programme involvement with a standardized methodology for measuring patient progress.

Increasingly, medical experts specializing in bariatric surgery are publicly acknowledging the need for a comprehensive psychological treatment programme managed by a mental healthcare expert trained to work with bariatric surgery patients. Professional medical organizations that have recognized the value of the bariatric mental health specialist include the American Society for Metabolic and Bariatric Surgery (ASMBS), formerly known as the American Society of Bariatric Surgery (ASBS), the International Federation of Surgery for Obesity (IFSO) and recently, the American College of Surgeons (ACS).

Research suggests that a professionally structured and managed recovery programme is an important key to successful long term surgical results. Typically, morbid obesity is a chronic disease shaped by years of what some patients refer to as 'addictive' behaviours, and it is common to hear participants in a programme characterize themselves as 'food addicts'. Although surgery can help bring about life-saving weight loss, medical improvement and a better quality of life, some patients' underlying psychological dynamics can undermine even the most encouraging short-term results. The return of deeply ingrained self-defeating attitudes can revive the destructive behaviours that first engendered or contributed to the disease of the patient's morbid obesity. (It is very important to be cautious when connecting addiction or addictive behaviours to morbid obesity because there is so much discrimination, prejudice and ignorance surrounding these subjects.)

Further support for a comprehensive mental healthcare programme is found in the increasing evidence that the disease of morbid obesity is partially driven by psychological dynamics — affective and physiological — similar to those known to characterize addiction. Salient among psychological factors is the potential of transference, a possibility that, in the absence of a return to overeating, patients may transfer or substitute their addictive approach to food to alcohol, substance abuse or other self-destructive behaviours.

The resurgence of life-long psychological habits can overwhelm even the powerful hope that arises when patients experience dramatic postoperative weight loss. Professional healthcare specialists must counsel patients beforehand in preparation for the potential emotional impact of surgery. Frequently, this approach helps avoid greater risk of shock and destruction should a relapse in behaviour occur.

The author's clinical experience suggests that the most promising post-operative outcome is seen when each patient's unique psychological profile is identified and incorporated in the very structure of postoperative care. This individualized regimen is then integrated into overarching guidelines of a standardized, multidisciplinary/interdisciplinary treatment programme. Once, the value of psychological services was limited to evaluating patients for surgery and predicting who would succeed or who would fail. This seems like a truncated view of psychological services because the inability to predict individual human behaviour, the value of the initial evaluation and the role of psychology, on a routine basis, has not been fully recognized. In fact, psychological services are of critical benefit, not only in enhancing patient compliance but also in ensuring a significant improvement in longer term quality of life.

Although research is referenced, this chapter does not attempt a comprehensive review of scientific findings. The author relies on relevant clinical data to elucidate the philosophy behind the research discussed here and better clarify assessment and treatment. Clinical data and observations draw upon a biomedical literature review and more than twenty years of clinical experience in the design and implementation of the psychological standardized protocol articulated by the author at ASMBS/ASBS and IFSO presentations. Hopefully, the information here will make it easier for medical professionals, as well as patients, their friends and loved ones, to understand and appreciate some of the challenges faced by bariatric surgery patients.

Results from a variety of bariatric procedures, including Vertical-Banded Gastroplasty, Roux-en-Y Gastric Bypass, Adjustable Banding and a clinical trial of Gastric Stimulator cases comprise the main body of the supporting data. The psychological sequelae of depression and destructive or addictive behaviours focus primarily on stress that is triggered by social factors, plus the patient's unique psychological characteristics. This includes the nature and extent of patient coping skills, as well as behaviours frequently observed in morbidly/super-obese people. The psychological impressions presented here are taken from direct practice or reflect collaborative research efforts over the last decade.

Bariatric Surgery is a Behavioural Surgery Too

Before discussing a basic recovery programme protocol that promotes a hopeful attitude in bariatric surgery patients, it is useful to describe in more detail the characteristics of this special patient population. Again, each recovery programme must be tailored to the individual, but to some extent, observed generalizations can be useful. Patients presenting for bariatric surgery are apt to be courageous, brave and complex. Often they have demonstrated the willpower to endure such humiliating treatments as jaw wiring and demanding regimes of self-imposed starvation diets in their efforts to control their obesity. Yet they can also be deeply troubled individuals suffering from negative family influences exacerbated by brutal social pressures. Additionally, profound alienation and addictive behaviours interact in complex and pernicious ways, making an integrated long-term psychological component essential within the multidisciplinary/interdisciplinary team approach for sustaining success after surgery. Bariatric surgery patients are a self-selecting minority among the countless people who might benefit from this procedure. Those who undergo bariatric surgery typically respond afterward with a powerful resurgence of hope as body weight falls away in the first period of recovery. The concept of recovery is a useful model in the work we, as healthcare specialists, do. Unfortunately, as specialists we recognize that the insidious disease of obesity cannot be cured by surgery alone. Thus, the concept of recovery work helps reduce the understandable yet defeating 'magical thinking' that some people often attribute to bariatric surgery. Furthermore, the basic concept of recovery empowers patients to address their involvement in the ongoing process of healing, and relinquish their false belief that surgery will do all the work. This sudden emotional rebirth taps into a wellspring of inner strength, often facilitating their commitment to a long-term psychologically oriented post-operative programme. Conversely, the persistence of denial after surgery quickly becomes a contributing factor to the disease, sometimes initiating a return to familiar counter-productive behaviours. This is one important reason why all the members of the team must share the philosophy and reinforce it to their patients. Literature reflects the clinical recognition that there is no archetypal obese personality. However, there are important similarities among obese patients, and these shared characteristics permit important generalizations for structuring treatment programmes for a variety of patients and surgical procedures. But over-generalization can be detrimental. Professionals cannot forget that each patient's unique psychological profile is a major factor in individual pre/post-operative planning.

Research and clinical experience suggests that the psychological dynamics of the morbidly/super-obese patient differ significantly from those observed among people who are less severely overweight or not overweight. While findings indicate that bariatric surgery patients are no more likely to suffer from serious conditions such as bipolar disorder or schizophrenia, affective disorders are more predictable, and increased intensity of conditions occurs as body mass index rises.

Emotional disorders such as depression and anxiety, and symptoms of somatization and the defence mechanisms of denial, distrust and loneliness occur with greater frequency among the morbidly obese. Some studies have reported that up to 95 per cent of morbidly obese patients described depressive symptoms matching those in the Diagnostic and Statistical Manual of Mental Disorder (DSM IV).[1] This is a startling number, especially since denial or other self-defence mechanisms frequently prevent patients from recognizing and reporting any signs of depression.

My European colleague, Elisabeth Ardelt-Gattinger PhD, and I have identified two potent factors affecting the beliefs, attitudes and behaviours of severely obese and super-obese individuals seeking surgical treatment. For those interested in greater detail and the history of this line of discussion, please refer to www.bariatrictimes.com and the two-part article by Moorehead and Alexander.[2,3] Briefly, while validating the Moorehead–Ardelt

Quality of Life Questionnaire[4] (MA II) and researching what we call the addiction component contributing to the disease of obesity, we confirmed the presence of the self-descriptive 'craving' and 'inability to control' factors.

These correspond to two of the three factors described in the well known 'Three Factor Eating Inventory'[5] developed by American psychiatrists and psychologists, Drs Albert Stunkard and Samuel Messick. The factors that they call 'hunger' and 'disinhibition' are consistently similar to our own 'craving' and 'inability-to-control'. In both cases these factors speak to patients' feelings about being hungry and about a perceived inability to resist the sight or tempting smells of food.

The real surprise was the absence of a correlation between the 'craving' and 'inability to control' factors, and Stunkard and Messick's third factor, 'cognitive restraint'. This indicated to us that for the morbidly/super-obese patient seeking surgery, experiencing 'craving' and 'inability to control' food consumption was an affective reaction — a response to their feelings, and emotions, rather than rational, cognitive thought processes.

The comparative ineffectiveness of conscious, cognitive efforts may explain why attempts to control eating behaviour through 'will' alone often fail. Such failure invariably exacerbates patients' psychological distress. The healthcare professional needs to make it clear to patients that all those dramatic vows to reform were doomed before given voice simply because conscious mental processes are not really in control here. Understanding even this much may allow patients, some for the first time, to stop blaming themselves for 'lack of willpower' or 'failing to face reality'. Such self-accusations are commonplace and are apt to deepen patients' shame for having failed to control deadly obesity 'on their own'. Similarly, acknowledging the limitations of conscious resolutions may relieve patients of shame for 'taking the easy way out' by choosing surgery. For that matter, the surgical route may not seem all that easy after the patient and family members realize that it implies a lifetime commitment to a rigorous recovery support programme.

Reduction or removal of shame is highly desirable when working with the severely/super-obese person. We need to understand the maturation and development of our patients in order to appreciate how their thoughts can trigger dangerously negative thought processes in the affective response system of the brain.

Many of our bariatric surgery patients have been obese since childhood and it is commonly known that obese children receive less attention and affection from caregivers, parents and teachers than do their leaner siblings and friends. Studies also suggest that obese children easily learn to dislike or even hate themselves because of the cultural prejudice and discrimination linked to severe obesity.

Research conducted by Stunkard and Wadden[6] underscored this self-hatred. In their study, they showed young children silhouettes of an obese child and asked them to describe the person portrayed by the image. The subjects described the child represented by the silhouette as 'lazy, dirty, stupid, ugly, cheats and liars.' Then drawings of children of various weights and disfigurements were shown to a variety of audiences, both adult and children. The audience, including obese people, rated the drawing of the obese child 'least likeable'.

We also know from research that the highest depression scores on pre-surgery, written psychological tests come from adults who have been obese since early childhood. Scores decrease somewhat among those who became obese in middle childhood and adolescence. The lowest depression scores were found among those who were adults at the onset of obesity. Interestingly, this stair-step of test results also occurs in preliminary findings on 'addiction factor' or 'inability to control' scales currently under investigation.

Consistently high depression scores coincide with a high frequency of reports of childhood abuse among obese patients. Research gathered and analysed, then reported at professional international bariatric conferences, identifies that fully two thirds of gastric-bypass patients report early childhood abuse. Further, a third of these same patients stated that they grew up in, or currently reside in a household permeated with alcoholism.

Add to this complex psychological background a credible genetic component, and it becomes clear that surgery alone cannot address the multiple contributing factors of this disease. Bariatric surgery is a behavioural surgery.

Although the psychological genesis of obesity varies, many patients typically develop in childhood (some in their pre-verbal state of development) what might be usefully described as a negative 'diet of thoughts'. Self-defeating mental refrains ('I'm not good enough, not lovable enough, not deserving enough of attention to meet my needs, etc.') can starve even the staunchest heart. Such psychological deprivation must be supplanted by a solid sense of inner fulfilment or, as I call it, psychological satiety, if the patient is to succeed beyond initial weight loss following bariatric surgery.

As soon as possible, patients must be fully apprised of the psychological hurdles that are intimately bound into this kind of surgical procedure, and be fully aware of the issues related to why eating for reasons other than physical hunger must be confronted early on. Literature is beginning to point out that pro-active transformational coping skills typically must be learned and actively practised if they are to replace eating as a way to manage chronic or acute stress.

Among the most pressing issues is a discussion of patients' motives for eating. Many pre-operative bariatric patients report that they eat for reasons other than physical hunger or a visceral need for satiety. Patients must quickly come to terms with the fact that weight loss, and more importantly weight loss maintenance, requires a lifetime commitment to all recovery programme guidelines. From the start, prospective patients are wise to understand that this means acknowledging and taking responsibility for their decisions, choices and lifestyle behaviours while also being reassured that neither perfectionism nor flawless adherence to guidelines are the desired behaviours.

Identifying negative self-fulfilling prophecies, e.g. 'I am not good enough, worthy enough ... etc.', or inability to put into place natural human legitimate rights such as, 'I have the right to put myself first sometimes or I have the right to say no without losing your love' are among the initial tasks for the mental health care professional. It is best to start this process before surgery and it is also an integral part of the post-operative programme. Fortunately, teaching the patient how to acquire a 'taste' for a healthier diet of thoughts can help derail such self-defeating mantras.

In an integrated, multidisciplinary/interdisciplinary team, patients receive psychological support during each follow-up visit to the surgeon's office, yet the preponderance of the mental health professional's job occurs in the period of time preceding surgery, when patients are highly motivated, and just after surgery — the time when the patient can be most vulnerable and receptive to supportive behavioural and conceptual changes. The optimal time to come to terms with obesity's most powerful psychological currents is between the first preoperative psychological evaluation and the first eighteen months immediately after surgery. The bariatric team has an opportunity to help patients address their most repetitious psychological issues at this time. Challenged patients who have not learned alternative, healthy ways of coping with stress are at risk of returning to a pre-operative, regressive style of eating. Often patients must learn new ways to manage their feelings, as well as the changing demands of ongoing relationships. Counter-productive hunger behaviours are apt to resurface even though patients' newly constructed bodies may report feeling physical satiety. Ultimately, cognitive recognition of the consequences of regressive coping behaviours does not deter patients as long as underlying emotional issues remain intact.

Before surgery, the patient gains a cognitive understanding of the need to find new ways to feel 'full or satisfied'. After surgery, guided by the mental health professional on the recovery team, the patient must learn *how* to satisfy the need for emotional, psychological satiety by means other than food consumption. The successful bariatric patient may develop a motto such as, 'I eat to live, rather than, I live to eat'. Such maxims become part of the healthy 'diet of thoughts', a key ingredient for a successful long-term recovery programme.

Initial patient evaluations include a section that offers psycho-education and post-operative objectives focused on an action-oriented replacement of negative thoughts or behaviours with more appropriate positive ones. Clearly, this requires the skill and commitment of a well-trained mental health care professional. In this way, the mental health specialist provides a valuable role not only to the patients, but also to the integrated team whose time is thereby freed from this needed focus, which in turn helps them address other necessary medical issues often faced by bariatric patients.

The healing psychological milieu most helpful to bariatric surgery patients and their loved ones is dynamic in nature, founded on relationship and rapport. Cognitive, affective, behavioural, somatic and even spiritual methods (medical hypnosis, desensitization, relaxation/breathing and body therapies) can be tailored to patients' maturational needs. Given the nature of modern culture, patients' personal history, their strengths and distress (e.g. stigmatization and isolation) and the consequent specific maturational needs, all therapeutic exchanges can provide a full range of potential interventions to be used for effective treatment. An effective mental health specialist will be familiar with a wide range of therapeutic methodologies; however, a key element becomes the purposeful use of authentic empathy and genuine warmth in the doctor/patient exchange. This requires the conscious planning and implementation of a 'good parent' transferential treatment environment. Responding in what is known in psychology as an anaclitic response, or a 'good parent' manner, rather than in a reactive authoritative fashion, will evidence a more useful approach with this particular patient population. Throughout the programme, a strong structural consistency in a multidisciplinary/interdisciplinary learning model will contribute to positive healing since some patients may attempt a necessary and needed recapitulation of their original family dynamics. A good bariatric programme will provide an environment where emotional healing can take place in every setting and discipline visited.

A Holistic Approach to Bariatric Surgery: Recovery Managed by Healthcare Specialists

A brief overview of the role and benefits of bariatric surgery psychology includes a description of a holistic approach to treatment and the crucial role played by the professional mental health specialist within the context of a multidisciplinary or interdisciplinary team.

The current literature review of bariatric surgical outcomes, where a broad spectrum of care was implemented, shows an admirable record of short-term success and some successful long-term outcomes. True successes deserve full marks. But what constitutes success? For that matter, do patients and bariatric teams define success or failure in the same way? These questions will be addressed shortly. Right now I would like to express what I consider a 'Best Practice of Care Model' that drives positive long-term outcomes and delivers services to bariatric surgery patients and their loved ones.

Throughout my professional travels, I have had privileged exposure to the emotional aspect of care provided within bariatric programmes particularly in the United Sates, Brazil, Europe and Japan. The emotional support provided to patients within these programmes has included, among other important medical services, the education of patients before surgery. This includes attentive and positive support offered both pre- and post-operatively by talented, often over-worked nurses and nutritionists, along with routine visits by the surgeons' or physicians' assistant at various prescribed intervals of time. Additionally, medical personnel within the programme may provide referrals for psychological evaluations or, when needed, suggest individual psychological treatment outside of the programme. Fortunately, our bariatric community has increasingly seen more hospitals and surgically based programmes provide in-house psychological evaluations and brief ongoing psychoeducational and behavioural support, on both a pre- and post-operative basis.

Unfortunately, this improving model of care is not universal. Throughout the world, treatment before and after bariatric surgery still varies widely. So do long-term outcome results. Even when recovery is carefully monitored using a standardized method of measuring patient progress, the full value of a professionally designed psychological recovery programme is yet to be fully appreciated. Well planned programmes need to be administered by a multidisciplinary/interdisciplinary team that includes at least one professional mental health care specialist.

The concept of a team approach is crucial, and we have primarily used a multidisciplinary model of care. A multidisciplinary team programme may have all the necessary team players involved in the basic care of the surgical patients, yet all team members primarily work in ways independent from each other, and perhaps communicate by written reports or progress/chart notes in the medical record or even have brief telephone conferences for more urgent matters. I have worked in this multidisciplinary manner with several wonderful bariatric surgeons; however, it is my experience that all parties involved are served to a higher degree in an integrated interdisciplinary programme of care. I suggest that this interdisciplinary team model be regarded as a gold standard toward which we strive. This model, when implemented with good leadership, provides the optimal recovery methodology and environment to work, while providing services that offer observable standards and results for measuring patients' values through communication.

Communication and superior co-ordination of care distinguishes this team approach. While pre-surgery preparation and post-surgical recovery are typically monitored by a variety of medical specialists, a designated professional manager or director can aid this team approach. This specialist, whether identified as a manager, director or coordinator, ensures that the different service providers develop a *shared understanding of each patient and their goals and coordinate an agreed-upon plan of care*. This individual coordinates and directs the unified team while maintaining fiscally sound business practices and functioning as the liaison to head administrators and Chief Executive Officer of the hospital or clinic. Each specialist has an essential role, and each reinforces the team's overall shared care goals to support the patient. Team members are aware of and emphasize to patients the inter-connectedness among the different clinical specialties — surgery, nursing, physical activity, nutrition and psychology — all members of the team including the patient, pulling together in the same direction and *under one roof*.

Psychologists are well suited to the advanced specialty training and delivery of services to the bariatric surgery patient population, though psychiatrists, psychiatric nurses and social workers have also proved invaluable to a comprehensive programme. Key characteristics of a skilled mental health specialist include empathy, authenticity, passion, willingness to learn and a solid understanding for the needs of the severely obese people seeking surgical intervention, and their loved ones.

Paramount is the specialist's ability to reflect deeply and to inventory meticulously his/her prejudices regarding this insidious disease. Above all, professionals must never pathologize their patients. Clinical interviews routinely show that many patients attempt twenty or more diet programmes before seeking bariatric surgery. Such strength of character may bode well for a commitment to a lifelong health maintenance programme that is properly administered by a sensitive team. However, clinical interviews also reveal quite honestly that many patients do not attempt earnest weight loss efforts before seeking bariatric surgery, or that when they do the effort is often short-lived and entered into without conviction. These people often foster a hidden belief that surgery will stop them from eating indefinitely, while finally bringing a sense of satisfaction and fulfilment to life. So while it is paramount to guard against personal prejudice, it is also essential not to attempt being politically correct by holding an erroneous belief that all bariatric patients are pioneering and courageous. Philosophically, to reverse a well-documented, long-standing trend of medical prejudice found against obese people, it might be useful to highlight and hold in mind a basic common denominator often identified in the motivation of bariatric candidates. Even for people who hold unrealistic expectations of surgery, core desires are to: prevent premature death, improve his/her medical condition and increase quality of life.

By recognizing through effective psychological evaluations those patients who might be unconsciously seeking the 'magic' of surgery, the team can focus on the underlying *healthy* motives for an improved life, while providing the needed adjuncts to surgery. This approach may help patients take greater responsibility in preparing realistically for their needed lifestyle changes. Pre-surgery classes for groups of bariatric surgery patients may further demystify the medical procedure and promote awareness of the value of building stress management skills and altering personal perceptions. Teaching people to feel empowered as they experience greater control of their lives will soften the changes in their relationship to food after surgery. Helping establish and strengthen patients' positive inner perceptions of themselves is of vital importance to 'changing the diet of thoughts' or inner dialogue to minimize self-sabotage and foster sustainable success following bariatric surgery.

Establishing a Three-Stage Psychoeducational Recovery Programme

Within the treatment team, the psychological professional must address a variety of issues recognized as common to many bariatric surgery patients before surgery, immediately following surgery and in the recovery years thereafter. One goal the author holds, that is yet to be an accepted norm of treatment, is to offer ongoing pre- and post-operative psycho-educational support. This level of attention can take different forms depending on how busy a particular practice is or on the degree of resources and personnel available. It has been reported that patients are often not motivated to attend their pre-surgery psychoeducational class, even when it is mandatory. For this plan to be viable and workable, in the real world, it would have to meet patients' true needs and the team would have to completely buy into its value. It is also recognized that healthcare professionals are sometimes called away on emergencies. To minimize any potential harm due to the interruption of routine care protocols, the following three conceptualized stages of programme care are offered as a flexible, best practice care recovery model:

1. The initial psychological, mental health or psycho-educational evaluation: specialized assessment tools and preoperative psychological recommendations may be offered that might advance the patient's safety and the efficacy of bariatric surgery;
2. In-hospital psychological support surrounding the surgical event: a wonderful means for enhancing the development of the therapeutic alliance because it helps people feel special and cared about during a very vulnerable time. After surgery, the psychological health care specialist's role changes somewhat from largely assessment and educational to one of active leadership, encouragement and support;
3. Over the course of the author's career this third step of specialized care has taken the form of routine brief (5–20 minute) post-operative follow-up sessions occurring directly in the surgeon's office or surgical programme's centre. Support may also take other forms such as offering six group classes before surgery, or several time limited one-on-one sessions after surgery, with the flexibility to include loved ones in any session. A comparatively new concept for high-volume practices is Shared Medical Appointments (SMAs). (Similar material may be provided in a different format of care.)[7] SMAs have been shown to offer patients and their loved ones prompt access to medical care. These ongoing contacts, regardless of the modality, are contained within the parameters of the full programme. They help keep patients ever mindful of their responsibility to alter their lifestyle, avoid behavioural choices that may interfere with healthy priorities, and practice stress management skills to improve self-care. Support group facilitation would be another duty of the mental healthcare

specialist. Having a provider who specializes in group-process dynamics is another invaluable way of improving patient compliance, encouraging programme attendance and helping patients stay on track. The above duties, when provided by the programme's mental health specialist, provide cost-effective services and save the time and energy of other team members. The other members of the interdisciplinary team are thereby freed to attend to other important matters of aftercare that are within their particular specialty. Under one roof, all these services become a routine for follow-up care as patients report to their surgeon or bariatric centre.

After a period of time, as strictly medical/surgical interventions and concerns fade, the psychologically oriented programme that enhances relationship development between patients and service providers will promote motivation for long-term follow-up, which can be the mainstay of recovery. In this type of setting, if need arises for a more intense form of psychological intervention, the clinical health-related, mental health specialist can provide referrals for individual, group or family psychotherapy.

A more detailed review of the three-stage system reveals that the first step focuses on both pre-surgical screening services for peri-operative psychological planning purposes and the development of adequate pre/post-operative psychosocial therapeutic support services. From the start, the mental healthcare professional creates an enduring climate of emotional healing. The principal goal is to facilitate patient cooperation and adjustment to long-range treatment goals. Further, the programme enhances sustainable quality-of-life modifications tailored to each patient's psychological characteristics, emotional vulnerability and detected obstacles or social withdrawal tendencies.

Before surgery, the programme emphasizes identifying patient's behaviours and attitudes that may lead to old behavioural habits. These habits often act as obstacles to the patient's identified goals. Once our patients become aware of the obstacles, positive choices that promote transforming old habits into new behaviours can be made. Ironically, though bariatric surgery is not, as some wags say, brain surgery, with this kind of mental health service in place, the desired bio/psycho/social medical changes can occur, giving the lie to this long-standing joke because the brain must change too. That is why it is paramount for us to accept that in part, bariatric surgery is a behavioural surgery. A harmful 'diet of thoughts' must be supplanted with a new way of thinking. This is not an easy task. The opposition is nothing less than chronic psychological co-morbidity. To overcome old habits and achieve behavioural and attitudinal changes, we must approach patients with comprehensive and pragmatic psychological programmes of care. Unsurprisingly, the best post-operative care begins with pre-operative care.

All members of the treatment team must understand that even making the decision to have bariatric surgery is transformational. For most patients, their mental health evaluation is the first chance they have to tell 'their story' fully to attentive listeners. And the team must be attentive because the weight-related challenges and losses endured while coming to this transformational decision can later be a source of strength for building upon much-needed future decisions and actions that will support overall recovery. Thus, the opportunity to detail one's history in a safe, non-judgmental environment with the support of an understanding specialist can be a pivotal step in the process of helping the patient let go of a life-long history of personal shame and self-blame.

Therefore, the initial evaluation is formulated on a broad psycho-educational model rather a narrower, traditional clinical psychological or psychiatric evaluation. In this context, the evaluation provides valuable patient education while simultaneously serving as a consultation to the bariatric surgeon and other team members. This evaluation is, for the entire team, more useful than the standard red light/green light checklist before surgery. An immediate advantage of the more detailed psycho-educational evaluation is the enhancement of the entire team's understanding of the patient's needs, strengths and vulnerabilities. With this added detail, team members can help put in place a safety net to address potential specific post-operative adjustment difficulties.

When the team plans ahead to address life events, issues and symptoms known to undermine a patient's efforts to comply with needed protocols, it collectively exerts a positive effect on post-operative adjustments. Items likely to arise from a thorough pre-surgery evaluation that can sound an alarm for potential postoperative patient adjustment issues may include:

- A chaotic or unstable lifestyle;
- Active bulimia nervosa;
- Dangerous or non-compliant behaviour in psychiatric or medical treatment;
- Active substance abuse/compulsive gambling;
- Untreated psychiatric symptoms or symptoms not stabilized by medication;
- Suicide attempts or psychiatric hospitalizations within the previous twelve months;
- Unresolved/untreated childhood abuse or neglect.

When such impediments are identified, the mental health specialist is more alert to specific behaviours and is better prepared to direct the patient to services necessary to reduce or stabilize problematic symptoms. The three most common services I have found valuable to refer to in problems such as the examples described above include a psychiatric referral for psychotropic medication evaluation or review, a recommendation for pre-surgical psychotherapeutic alliance (therapy) with a mental health specialist outside of the surgical programme and the 'Alanon Family Group'. Alanon is a wonderful worldwide fellowship and resource that can be utilized in order to help patients or those whose lives have been negatively impacted by a loved one or friend's alcohol or drug usage. This programme is free of charge and offers valuable opportunities for building stress management skills to people in need.

Additionally, it is essential for the surgical programme's mental health specialist to understand the surgeon and team's philosophy and expectations. For example, if a surgeon prefers only minimal post-operative involvement, the specialist will design a programme to compensate for less medical follow-up. If the patient has been described before surgery as having serious psychiatric conditions known to thwart recovery, the mental health specialist must adjust the recovery programme accordingly.

Surgeons may choose to proceed with surgery even when a comprehensive pre-surgical evaluation indicates only a modest chance of long-term success. Pre-surgical conditions I have encountered that, at times, evidenced a complicated recovery include: severe (non-psychotic) depressions (particularly where there was a history of childhood abuse without therapeutic attention), untreated anxiety conditions or attention deficit disorders that become interruptive to life, active substance abuse or dependency, post-traumatic shock disorder, schizophrenia and what was once known as multiple personality disorder not properly managed or stabilized with appropriate medications and treatment, bipolar disorder with or without psychotic episodes also not stabilized and extreme body image distortion/severe eating disorders. Though seen infrequently in surgical candidates, even these worrisome conditions do not necessarily preclude success. Rather, these more serious circumstances require increased team awareness of the specific dynamics of the individual's mental processes. I have had the opportunity to provide consultations to such patients for surgeons before full preoperative services were fully in place. While at times these cases can be managed with great difficulty postoperatively, it has been my experience that implementing pre-operative recommendations often provides the extra help some people need to safely undergo bariatric surgery, and increases their chances for improved medical conditions and a better quality of life. Team members need to apply a psychodynamic understanding within their sub-specialty, so that the possibility for providing a safe, therapeutic environment for the patient's life-long success increases.

Incorporating a patient's particular psychological dynamic into each subspecialty on the recovery team begins with the rejection of a morbid obesity stereotype. Patients may present similar symptoms, but the psychological healthcare specialist must make sure that all professionals focus on the individual being interviewed. No team member can be permitted to lapse into prejudice; patients are hyper-sensitive to adverse first impressions. An inadvertent slip before surgery is likely to increase the risk of post-operative iatrogenic complications.

By rejecting stereotypes, the professional builds a bridge of empathy to the individual with targeted clinical pathways for specialized service delivery. It is at this juncture that the team psychologist, in consultation with team members, can refine and enrich the contributions of each team specialist, enabling him/her to provide the most efficacious care.

The Initial Psychoeducational Interview

With the aid of other dedicated colleagues, a comprehensive paper was created on this topic and is available from the ASMBS.[8] The ASMBS paper expounds further on the various aspects of a pre-surgery mental health evaluation that can be covered by the mental health specialist, as well as considerations for the choice and use of psychological instruments. (For those interested in obtaining a copy of the nine-page skeleton work sheet used and created by members of my office simply visit our website, Drmoorehead.com.)

Briefly, the pre-surgery evaluation is a comprehensive, structured psychological and educationally oriented clinical interview. The goal is to collect a thorough psychosocial history of the individual, including his/her perception of past and present family life. Among items of special interest is the body-weight history with specific emphasis on the patient's psychological relationship to food, dieting and frustration-tolerance. A weight history assessment includes an evaluation of the patient's family weight and food-use rules and patterns.

The clinical evaluation measures the level and depth of psychological functioning for each surgical candidate, including emotional stamina, ego strength, defence and personality structure, intact coping strategies, characteristic cognitive and behavioural patterns, reasoning styles/ problem-solving methods, body image and self-esteem profiles. Medical and psychological co-factors, including pertinent psychiatric history, early abuse history, chemical substance abuse or dependency issues are also important, as is a description of the existing social support for each patient.

Also of diagnostic relevance are an assessment of the patient's *ad hoc* problem-solving skills, a mental status exam and an evaluation of the patient's typical pain management thresholds. The assessment and evaluation of each patient's suggestibility should be conducted with an eye to pain-management training. The initial interview needs also to delineate the patient's motivation for, and understanding of the details of surgery and the after-care regimen.

When structured as a psycho-educational model, the interview provides patients with a detailed understanding of some of the dramatic changes that may lie ahead. While improvement in quality of life is a reasonable expectation following surgery, altering consequences may also include:

- Radical and unexpected changes in the dynamics of important relationships (workplace or domestic);
- Spiking in pre-operative depression or anxiety as patients lose the ability to turn to food for emotional comfort;
- Potential for substitution of food with another form of destructive behaviour such as smoking, excessive alcoholic consumption, shopping leading to financial difficulties, gambling etc. (what the mass media refers to as 'transfer of addiction').[9]

Thorough pre-surgery education and evaluation are the main components of securing psychological informed consent. In the course of the evaluation, patients can gain a clearer understanding of the victories and challenges that some people encounter before, during and after bariatric surgery. Psychologically informed consent is essential for helping prevent the patient from feeling overwhelmed, neglected or deprived after surgery–feelings that can undermine programme involvement. Additionally, the evaluation process itself can be of therapeutic value. The mental health professional can address the patient's immediate fears, while establishing a rapport through the use of didactics with combined empathic treatment.

This initial face-to-face contact cannot be underestimated. Professionals specializing in the surgical treatment of severely/super-obese patients often agree that many who struggle with the disease of morbid obesity experience predictably similar forms of acute and chronic psychological distress. While the rapid changes that come with surgery are most frequently welcomed, they can also easily topple a fragile personality. When the dramatic body weight reduction following surgery is considered in light of the extreme, pre-treatment psychological stressors described by some patients, it becomes abundantly clear that post-surgical attitudinal changes and behavioural modifications can destabilize some patient's fragile ego status.

Moreover, readily apparent radical changes may serve as precipitants to a period of even more pronounced psychological vulnerability. It is important to remember that bariatric surgery, unlike gall bladder surgery, often changes the way people cope with their feelings. Bariatric surgery most often takes away or interrupts the way some people deal with life–by eating, eating and eating. Many patients go into surgery excited for this change. Others are fearful of the change, and some do not come to the awareness until after the surgery. Ironically, the direct experience of this potent change is sometimes experienced as a profound loss. The point is that when we threaten or take away a coping mechanism, we foster vulnerability that causes some patients to experience a regressed state of emotion. During this brief window of time, when the regressed psychological maturation level is evidenced, there is definitive indication for hand-in-hand psychological care concurrent with the surgical intervention. The vast majority of the world's bariatric programmes do not offer this service. Our programmes will improve as we do.

When evaluating any candidate for weight-loss surgery, it is important to remember that the disease of morbid or severe obesity kills and/or substantially reduces the quality of life of the afflicted, and dramatically, often adversely, affects the lives of their loved ones. Because a lifelong transformation is at stake, as well as the very life of the patient, the evaluator must never lose sight of the two purposes of the pre-surgery interview: educating the patient and providing the surgeon and team members with a comprehensive report on the patient's underlying strengths and challenges.

In this respect, it may be instructive to liken the mental health specialist in the bariatric arena to the child custody evaluator in a divorce proceeding. While the judge or attorneys may want the psychologist to determine which parent might provide better care, the decision is a legal matter that lies with a higher authority. As such, it falls to the judge; the custody evaluator merely advises. Similarly, before surgery an in-depth evaluation can assist the surgeon in appreciating patient psychosocial dynamics so that the surgeon, as head of the team, can make a more informed medical/surgical determination for a particular patient regarding the appropriateness of surgery and weighing potential surgical benefits against possible psychological challenges. Ultimately, just as the judge decides matters of law, the surgeon remains responsible for surgical decisions concerning patient care.

Because surgery is the central element of the entire transformation from obesity to manageable weight, some have questioned whether there is a meaningful role for psychology during the hospital stay and subsequent outpatient medical follow-up visits. I would urge that psychological support at every stage is invaluable, and I know that many of my peers share this view, favouring active involvement that helps patients manage the emotional stress, behavioural transitions and even physical demands that often arise during and after bariatric surgery. This provides an excellent opportunity for healing and nurturing the spirit of our patients during the dramatic weight loss process.

It is no small accomplishment for the patient to plan and arrange for surgery; however, the full psychological impact of entering the hospital, enduring surgery and facing the challenges of successful recovery are an altogether distinct experience that requires consideration. Most patients readily grasp the basic science of their surgery, but what they face afterward, often in silence, is unknown territory. After surgery they must cope with the frequently frightening uncertainties that accompany behavioural and lifestyle changes, including learning an entirely different way to feel about and approach food. Moreover, to an extraordinary degree, some people in support group settings talk about their new relationship to food as comparable to an ex-smoker's memories of nicotine or a former addict's cold flame for drugs.

Post-surgical support must be immediate. As a member of a larger, multi-disciplinary/interdisciplinary outpatient team, the mental health specialist can contribute a great deal even when medical concerns take precedence. This includes follow-up exams or 'fills', for adjustable band surgery patients. Though the purpose of the office visit is largely medical, the mental health professional can provide counsel and comfort for patients, which in turn enhances further participation in their programme, as patients learn and practice new coping and behavioural skills. As part of a coordinated team effort, such services and expertise greatly improve the patient's chances of implementing the positive behaviours necessary to achieve lifelong success.

Creating this kind of positive period of time *before* surgery can provide a 'golden window of opportunity' period of time *after* surgery. During this 'honeymoon' time, patients experience their maximum weight reduction, which makes them motivated and receptive to overriding even deeply ingrained behaviours with new, life-affirming ideas and actions. Providing skills-building activities such as positive affirmation work and structured progressive relaxation can be particularly effective during these phases of time when patients are preparing to discover or are rediscovering their new bodies, in effect, their new self. This is the best time to systematically supplant the morbid 'diet of thoughts'. Familiar negative thoughts now must give way to behaviours and thoughts that reinforce life-saving, long-lasting behaviours, transferring from a pleasant honeymoon experience to a health satisfying marriage with their surgery.

Clearly, this is not solely about giving up the lifelong habit of turning to food for comfort. A well designed recovery programme also shows patients how to acknowledge, appreciate, and take ownership of all the positive changes that have occurred: 'I am good enough. I am loveable. I deserve the attention I need'. At every step along the way, the mental health specialist assists patients in making the smoothest transition possible to their new life. And for virtually every bariatric surgery patient, the resulting weight loss resolve, improvement of medical condition and enhancement in quality of life may also be regarded as a medical resurrection.

In addition to the above range of psychological and mental health services, the bariatric support group is a crucial component of the patient's psychological and emotional journey toward full recovery. For many, these meetings provide patients with their first opportunities to free themselves from a profound social and emotional isolation and become a valued member of a community of hope. It is quite common for our patients to feel misunderstood and even blamed for seeking bariatric surgery, which is frequently and erroneously viewed as the 'easy way out'. The support group confronts these hurtful misconceptions head-on, and supplants them with well-deserved praise for embracing the difficult and varied challenges that can arise before and after surgery.

In light of many patients' histories of despair, discrimination, hopelessness, depression and anxiety, the overarching theme of the support group raises feelings of personal life-transformation and pride in accomplishment. So pervasive is this sense of a second chance at life that many bariatric surgery patients declare that they now have two birthdays — the day of their birth and the day of their surgery.

What is it about the concept of rebirth that makes it such a common theme among these patients? The answer becomes evident when patients share their life stories and the changes resulting from surgery and group support. Abusive relationships end as patients no longer accept victimization; diabetes, chronic debilitating pain and other life-threatening conditions disappear; parents become more actively engaged in their children's development; infertile couples give birth to long-dreamed-of babies. Many mundane daily activities become small celebrations of a new life. Patients find they are suddenly comfortable in public seating, walk easily down store aisles, and attract no more attention than anyone else in public forums. Many discover new job prospects and entirely new economic or social opportunities. Exhilarated patients admit they are so pleased with their success that if needed, they would undergo the surgery again. Even patients who experience significant complications and setbacks after bariatric surgery say they would do it again 'in a heartbeat'.

The healing process comes full circle when support group members take the added therapeutic step of comforting and counselling others who are considering or preparing for bariatric surgery. This service by group members gives prospective patients a valuable opportunity to interact with those for whom surgery was successful. Plus, the pre-operative patient can meet people in several different stages of recovery. This becomes an especially effective tool for managing patient expectations and reducing anxiety. Interactions with other group members can become a key component of informed psychological consent.

Another significant role of the support group involves encouragement and education after surgery. Patients often experience a rise in self-esteem just from 'giving back' to the group by sharing their personal stories of triumph and tribulation. By trusting and sharing their experiences in a group, people can learn that slips or lapses in following programme protocols do not have to end in collapse or failure. Meetings provide opportunities to learn how to handle feelings in new ways other than turning to food. They can help individuals understand that while it is natural to fear the regaining of weight, the power to sustain their weight loss is always within their grasp.

What is the Value of Speaking the Same Language in Outcomes?

How can we ensure that a programme is really working to help patients succeed and feel successful? After all, psychological wellbeing can be greatly impacted by perceived success or failure. For that matter, what determines success or failure? How can we, as a worldwide bariatric community, help patients re-define what it means to be successful or to have failed after bariatric surgery, rather than simply reading numbers on a scale? How can bariatric programmes improve the reporting and comparing of outcomes by including the patient's input in the process? How can we come together universally to report our findings in meaningful ways, particularly as we speak so many different languages?

A reliable, standardized easy method for measuring patient progress is a key to understanding success for any widely applicable recovery programme. The Bariatric Analysis and Report Outcome System (BAROS), described and published in 1998 (Oria and Moorehead[10]) is such a tool. BAROS, in an effort to respond to the 1991 National Institute of Heath Consensus report, organizes acknowledged definitions and stages of recovery into three categories to create a concise, clear accounting of an individual's progress.

As recovery proceeds, the healthcare professional continues to measure and chronicle progress using the BAROS system. BAROS provides objective definitions and standards for measuring recovery, including percentage of excess weight loss, improvement in co-morbidities related to obesity and patient perceived quality-of-life as measured by The Moorehead–Ardelt Quality of Life Questionnaire II (MA II).[11]

Briefly, BAROS defines five outcome groups–failure, fair, good, very good and excellent–by results on a scoring table that adds or subtracts points for percentage of excess weight loss, changes in medical conditions and QOL ratings (Fig. 1).

To assess quality of life before and after treatment, BAROS incorporates the MA II (Fig. 2), also designed for independent use, specifically to address self-esteem, physical activity, social life, work conditions, sexual activity and relationship to food. The one-page questionnaire uses simple

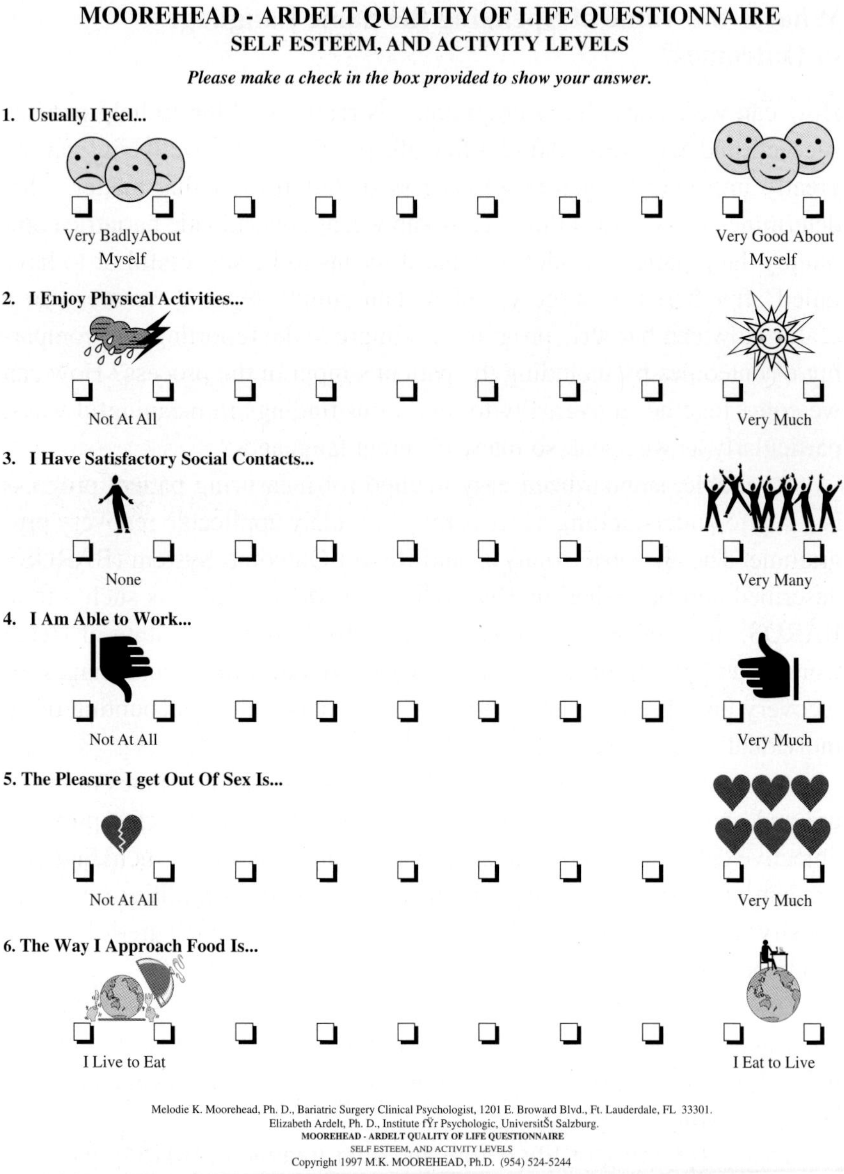

MOOREHEAD - ARDELT QUALITY OF LIFE QUESTIONNAIRE
SELF ESTEEM, AND ACTIVITY LEVELS

Please make a check in the box provided to show your answer.

1. **Usually I Feel...**

   ☐ ☐ ☐ ☐ ☐ ☐ ☐ ☐ ☐ ☐
   Very Badly About Myself ··· Very Good About Myself

2. **I Enjoy Physical Activities...**

   ☐ ☐ ☐ ☐ ☐ ☐ ☐ ☐ ☐ ☐
   Not At All ··· Very Much

3. **I Have Satisfactory Social Contacts...**

   ☐ ☐ ☐ ☐ ☐ ☐ ☐ ☐ ☐ ☐
   None ··· Very Many

4. **I Am Able to Work...**

   ☐ ☐ ☐ ☐ ☐ ☐ ☐ ☐ ☐ ☐
   Not At All ··· Very Much

5. **The Pleasure I get Out Of Sex Is...**

   ☐ ☐ ☐ ☐ ☐ ☐ ☐ ☐ ☐ ☐
   Not At All ··· Very Much

6. **The Way I Approach Food Is...**

   ☐ ☐ ☐ ☐ ☐ ☐ ☐ ☐ ☐ ☐
   I Live to Eat ··· I Eat to Live

Melodie K. Moorehead, Ph. D., Bariatric Surgery Clinical Psychologist, 1201 E. Broward Blvd., Ft. Lauderdale, FL 33301.
Elizabeth Ardelt, Ph. D., Institute fÿr Psychologic, Universitšt Salzburg.
MOOREHEAD - ARDELT QUALITY OF LIFE QUESTIONNAIRE
SELF ESTEEM, AND ACTIVITY LEVELS
Copyright 1997 M.K. MOOREHEAD, Ph.D. (954) 524-5244

Figure 1. Moorehead–Ardelt quality of life questionnaire.

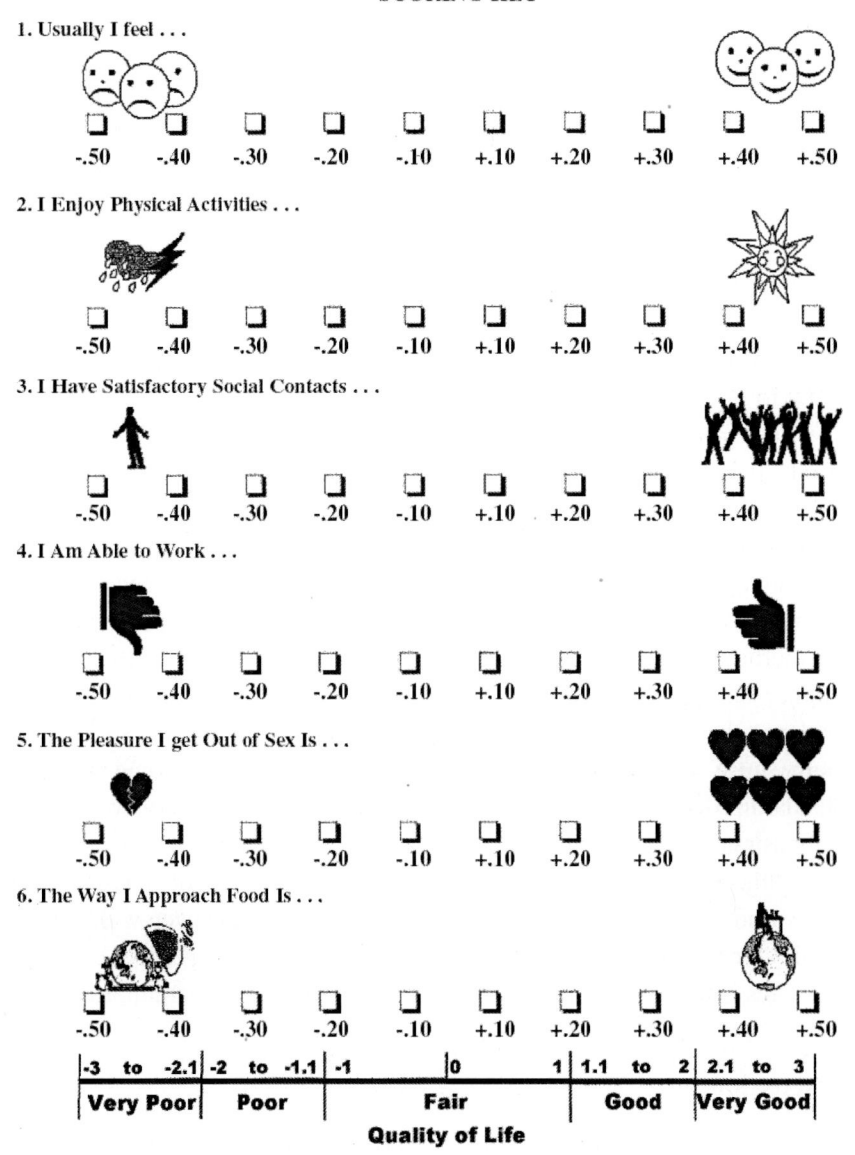

Bariatric Surgery: When the Miracle is Not Enough 319

M-A QoLQ II
Self Esteem and Activity Levels
SCORING KEY

1. Usually I feel . . .

| -.50 | -.40 | -.30 | -.20 | -.10 | +.10 | +.20 | +.30 | +.40 | +.50 |

2. I Enjoy Physical Activities . . .

| -.50 | -.40 | -.30 | -.20 | -.10 | +.10 | +.20 | +.30 | +.40 | +.50 |

3. I Have Satisfactory Social Contacts . . .

| -.50 | -.40 | -.30 | -.20 | -.10 | +.10 | +.20 | +.30 | +.40 | +.50 |

4. I Am Able to Work . . .

| -.50 | -.40 | -.30 | -.20 | -.10 | +.10 | +.20 | +.30 | +.40 | +.50 |

5. The Pleasure I get Out of Sex Is . . .

| -.50 | -.40 | -.30 | -.20 | -.10 | +.10 | +.20 | +.30 | +.40 | +.50 |

6. The Way I Approach Food Is . . .

| -.50 | -.40 | -.30 | -.20 | -.10 | +.10 | +.20 | +.30 | +.40 | +.50 |

-3 to -2.1	-2 to -1.1	-1 0 1	1.1 to 2	2.1 to 3
Very Poor	Poor	Fair	Good	Very Good

Quality of Life

© 2003, Melodie Moorehead, Ph.D., and Elisabeth Ardelt, Ph.D.

Figure 2. MA QoLQ II self esteem and activity levels scoring key.

drawings to represent the patients' choices among perceived degrees of change, and points are awarded to the responses that help determine the score. BAROS also accounts for complications and re-operative surgery. Points are merely deducted from the final tally of the scoring, thus avoiding the controversy of considering re-operations as failures.

BAROS analyses outcomes in a simple, objective, unbiased and evidence-based fashion. While it is not a perfect system, it helps provide a common understandable language for our international community. Additionally, it can be adapted to evaluate other forms of medical intervention for the control of obesity. This method merits further consideration by all international organizations seeking an adoption of standards that will measure the success and impact of bariatric treatments and will provide the comparison of results among surgical series.

Standardized outcomes measuring the three fields identified in BAROS also help bring quantitative support to qualitative terms, such as success and failure. This can help patients broaden their view of what constitutes success while reducing their fear of weight regain. Used in this context, BAROS can be valuable, clinically, for helping patients remain accountable. Quantification of specific changes and results on the Improvement of Co-morbidities and QoL sections of BAROS can be used to provide reassurance to patients returning to their surgeons by providing concrete evidence that helps to decrease feelings of shame and anxiety and reduce their sense of 'failure' simply because they gained some weight. Standardized outcomes that quantify a range of success very well could demonstrate a 'good' or 'fair' result even when there is weight *gain* after surgery. Objective measurements of quality-of-life-improvement and resolve of co-morbidities may well maintain their high scoring value even with weight regain! One value for speaking a standardized language regarding outcome measures is that we can better help our patients and our programmes.

Discussion

Bariatric surgery continues to be on the rise worldwide. One thing we can all agree on is that there is still much to be learned about the disease of obesity. Research is warranted and currently under way that demonstrates the need for evidenced-based practice (EBP) in healthcare. Fortunately, the field of bariatric surgery psychology is growing strong in the face of the advancing problem of morbid/super-obesity. The participation of major medical and internationally recognized academic institutions will help to determine scientifically what specialized bariatric mental health services are needed in every comprehensive bariatric surgery programme. These services can help patients build and strengthen healthy coping skills while advancing their legitimate rights. EBP involves a process of clinical decision-making based on research, clinical expertise, patient preferences and characteristics. They are trans-disciplinary and promote a lifelong learning process. While empirically supported treatments are a driving force of EBP, they must not be reduced to such. We as helping professionals must also be free to act as creators, acting within the scope of our licences and expertise while engaging patients in the shared decision making process.[12] Helping to change the patient's inner 'diet of thoughts', accompanied by progressive relaxation for stress management, can supplant regressive coping behaviours that often leave bariatric surgery patients vulnerable.[13]

Beyond working directly with patients and their loved ones, development of a superstructure for cost-effective psychological practice standards that responds specifically to the needs of bariatric surgery patients is another area worthy of research. Such inquiry must lead to the development of sound clinical pathways aimed to increase patient cooperation that maximizes successful weight reduction and quality of life while minimizing the litigious impact often seen in bariatric surgery.

Acting as political change agents, bariatric healthcare providers all over the world have an opportunity and responsibility to provide leadership in this ever-shrinking planet by participating in venues that focus on prevention of obesity. An example of this occurred in May 2007 when major stakeholders gathered in Washington DC.[14] More than 100 leaders from the public health, academic, industry and government communities came together to discuss and identify a common list of urgent federal policy actions needed to reverse the American obesity epidemic. Six recommendations were identified as essential policy changes to be made, and were provided in a report offered to Congressional leaders in Washington DC. This agenda promises to become the central platform for the newly formed Collaborative Campaign to End Obesity (CCEO), through which leaders and advocates can work together to reduce obesity in North America. Helping to facilitate this gathering and establishing a common agenda proved immediately fruitful and focused on three primary core panel areas:

- Promoting active lifestyles;
- Promoting better nutrition;
- Change in the health care sector.

Six identified policies changes were offered to Congress that can be translated quickly into 'critical and realizable' actions:

1. Expand coverage for prevention, diagnosis and effective treatments of obesity;
2. Increase federal support for research services focused on obesity;
3. Ensure that all foods in schools meet the *Dietary Guidelines for Americans.* See http://www.health.gov/dietaryguidelines/;[15]
4. Reduce the marketing of unhealthy foods and increase the marketing of healthy, culturally relevant foods;
5. Increase physical activity in schools;
6. Create a built environment that supports physically active lifestyles.

For the complete report go to: www.obesitycampaign.org.

I close this chapter with a remark made to me by a patient many years ago that remains relevant in our discussion regarding the role and value of psychological services in a bariatric programme:

> 'I know that for me, obesity surgery probably saved my life and most definitely improved the physical quality of my life. At the same time, I believe that the vast majority of patients who need obesity surgery have psychological/emotional issues, such as low self-esteem that need to be addressed and would benefit from psychological counselling and intervention. I believe that the psychological intervention is just as important as every incision, pouch, suture, band or staple.'

Acknowledgements

I would like to give my appreciation to Drs Nadey S. Hakim, Franco Favretti and Gianni Segato, for the opportunity to offer my talents and views regarding perspectives held on the subjects discussed in the chapter. I honour the relationships with Drs Norman Samuels and Emanuel Hell for inviting me into the field of bariatric surgery and introducing me to the worldwide community. Recognition is given to Drs Elisabeth Ardelt-Gattinger, Cynthia Buffington, Florence Kaslow and Cynthia Alexander for enduring stimulation and vitality to my career. Gratitude is acknowledged to my former business colleagues, Drs Joan M. DiGregorio and Michael S. Parish, and to William C. Banks, formerly of Money Magazine, for his outstanding and extensive editing efforts. Lastly, I would like to simply thank Mr and Mrs Maurice and Joyce Williams, my Mom and Dad, for their undying support and understanding. Happy 80th Birthday Mom and Dad!

References

1. American Psychiatric Association (1994). *Diagnostic and Statistical Manual of Mental Disorders*, 4th ed., American Psychiatric Association, Washington, DC.
2. Moorehead, M.K., Alexander, C.L. (2007). Transfer of addiction and considerations for preventive measures in bariatric surgery, Part 1. *Bariatric Times* 4(1): 22–25.
3. Moorehead, M.K., Alexander, C.L. (2007). Transfer of addiction and considerations for preventive measures in bariatric surgery, Part 2. *Bariatric Times* 4(4): 18–21.
4. Moorehead, M.K., Ardelt-Gattinger, E., Lechner, H. et al. (2003). The validation of the Moorehead-Ardelt Quality of Life Questionnaire II. *Obes Surg* 13: 684–692.
5. Stunkard, A.J., Messick, S. (1986). *Eating Inventory Manual*, The Psychological Corporation, Toronto.
6. Stunkard, A.J., Wadden, T.A. (1992). Psychological aspects of human obesity. In: Bjorntorp P., Brodoff B.N. (eds). *Human Obesity: General Aspects*, pp. 352–358, Lippincott, Philadelphia.
7. Kaidar-Person, O., Wong Swartz, E., Lefkowitz, M. et al. (2006). Shared medical appointments: new concept for high-volume follow-up for bariatric patients. *Surg Obes Relat Dis* 2: 509–512.
8. LeMont, D., Moorehead, M.K., Parish, M.S. et al. (2004). Suggestions for the Pre-Surgical Psychological Assessment of Bariatric Surgery Candidates, American Society for Bariatric Surgery, Gainsville, Florida, USA.

9. The new science of addiction: emergence of alcoholism after weight-loss surgery offers clues to roots of dependency. (July 18, 2006). *The Wall Street Journal*, D1–3.
10. Oria, H.E., Moorehead, M.K. (1998). Bariatric Analysis and Reporting Outcome System (BAROS). *Obes Surg* 8: 487–499.
11. Moorehead, M.K., Ardelt-Gattinger, E., Lechner, H. et al. (2003). The validation of the Moorehead–Ardelt Quality of Life Questionnaire II. *Obes Surg* 13: 684–692.
12. Spring, B. (2007). Evidence-based practice in clinical psychology: what it is, why it matters; what you need to know. *J Clin Psychol* 63: 611–631.
13. *The Gift and the Tool©: A Personal Guide for a Lifelong Journey.* A two-CD audio set for those living with the disease of severe/super obesity. Dramatically presented, it is a complete emotional guide for the bariatric surgery patient and their loved ones. CD 1 is an inspirational presentation helping to promote psychological informed consent. CD 2 contains a combination of relaxation techniques and positive affirmations to help prepare patients for surgery, the surgery itself and for facing life and its challenges after surgery. Also included are five Quality of Life Questionnaires that will help measure progress from pre-surgery, to recovery and to maintenance. Melodie K. Moorehead PhD (Drmoorehead.com).
14. National Summit on Obesity Policy, 8–9 May 2007, Ronald Reagan Building & International Trade Center. Sponsored by Johnson & Johnson and Discovery, coordinated by Venn Strategies.
15. http://www.health.gov/dietaryguidelines/ Accessed 31 March 2010.

Suggested Reading

DiGregorio, J.M., Moorehead, M.K. (1994). The psychology of the bariatric surgery patients: a clinical report. *Obes Surg* 4: 361–369.

Al-anon (1995). *How Al-anon Works for Families and Friends of Alcoholics*, Al-anon Family Group Headquarters Inc., Virginia Beach, Virginia, USA.

Kleiner, K.D., Gold, M.S., Frost-Pineda, K. et al. (2004). Body mass index and alcohol use. *J Addict Dis* 23: 105–118.

Kolotkin, R.L., Crosby, R.D., Pendelton, R. et al. (2003). Health-related quality of life in patients seeking gastric bypass surgery vs. non-treatment-seeking controls. *Obes Surg* 13: 371–377.

Maddi, S.R., Fox, S.R., Khoshaba, D.M. et al. (2001). Reduction I psychopathology following bariatric surgery for morbid obesity. *Obes Surg* 11: 680–685.

Mahoney, M.J. (2003). *Constructive Psychotherapy: A Practical Guide*, Guilford Press, New York.

Moorehead, M.K., Ardelt-Gattinger, E., Lechner, H. et al. (2003). The validation of the Moorehead–Ardelt quality of life questionnaire II. *Obes Surg* 13: 684–692.

Sogg, S., Mori, D. (2004). The Boston interview for gastric bypass: determining the psychological suitability of surgical candidates. *Obes Surg* 14: 370–380.

Stunkard, A.J., Wadden, T.A. (1992). Psychological aspects of human obesity. In: Bjorntorp P., Brodoff B.N. (eds). *Human Obesity: General Aspects*, pp. 352–358, Lippincott, Philadelphia.

Oria, H.E., Moorehead, M.K. (1998). Bariatric Analysis and Reporting Outcome System (BAROS). *Obes Surg* 8: 487–499.

Wadden, T.A., Sarwer, D.B., Arnold, M.E. et al. (2000). Psychosocial status of severely obese patients before and after bariatric surgery. *Prob Gen Surg* 17: 13–22.

Wadden, T.A., Stunkard, A.J. (eds.) (2002). *Handbook of Obesity Treatment*, Guilford Press, New York.

Wang, G.J., Volkow, N.D., Thanos, P.K. et al. (2004). Similarity between obesity and drug addiction as assessed by neurofunctional imaging: a concept review. *J Addict Dis* 23: 39–53.

Wolf, A.M., Falcone, A.R., Kortner, B. et al. (2000). BAROS: an effective system to evaluate the results of patients after bariatric surgery. *Obes Surg* 10: 445–450.

Chapter 12

Effects of Bariatric Surgery on Co-Morbidities

Sebastiaan Van Cauwenberge and Bruno Dillemans

Introduction

Much has been written about the medical conditions that are associated with morbid obesity and their response to bariatric surgery. Diabetes, hypertension, hypercholesterolemia and obstructive sleep apnoea are among the commonly reported co-morbid conditions which tend to improve significantly or resolve completely following weight loss surgery.

This chapter gives an overview of the positive effects of bariatric surgery on the previously mentioned co-morbidities. It will focus on adjustable gastric banding (AGB), Roux-en-Y gastric bypass (RYGB) and biliopancreatic diversion/duodenal switch (BPD/DS). We describe in detail the evidence of their beneficial properties on those various co-morbid conditions based on the current available literature.

Other co-morbidities such as gastro-oesophageal reflux disease (GORD), musculoskeletal problems and polycystic ovary syndrome will also be discussed. At the end of the chapter, the quality of life changes after bariatric surgery will be reviewed.

Hypertension

One of the most frequent complications of obesity is hypertension.[1] Hypertension is a risk factor for cardiovascular disease and stroke. It has long been known that even a modest reduction in body weight (10 per cent) will help reduce blood pressure (BP).[2] However, in the Swedish Obese Subjects (SOS) study no long term difference was observed in the frequency of hypertension between the operated patients and obese controls, due to long-term increase in hypertension prevalence irrespective of weight changes.[3]

Pathogenesis of hypertension in obesity

Obesity-induced hypertension has multiple potential etiologic pathways, the most well established being increased renal sodium reabsorption with impaired pressure natriuresis via (1) activation of the renin-angiotensin system; (2) stimulation of the sympathetic nervous system; and (3) altered intrarenal physical forces.[4] When the metabolic syndrome is present, insulin resistance and hyperinsulinemia may contribute to hypertension through diverse mechanisms.[5] The sleep apnoea syndrome is an additional contributing factor to the development of hypertension in a subgroup of obese patients. Activation of the sympathetic nervous system, enhanced aldosterone levels, and increased levels of endothelin by repeated episodes of hypoxia are thought to be responsible in part for the elevation in BP in this disorder.[6,7]

Effects of RYGB on hypertension

Weight loss is the best means to reduce obesity-related hypertension.[4] The diet-induced decline in BP was assessed in a 2008 meta-analysis of 38 randomized controlled trials that found a mean fall in BP of 6.3/3.4 mmHg with weight loss diets.[8] RYGB surgery is not only one of the most effective methods for obesity treatment, but it also exerts the most significant effect on obesity-related co-morbidities such as hypertension resolving it in some 60 per cent[9] of patients while improving control in others.[10–15] Furthermore, the normal diurnal variation in BP which is lost in obese hypertension is restored after RYGB.[16] Weight loss associated with RYGB substantially improves and/or resolves hypertension in the majority of patients. In a study, 95 obese patients with documented hypertension and being treated with antihypertensive medication(s) underwent RYGB. The mean systolic BP decreased significantly from 140 ± 17 mmHg preoperatively to 120 ± 18 mmHg at 12 months ($p < 0.01$). The mean diastolic BP also significantly decreased from 80 ± 11 mmHg preoperatively to 71 ± 8 mmHg at 12 months ($p < 0.01$). At 12 months follow-up, 44 (46 per cent) patients had complete resolution of hypertension while 18 (19 per cent) patients had improvement. Patients with complete resolution had a shorter duration of disease as compared to patients without resolution (53 versus 95 months, respectively, $p = 0.01$).[17] Carson et al. evaluated the relationship between weight loss and BP in patients with diastolic hypertension who had RYGB surgery for morbid obesity. They concluded that postoperative weight loss in patients undergoing RYGB surgery was associated with resolution or improvement of diastolic hypertension in approximately 70 per cent of cases. Resolution or improvement of hypertension occurred more often in patients with a lower postoperative body mass index.[10]

Ahmed et al. analysed 89 women and 11 men who underwent RYGB, and monitored their BP monitored for one year. There was an 85 per cent follow-up rate with mean percentage excess body weight loss of 60. Reductions in systolic (9 mmHg) and diastolic (7 mmHg) BP measurements were seen as early as week one postoperatively and maintained for the duration of 12 months ($p < 0.05$). Furthermore, postoperative usage of antihypertensive medication was reduced to a third of preoperative use. This early impact on BP occurs before any significant weight loss is achieved, thereby suggesting a hormonal mechanism that may be involved for the changes observed.[18]

Even super-obese patients experience significant improvements in co-morbidities and quality of life after RYGB even if their BMI remains > 35 kg/m². Patients who had undergone RYGB and who had a preoperative BMI > 50 kg/m² and postoperative BMI > 5 kg/m² were identified. The records of 120 patients were reviewed for the presence of diabetes, hypertension, hyperlipidemia and gastro-oesophageal reflux disease. The average preoperative and postoperative BMI was 63.2 and 43.7 kg/m². Of the 120 patients, 77 responded to the survey. In the preoperative group, the rate of diabetes, hypertension was 50.8 per cent. Postoperatively 62.3 per cent of patients had been cured of their hypertension. The change in the incidence of hypertension was significant at $p = 0.037$.[19]

Effects of AGB on hypertension

Forty hypertensive and 55 normotensive obese subjects were studied under basal conditions and again one year after significant weight loss obtained through AGB. BP decreased in hypertensive subjects, with a concordant decrease in PRA and supine aldosterone levels, not observed in normotensive patients.[20]

Brancantisano et al. prospectively analysed 838 consecutive morbidly obese patients who underwent AGB. After a median follow-up of 13 months (range 6–36 months), resolution and/or improvement of hypertension was 67 per cent.[21] Weiner reports similar results on 954 patients with improvement or resolution of hypertension in 50 per cent of the hypertensive patients.[22] In a retrospective study on 454 patients with a mean follow-up of 30 months, hypertension was present in 73.4 per cent of the patients. After AGB, hypertension markedly improved in 74.9 per cent of these patients.[23] In a study of 88 patients with hypertension followed for 12 months after AGB placement, 59 per cent had normal BP (without any treatment) and a further 33 per cent had improved BP control with less therapy.[24] AGB can also play a role in the primary prevention of arterial hypertension.[25]

Effects of BPD on hypertension

In the well-known meta-analysis of Buchwald et al. hypertension improved or resolved in 91.8 per cent of the evaluated patients after BPD/DS.[9] Scopinaro followed 312 patients who underwent BPD. Hypertension was present in 86 per cent of the diabetic obese patients before BPD. A significant reduction of the frequency of hypertension following the operation was observed. At one year after the operation (follow-up on 305 patients) 50 per cent of the operated patients showed a normal arterial pressure. The percentage of normal values rose to 64 per cent at five years and to 74 per cent at ten years (follow-up on 243 patients).[26] Similar results were reported by Adami et al. [27,28] BPD was more effective than AGB on BMI, on almost all cardiovascular parameters and on cholesterol, although not on triglyceride and blood glucose. Disappearance of diabetes, hypertension and metabolic syndrome was similar with BPD and with AGB, and no new cases were observed.[29]

Obstructive Sleep Apnoea

Prevalence and pathophysiology of obstructive sleep apnoea in obesity

Obstructive sleep apnoea is a common chronic disease in Western society whose prevalence is estimated at two per cent of women and four per cent of men in the general population.[30]

Obstructive sleep apnoea–hypopnea syndrome (OSA) involves recurring episodes of total obstruction (apnoea) or partial obstruction (hypopnea) of airways during sleep. OSA is defined by an apnoea-hypopnea index (AHI) of five or more episodes per hour associated with daytime somnolence.[31] Definite risk factors for OSA include obesity and craniofacial or upper airway soft tissue abnormalities, while potential risk factors include heredity, smoking and nasal congestion.[32,33] Among these, obesity is one of the strongest sleep apnoea risk factors. Mild to moderate obesity has been associated with markedly increased sleep apnoea prevalence. In severe obesity (BMI > 40 kg/m^2), the prevalence of sleep apnoea was estimated to vary between 40 and 90 per cent, and the severity of sleep apnoea was generally greater than that found in leaner clinical populations.[34]

Although it is clear that obesity is a key risk factor for the development of OSA and modest reductions in weight lead to improvement in OSA severity, the physiological mechanisms remain less than certain. Deposition of fat around the pharyngeal airway is likely to increase the collapsibility of the pharyngeal airway. Fat deposition around the abdomen leads to reductions in functional residual capacity, which would be predicted to reduce lung volume tethering effects on the upper airway. Low lung volumes are also associated with diminished oxygen stores, which would contribute to ventilatory control instability (high loop gain). Finally, obesity has been associated with functional impairment in upper airway muscles.[35]

Nasal continuous positive airway pressure (CPAP) is the primary form of treatment of OSA. The concept is to deliver positive pressure through a nasal mask to the pharynx, thereby creating a pneumatic stent. Excessive daytime sleepiness is reversed, and the cardiopulmonary sequelae are eliminated with nasal CPAP.[36]

One problem with nasal CPAP is the issue of long-term patient compliance. Objective data suggest that nasal CPAP compliance is less than 50 per cent.

Surgical treatment of OSA is limited and is usually reserved for those persons in whom a trial of nasal CPAP fails. The first surgical procedure for the treatment of OSA was a tracheostomy, but is now rarely done, partly because it is poorly tolerated and there are other surgical procedures that better correct the problem. In 1979 the initial use of uvulopalatopharyngoplasty as a primary treatment of OSA was reported. It was the treatment of choice in the early 1980s and proved to be an excellent method of controlling snoring; however, several retrospective reviews reported improvement in only 50 per cent of the patients and complete control of the syndrome in only about 30 per cent.[37]

Weight loss remains a highly effective strategy for treating OSA. Schwartz *et al.* showed that weight loss is associated with decreases in upper airway collapsibility in OSA.[38] On its own, moderate weight loss can alleviate OSA, improve sleep architecture and decrease daytime hypersomnolence.[39]

Improvements in sleep apnoea with weight loss have been related to effects of adiposity on upper airway function during sleep. In controlled weight loss intervention studies, a decrease in upper airway collapsibility was demonstrated during sleep with weight loss, which can be attributed to reductions in mechanical loads or improvements in pharyngeal neuromuscular control. These mechanisms may be related to alterations in humoral factors, including ghrelin, adiponectin and leptin, which have been linked to changes in body weight and regional adiposity.[34]

Effects of RYGB on OSA

In a meta-analysis of 22,094 patients who underwent bariatric surgery, Buchwald *et al.* clearly demonstrated dramatic improvement in the vast majority of patients after surgery, with reductions in AHI of 33.9 episodes/hour and OSA resolution in 85.7 per cent of patients.[9]

Varela *et al.* determined the clinical outcome of a cohort of morbidly obese patients with documented sleep apnoea who underwent RYGB. Fifty-six morbidly obese patients with documented sleep apnoea by polysomnography underwent RYGB. The Epworth sleepiness scale (ESS) scores and the number of patients requiring the use of CPAP therapy were recorded preoperatively and at three-month intervals. The ESS is a validated questionnaire. It asks patients their likelihood of falling asleep in eight situations ranked from zero (would never fall asleep) to three (high chance of dozing). An ESS score of seven or higher is considered as abnormal with a high likelihood of a clinical diagnosis of sleep apnoea.

The mean ESS score decreased from 13.7 preoperatively to 5.3 at one month postoperatively ($p < 0.05$) and maintained below the threshold level (< 7) for the entire 12 months of follow-up. Of the 29 patients requiring preoperative CPAP, only four (14 per cent) patients required CPAP at three months postoperatively and none required CPAP at nine months. The authors conclude that weight loss associated with RYGB significantly improves the symptoms of sleep apnoea and is effective in discontinuation in the clinical use of CPAP therapy. Improvement of OSA symptoms occur as early as one month postoperatively.[40] In a study by Rasheid et al. there is evidence that weight loss following RYGB results in profound improvement in OSA. The severity of apnoea cannot be reliably predicted by preoperative BMI and ESS; therefore, patients with symptoms of OSA should undergo polysomnography.[41]

Lankford evaluated the CPAP pressure requirements in a group of patients undergoing rapid weight loss following RYGB. All patients experienced a reduction in required optimal pressures. Pre-surgical optimal CPAP pressures ranged from 7 to 18 cm H_2O, with an average of 11 ± 3.0 cm H_2O. The average BMI was 48 ± 7.4 kg/m^2. Post-RYGB, the average BMI dropped to 32 ± 7.8 kg/m^2. The post-surgical CPAP pressures ranged from 4 to 12 cm H_2O, with an average pressure of 9 ± 2.7 cm H_2O. This represents an overall reduction in CPAP pressure requirements of 18 per cent.[42]

Postoperative CPAP/BiPAP can be safely omitted in laparoscopic RYGB patients with known OSA, provided they are observed in a monitored setting and their pulmonary status is optimized by aggressive incentive spirometry and early ambulation.[43]

Effects of AGB on OSA

Dixon et al. studied 313 consecutive patients with severe obesity who received AGBs. The patients completed a preoperative sleep questionnaire and clinical assessment. Twelve months after AGB the same assessment was completed by 123 patients. There was a significant improvement in the responses to all questions at follow-up, with habitual snoring reduced to 14 per cent (preoperative value, 82 per cent), observed sleep apnoea to two per cent (preoperative value, 33 per cent), abnormal daytime sleepiness to four per cent (preoperative value, 39 per cent), and poor sleep quality to two per cent (preoperative value, 39 per cent) ($p < .001$ for all).[44] Also patients > or = 60 years of age can experience a significant improvement: they showed improvement one year after surgery in 100 per cent of cases of OSA.[45]

In a recent study on Asian patients who had AGB surgery, the authors demonstrate an improvement in sleep architecture in addition to a reduction in AHI, in association with weight loss. After the set target weight loss of 20 kg and one year post-procedure, AHI showed an average improvement of 50 per cent, with a cure of OSA (AHI < 5) in many preoperatively severe cases in the repeat studies pool ($p < 0.001$).[46]

Effects of BPD on OSA

In a consecutive series of 19 patients who have been followed-up for more than four months after open BPD, three patients had OSA, and overnight CPAP was able to be stopped in two patients by four months, showing the early effect of the surgery.[47]

Simard *et al.* determined the prevalence of asthma and OSA in morbidly obese patients and the effect of BPD/DS on these conditions. For the cohort of 398 patients OSA was improved in all but one with this condition; among 29 SAS patients using CPAP before surgery, only four were still using this treatment after two years.[48]

Dyslipidemia

Dyslipidemia in obesity is characterized by hypertriglyceridaemia, low high-density lipoprotein (HDL) cholesterol, and increased prevalence of small dense low-density lipoprotein (LDL) particles.[49,50] Small, dense LDL particles are atherogenic and associated with an increased risk of coronary heart diseases.[51,52]

Modification of diet is the first line intervention for hypercholesterolaemia, but it has limited efficacy.[53,54] The meta-analysis of Buchwald confirmed that effective weight loss obtained by bariatric surgery in morbidly obese subjects lead to an improvement of hyperlipidemia in more than 70 per cent of patients.[9] In the SOS study, bariatric surgery induced improvement of hypertriglyceridaemia and low HDL cholesterol levels, but not of hypercholesterolemia, in comparison with conventional therapy.[3] In 11 studies evaluated by Maggard *et al*. improvement or resolution of dyslipidemia was seen in 60–100 per cent of surgical subjects.[55]

Effects of RYGB on dyslipidemia

Zlabek *et al*. retrospectively analysed 168 patients after RYGB and had lipid analyses performed preoperatively and at one and two years postoperatively. RYGB improved all lipid parameters studied and decreased the percentage of dyslipidemic patients. Furthermore, fewer patients were taking lipid-modifying medications postoperatively, suggesting a substantial medication cost savings over time.[56] Moreover, the improvements in lipid profiles can be observed as early as three months postoperatively.[57] Those effects seem to be sustained in the long term. In a five year follow-up study on 193 patients, the prevalence of hypercholesterolemia, hypertriglyceridaemia and low HDL decreased from 41.6 per cent to 15.2 per cent, from 45.2 per cent to 4.4 per cent and from 65.8 per cent to 28.9 per cent respectively after RYGB.[58] In the SOS study, after ten years, the subjects who had undergone RYGB had greater improvements in triglycerides (28.0 per cent versus 18.0 per cent decrease), total cholesterol (12.6 per cent versus 5.0 per cent decrease), and HDL levels (47.5 per cent versus 20.4 per cent increase) than those who had AGB.[3]

Effects of AGB on dyslipidemia

Zambon *et al*. recently demonstrated that AGB produces an important body weight reduction in morbidly obese subjects associated with an improvement of the plasma lipoproteins, with significant reduction of triglycerides and significant increase of HDL, reducing the small dense

LDL fraction. These latter modifications were not related to weight reduction nor to changes in phospholipid fatty acid composition (a marker of habitual dietary fatty acid intake), but they were most prominently associated with triglyceride reduction.[59]

In a prospective study, a total of 50 patients (17 men, 33 women) with type 2 diabetes were studied preoperatively and again one year after AGB surgery. There was a 43 per cent decrease in mean fasting triglyceride and a 20 per cent decrease in the mean total cholesterol/HDL cholesterol ratio, with an 18 per cent increase in mean HDL cholesterol levels.[60]

In a larger series of 709 patients, 34 per cent presented with elevated triglyceride levels. By 12 months after surgery, only nine per cent had elevated levels. Eighteen percent presented with low HDL-cholesterol levels and by 12 months only five per cent had low levels.[61]

Effects of BPD on dyslipidemia

Scopinaro had remarkable results on 312 BPD obese patients with type 2 diabetes. Before BPD, the serum triglyceride and total cholesterol were above normal values in nearly one-third and two-thirds of the patients, respectively. A marked and highly significant reduction of the mean value of serum triglyceride and total cholesterol concentration was seen by the first postoperative year, with only one subject showing a serum cholesterol value slightly above normal. The percentage of hypertriglyceridaemic patients showed a progressive decrease, reaching one per cent at five and ten years. In all subjects the serum total cholesterol level was in the normal range at the second year and at all subsequent follow-up times, all subjects being with no medication and on totally free diet. Since the simple reduction of cholesterol intestinal absorption alone cannot yield such an outcome, a specific action of BPD on cholesterol metabolism also has to be postulated. In fact, the enterohepatic bile salt circulation is partly interrupted after BPD, with the consequent loss of bile salts causing enhancement of hepatic bile acid synthesis at the expense of the cholesterol pool. Furthermore, a sharp reduction of endogenous cholesterol is likely to occur, along with other lipid absorption. The reduced availability of free cholesterol ultimately stimulates the synthesis of LDL receptors, thus resulting in an increased removal of LDL from the bloodstream. The normalization of serum total cholesterol at long term following BPD is accompanied by a rise of HDL cholesterol.[26] In addition, the reduction of gastric volume may also play a role in the lipid malabsorption, because a reduction in the passage of nutrients through the stomach, particularly amino acids and lipids, causes a decrease in the secretion of gastric lipase, an enzyme that represents one of the initial steps in lipid absorption. Another component is a reduction in the secretion of cholecystokinin, which normally stimulates the secretion of digestive enzymes (lipase, colipase and proteases).[62] These changes are responsible for a marked decrease in the hydrolysis of triacylglycerols to monoacylglycerols, diacylglycerols, and fatty acids, with consequent reduction of the absorption of free fatty acids.

Garcia-Diaz *et al.* found a spectacular decrease of 33 per cent of total cholesterol and 46 per cent of LDL levels in 58 patients after BPD. In addition to the decrease of lipids, they found simultaneous reduction of 37 per cent of apolipoprotein B. The decrease in triglycerides was more moderate, although also significant, while there were no significant change in HDL-cholesterol.[63]

Type 2 Diabetes

More than 80 per cent of the diabetic type 2 patients are obese; in the USA 50 per cent of the patients diagnosed with type 2 diabetes are obese (BMI > 30) and nine per cent morbidly obese (BMI > 40).[64] Diet, exercise, oral anti-diabetic drugs and insulin only establish glycemic control in less than one third of patients. The UK prospective diabetes study analysed the effect of diet, insulin and sulphonylurea on 4,075 newly diagnosed type 2 diabetes patients. HbA1c levels of less than seven per cent were attained respectively only in nine per cent, 28 per cent and 24 per cent of the cases after a follow-up period of nine years.[65] To date, however, there is growing evidence that surgery can effectively cure type 2 diabetes. Surgical induced diabetes resolution is not only due to weight loss but also through certain direct mechanisms.

In the Buchwald meta-analysis complete resolution of diabetes occurred in 76.8 per cent and resolved or improved in 86 per cent of the patients after bariatric surgery. Complete resolution of diabetes was demonstrated in 83.7 per cent of the patients after RYGB and in

98.9 per cent of the patients after BPD. This effect is maintained on the long-term and is independent of the weight loss.[9] The same author conducted a comprehensive review of all studies published in the English literature containing data on weight loss and type 2 diabetes-related outcomes for patients treated with any form of bariatric surgery. The dataset consists of 621 studies with 888 treatment arms and 135,246 patients; 103 arms with 3,188 patients reported on the resolution of the clinical and laboratory manifestations of type 2 diabetes. Nineteen studies with 43 treatment arms and 11,175 patients reported both weight loss and diabetes resolution outcomes separately for the 4,070 diabetic patients in these studies. The diabetic patients had an overall 78.1 per cent resolution of their clinical manifestations of diabetes, and diabetes was improved or resolved in 86.6 per cent. Diabetes resolution was greatest for patients undergoing BPD/DS (95.1 per cent resolved), followed by RYGB (80.3 per cent), gastroplasty (79.7 per cent), and then laparoscopic AGB (56.7 per cent). The proportion of patients with diabetes resolution or improvement was fairly constant at time points less than two years and two years or more.[66] One study suggested that insulin sensitivity improved in proportion to weight loss with the use of predominantly restrictive procedures but was reversed completely by predominantly malabsorptive approaches long before normalization of body weight.[67]

Mechanisms of diabetes control

Morbid obesity is associated with profound insulin resistance and marked insulin hypersecretion, but the dynamics of β-cell function (i.e. β-cell glucose sensitivity, rate sensitivity and potentiation) are preserved. On the other hand, overt diabetes and impaired glucose tolerance are characterized by a progressive loss of β-cell glucose sensitivity, independent of insulin resistance. It is well known that bariatric surgery leads to a large improvement in insulin sensitivity and absolute insulin secretion decreases significantly after bariatric surgery.[68]

Glucagon-like peptide-1 (GLP-1) is secreted by the L-cells that are primarily located in the distal ileum and colon. In response to glucose and satiety it induces insulin secretion. Since after RYGB and BPD/DS the L-cells are stimulated earlier, GLP-1 production and consequent insulin secretion could be enhanced ('hindgut hypothesis').[69] However, studies have questioned that GLP-1 is responsible for reversal of diabetes after surgery. Morinigo *et al.* have demonstrated that GLP-1 response to a meal is not a critical factor for the early amelioration in glucose homeostasis after RYGB. Six weeks after surgery, the GLP-1 increase was only significant in patients with normal glucose or impaired glucose tolerance, but not in the diabetic patients.[70] In a longitudinal study, fasting GLP-1 concentrations decreased and peptide YY levels increased independently of each other in morbidly obese patients two years after dramatic weight loss, indicating that the relationship between these gut hormones seems to be more complicated than assumed before.[71] In a three-year follow-up study in diabetic patients, Rosa *et al.* have shown that reversibility of diabetes is dependent on the improvement of skeletal muscle insulin sensitivity, mediated by changes in the expression of genes regulating glucose and fatty acid metabolism in response to nutrient availability.[72]

The alternative hypothesis ('foregut hypothesis') states that duodenal and proximal jejunal exclusion may prevent secretion of a putative signal that promotes insulin resistance and type 2 diabetes. Other studies demonstrated a decrease in plasma levels of leptin and insulin, with increased levels of adiponectin and peptide YY3-36 after RYGB or BPD.[69] The possible mechanisms for type 2 diabetes control after bariatric surgery are summarized in Fig. 1.

Effects of RYGB on type 2 diabetes

In 2003 Schauer *et al.* published their report of the effect of RYGB on type 2 diabetes. They analysed 191 patients with impaired fasting glucose and type 2 diabetes pre- and post-operative RYGB (mean follow-up of 19.7 months). Fasting plasma glucose and glycosylated haemoglobin concentrations returned to normal levels (83 per cent) or markedly improved (17 per cent) in all patients. A significant reduction in use of oral antidiabetic agents (80 per cent) and insulin (79 per cent) followed surgical treatment. Patients with the shortest duration (< 5 years), the mildest form of type 2 diabetes (diet controlled), and the greatest weight loss after surgery were most likely to achieve complete resolution of type 2 diabetes.[74] In the experience of Pories and Albrecht, the mortality risk from diabetes over

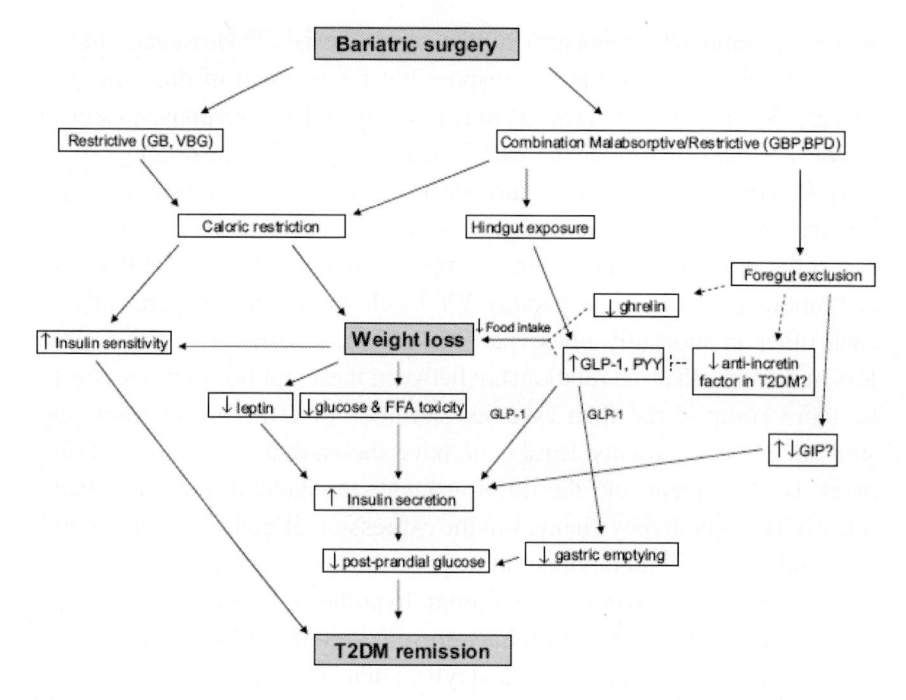

Figure 1. Proposed model for mechanisms of T2DM remission after bariatric surgery based on available studies. Dashed lines indicate hypothetical links.[73]

a ten year follow-up after RYGB was less than that in a cohort of diabetic patients matched for age, weight and BMI who were not operated on (1.0 per cent versus 4.5 per cent for every year of follow-up; $p < .0003$).[75]

Hickey *et al.* demonstrated significantly lower levels of fasting plasma glucose, plasma insulin, and serum leptins in a group of patients maintaining stable weight after RYGB compared to a group of patients matched in weight, age, and percentage of fat who did not undergo surgery.[76]

Table 1 summarizes the results of some large studies regarding the effect of RYGB on type 2 diabetes. In Fig. 2 the hypothesized mechanism responsible for the control of type 2 diabetes after RYGB is depicted.

Effects of AGB on type 2 diabetes

The diabetes remission after AGB occurs gradually and is correlated to the degree of weight loss. In an unblinded randomized controlled trial, 60 obese

Table 1. Effect of RYGB on type 2 diabetes.

Author	N	Patients with T2DM (%)	Follow-up	Resolved improved unchanged
Sugerman[15]	1025	15	1–10 years	R = 86%
Wittgrove[78]	500	17	5 years	R = 98%
				I = 2%
Pories[79]	608	27	10 years	R = 89%
				I = 7%
				U = 4%
Schauer[74]	1160	20	4 years	R = 83%
				I = 17%
Diniz[80]	31	100	27 months	I = 100%
Rubino[81]	10	60	3 weeks	R = 100%
Morinigo[70]	34	29.4	6–12 months	I = 100%

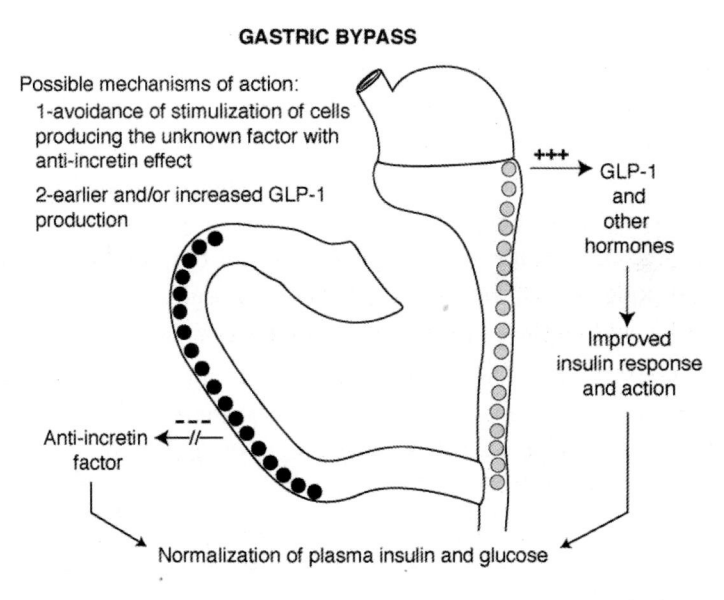

Figure 2. Hypothesized mechanism responsible for the control of diabetes after RYGB.[77]

patients (BMI > 30 and < 40) with recently diagnosed (< 2 years) type 2 diabetes were analysed. Patients either received either conventional diabetes therapy with a focus on weight loss by lifestyle change, or laparoscopic AGB with conventional diabetes care. Ninety-two percent of the patients completed the two year follow-up. Remission of type 2 diabetes was achieved by 22 (73 per cent) in the surgical group and four (13 per cent) in the conventional-therapy group. Remission of type 2 diabetes was related to weight loss and lower baseline HbA1c levels.[82] In a study of 838 patients undergoing AGB, 545 patients were identified with co-morbid illness at more than six months follow-up. After a median follow-up of 13 months (range 6–36 months), resolution and/or improvement of type 2 diabetes mellitus was 79 per cent.[21] One study examined the effect of AGB on metabolic profile of 122 diabetics. After AGB 93.1 per cent of the patients experienced an improvement in fasting glucose levels and 75.4 per cent had an improvement in HbA1c levels at the end of one year. All patients experienced a decrease in insulin requirements, and 36.6 per cent were able to totally discontinue using it.[83] Busetto *et al.* examined the effect of AGB in older patients and one year after surgery there was an improvement in 100 per cent of the diabetic cases.[45] Korenkov evaluated the impact of AGB on obesity-associated diseases and diabetes decreased from 10 per cent to four per cent in a group of 138 patients three to eight years postoperatively.[84]

Even the occurrence of type 2 diabetes can be prevented after sustained and long-lasting weight loss obtained through AGB.[25]

Table 2 summarizes the results of some large studies regarding the effect of AGB on type 2 diabetes.

Table 2. Effect of AGB on type 2 diabetes.

Author	N	Patients with T2DM (%)	Follow-up	Resolved improved unchanged
Dixon[60]	500	11	1 year	R = 64%
				I = 26%
				U = 10%
Pontiroli[85]	143	45	3 years	R = 80%
Dixon[82]	55	100	2 years	R = 73%

Effects of BPD on type 2 diabetes

In a series of 312 obese patients with type 2 diabetes, fasting serum glucose concentration fell to within normal values in all but two of the patients and remained in the physiological range in all but six for a mean follow-up of ten years.[26]

Palomar analysed 35 patients after BPD. Type 2 diabetes was present in 18 per cent of the patients, 18 per cent were on hypoglycaemic therapy and 25 per cent had impaired glucose tolerance. At 12 months after BPD, the prevalence of diabetes decreased to zero per cent ($p < 0.01$) and impaired glucose tolerance to three per cent ($p < 0.01$). Fasting glucose levels were reduced from 117 ± 25 mg/dl at baseline to 91 ± 15 mg/dl at one year ($p < 0.01$).[86]

In 1998, Scopinaro *et al.* reported normalization of glucose levels in 100 per cent of their morbidly obese patients after BPD with no need for medication and on a totally free diet as early as one month after operation, when excess weight was still more than 80 per cent.[87]

Other Co-Morbidities

Gastro-oesophageal reflux disease

Nearly all epidemiologic studies have found an association between increasing BMI and symptoms of gastro-oesophageal reflux disease (GORD). GORD symptoms have been reported in 35–70 per cent of obese patients requiring bariatric surgery.[88–90]

Changes in gastro-oesophageal anatomy and physiology caused by obesity may explain the association. These include an increased prevalence of oesophageal motor disorders, diminished lower oesophageal sphincter (LES) pressure, the development of a hiatal hernia, and increased intragastric pressure. Central adiposity may be the most important risk for the development of reflux and related complications such as Barrett's oesophagus and oesophageal adenocarcinoma. Weight loss, through caloric restriction and behavioural modification, has been studied infrequently as a means of improving reflux. Bariatric surgery and its effects on a number of obesity-related disorders have been studied more extensively.[91] Bariatric surgery has had an impact on the frequency of

GORD in obese patients, and GORD prevalence varies after each of the different types of bariatric surgery.

Some studies that included patients with morbid obesity and RYGB have reported complete improvement of symptoms in 80 per cent of the cases and discontinuation of anti-secretory therapy in 97 per cent of the patients.[92-96] RYGB improves the reflux symptoms, oesophageal exposure to acid, and oesophageal hypercontractility in patients with morbid obesity.[97] In addition, healing of oesophagitis and improvement in Barrett's oesophagus have recently been reported and some authors have proposed RYGB for severe reflux disease after vertical banded gastroplasty (VBG).[98-100]

AGB has been shown to have various effects on reflux. It can act as an antireflux procedure or it can enhance GORD.[101-106] AGB also rapidly alters oesophageal motility, with a decrease in the amplitude of contractions in the lower oesophagus as soon as nine months after surgery.[105] With increasing length of follow-up, however, a growing number of long-term complications arise, such as pouch dilatation with or without slippage, band erosion, progressive oesophageal dilatation with pseudoachalasia, food intolerance with gastro-oesophageal reflux and band leaks. These complications are sometimes difficult to manage and often lead to progressive weight regain. Reasons why some patients tolerate the band very well and others develop complications are essentially unknown, although eating behaviour, which shows abnormal patterns in the majority of morbidly obese patients, and pre-existing conditions of the upper gastrointestinal tract like hiatus hernia, GORD and oesophageal motility disorders have been incriminated. It would be of interest to be able to better select morbidly obese patients for AGB and exclude from this procedure those in whom long-term complications can be anticipated on the basis of preoperative factors.[107]

Musculoskeletal problems

A causative relationship between excess weight and musculoskeletal problems has been difficult to establish for many conditions. Nevertheless, weight loss can make a substantial difference in most musculoskeletal symptoms, as well as help prevent heart disease and metabolic syndrome. Some studies have looked at how major weight loss after bariatric surgery affects baseline musculoskeletal symptoms. McGoey et al. reported a prospective study of 105 patients who lost a mean of 44 kg after VBG. The prevalence of back pain decreased from 62 per cent to 11 per cent, hip pain from 11 per cent to two per cent, knee pain from 57 per cent to 14 per cent, ankle pain from 34 per cent to two per cent, and foot pain from 21 per cent to one per cent.[108] Peltonen et al. looked at work-restricting musculoskeletal symptoms in the general population compared with those in 2,010 surgically treated obese patients ages 37–60, and those in 2,037 age-matched and sexmatched obese patients not undergoing surgery. Obese patients had more work restricting neck, low back, hip, knee and ankle pain, and the prevalence increased with BMI. Patients who underwent VBG had a significant decrease in work-restricting low back pain at all five sites.[109] In a retrospective study of 400 consecutive RYGB patients, arthritis, back or extremity pain, and depression improved in 52–73 per cent of patients.[110]

Non-alcoholic steatohepatitis

The prevalence of obesity-related non-alcoholic steatohepatitis (NASH) has increased substantially in recent years. In a study by Mattar et al. there was a marked improvement in liver steatosis (from 88 per cent to eight per cent), inflammation (from 23 per cent to two per cent), and fibrosis (from 31 per cent to 13 per cent; all $p < 0.001$) after weight loss surgery (RYGB, AGB and sleeve gastrectomy). Inflammation and fibrosis resolved in 37 per cent and 20 per cent of patients respectively, corresponding to improvement of 82 per cent ($p < 0.001$) in grade and 39 per cent ($p < 0.001$) in stage of liver disease.[111] Dixon et al. analysed the effect of weight loss on 36 patients with NASH; 82 per cent had resolution of disease after AGB, nine per cent showed improvement, and nine per cent had no change. Furthermore, nine of ten patients who had stage three fibrosis before surgery had regression of fibrosis at a mean follow-up of 25.6 ± 11 months.[112]

Pseudotumor cerebri

Pseudotumor cerebri (PTC), also known as idiopathic intracranial hypertension, is a condition associated with headache, blurred vision and often pulsatile tinnitus (an annoying auditory swishing sound synchronous with the heartbeat). Cranial imaging studies are normal, with the exception of small ventricles and/or an empty sella. Cerebrospinal fluid (CSF) pressures are always elevated. These patients may also have other central nervous system and cranial nerve dysfunction, including visual disturbances and rarely Bell's palsy and trigeminal neuralgia. Increased intra-abdominal pressure associated with central obesity is the probable etiology of PTC, a condition that should no longer be considered idiopathic. Bariatric surgery is the long-term procedure of choice for severely obese patients with PTC and is shown to have a much higher rate of success than CSF–peritoneal shunting reported in the literature, as well as providing resolution of additional obesity co-morbidity.[113]

Polycystic ovary syndrome

Polycystic ovary syndrome (PCOS) was first described by Stein and Leventhal in 1935. It is a heterogeneous disorder of unclear etiology and it is an important cause of both menstrual irregularity and androgen excess in women. When fully expressed, the manifestations include ovulatory dysfunction, androgen excess, polycystic ovaries and obesity. It is recognized as one of the most common endocrine/metabolic disorders of women.[114]

In a study of 17 obese women with PCOS with a mean BMI of 50.7 kg/m^2, bariatric surgery was associated with a mean weight loss after 12 months of 41 ± 9 kg, restoration of ovulatory cycles, and improvements in insulin resistance, hyperandrogenemia and hirsutism scores.[115] Eid *et al.* studied 24 women with PCOS who underwent elective laparoscopic RYGB. All women resumed normal menstrual cycles after a mean of 3.4 ± 2.1 months postoperatively. Of the 23 women with hirsutism, 12 (52 per cent) had complete resolution at a mean follow-up of 8 ± 2.3 months; 6 (25 per cent) had moderate resolution at a mean of 21 ± 18 months; and three had minimal resolution at 34 ± 14 months. Five women were able to conceive after surgery without the use of clomiphene.[116]

Quality of Life After Bariatric Surgery

The SOS study found a dramatic improvement in the quality of life at two years among patients who had surgical treatment for obesity, particularly concerning psychological performance (also see Chapter 13). There is a strong positive correlation between the degree of improvement in quality of life and the degree of weight loss.[117] Schauer et al. reported improvement in quality of life in 95 per cent of 275 patients who underwent laparoscopic RYGB.[89] Similar results have been reported for laparoscopic AGB.[118] Several studies have attempted to validate quality of life instruments for assessment in bariatric surgery patients. Three instruments have been tested extensively: the Medical Outcome Study Short Form-36 (MOS SF-36, Rand SF-36 or SF-36), Bariatric Analysis and Reporting Outcome System (BAROS) and the Impact of Weight on Quality of Life-Lite (IWQoL-Lite). A total of 308 RYGB patients were compared with 253 individuals who sought but did not undergo RYGB and 272 population-based obese individuals using the weight-related IWQoL-Lite and general MOS SF-36 health related quality of life (HRQoL) questionnaires at baseline and two years of follow-up. Dramatic improvements had occurred in weight-related and physical health related quality of life for RYGB patients at two years after surgery compared with two severely obese groups who had not undergone surgery. These results support the effectiveness of RYGB surgery in improving patients' HRQoL.[119] Bond et al. suggest that RYGB patients who become active postoperatively achieve weight losses and HRQoL improvements that are greater than those experienced by patients who remain inactive and comparable to those attained by patients who stay active.[120] Psychiatrists and surgeons at the University of Chicago compared SF-36 scores before, immediately after and six months after RYGBP. Twenty out of 32 patients completed the follow-up evaluation. SF-36 scores significantly improved for physical functioning, general health, vitality and mental health.[121] O'Brien and colleagues compared SF-36 scores before and after AGB at one and two years with the Australian general community. They found highly significant improvements in QoL following AGB.[61] Favretti et al. used BAROS to follow 170 patients for at least 18 months after AGB. They were able to demonstrate improved results after a 'learning curve' in their first 50 AGBs.[122]

Adami et al. administered the IWQoL-Lite questionnaire to 50 obese patients prior to and at one year following BPD, to 150 post-obese subjects at three years following BPD and to 50 lean controls. At one year after the operation, the authors found a sharp improvement toward normality in the QoL, and the cross-sectional findings suggest that this result was maintained in the long term. Following BPD, patients' weight loss and long-term maintenance are accompanied by overall beneficial effects on their QoL.[123] Moneghini and his team followed 30 patients after BPD. The course and QoL were assessed using BAROS after a minimum follow-up of 18 months. According to the BAROS, the outcome was classified as Excellent in 10 per cent of cases, Very Good in 63.3 per cent, Good in 20 per cent, Fair in 6.7 per cent; no patients had Failure course. Ninety-three percent of patients had resolution of at least one of their major co-morbidities, and an improvement of the medical conditions was registered in all the cases. The QoL was greatly improved in 55 per cent, improved in 35 per cent and did not change in 10 per cent of the patients.[124]

References

1. Must, A., Spadano, J., Coakley, E.H. *et al.* (1999). The disease burden associated with overweight and obesity. *JAMA* 282(16): 1523–1529.
2. Goldstein, D.J. (1992). Beneficial health effects of modest weight loss. *Int J Obes Relat Metab Disord* 16(6): 397–415.
3. Sjostrom, L., Lindroos, A.K., Peltonen, M. *et al.* (2004). Lifestyle, diabetes, and cardiovascular risk factors 10 years after bariatric surgery. *N Engl J Med* 351(26): 2683–2693.
4. Frezza, E.E., Wei, C., Wachtel, M.S. (2009). Is surgery the next answer to treat obesity-related hypertension? *J Clin Hypertens (Greenwich)* 11(5): 284–288.
5. Singer, G.M., Setaro, J.F. (2008). Secondary hypertension: obesity and the metabolic syndrome. *J Clin Hypertens (Greenwich)* 10(7): 567–574.
6. Goodfriend, T.L., Calhoun, D.A. (2004). Resistant hypertension, obesity, sleep apnoea, and aldosterone: theory and therapy. *Hypertension* 43(3): 518–524.
7. Phillips, B.G., Narkiewicz, K., Pesek, C.A. *et al.* (1999). Effects of obstructive sleep apnea on endothelin-1 and blood pressure. *J Hypertens* 17(1): 61–66.
8. Horvath, K., Jeitler, K., Siering, U. *et al.* (2008). Long-term effects of weight-reducing interventions in hypertensive patients: systematic review and meta-analysis. *Arch Intern Med* 168(6): 571–580.

9. Buchwald, H., Avidor, Y., Braunwald, E. *et al.* (2004). Bariatric surgery: a systematic review and meta-analysis. *JAMA* 292(14): 1724–1737.
10. Carson, J.L., Ruddy, M.E., Duff, A.E. *et al.* (1994). The effect of gastric bypass surgery on hypertension in morbidly obese patients. *Arch Intern Med* 154(2): 193–200.
11. Fazylov, R., Soto, E., Merola, S. (2008). Laparoscopic Roux-en-Y gastric bypass in morbidly obese patients > or = 55 years old. *Obes Surg* 18(6): 656–659.
12. Fernstrom, J.D., Courcoulas, A.P., Houck, P.R. *et al.* (2006). Long-term changes in blood pressure in extremely obese patients who have undergone bariatric surgery. *Arch Surg* 141(3): 276–283.
13. Foley, E.F., Benotti, P.N., Borlase, B.C. *et al.* (1992). Impact of gastric restrictive surgery on hypertension in the morbidly obese. *Am J Surg* 163(3): 294–297.
14. Reinhold, R.B. (1994). Late results of gastric bypass surgery for morbid obesity. *J Am Coll Nutr* 13(4): 326–331.
15. Sugerman, H.J., Wolfe, L.G., Sica, D.A . *et al.* (2003). Diabetes and hypertension in severe obesity and effects of gastric bypass-induced weight loss. *Ann Surg* 237(6): 751–756; discussion 757–758.
16. Czupryniak, L., Strzelczyk, J., Pawlowski, M. *et al.* (2005). Circadian blood pressure variation in morbidly obese hypertensive patients undergoing gastric bypass surgery. *Am J Hypertens* 18(4 Pt 1): 446–551.
17. Hinojosa, M.W., Varela, J.E., Smith, B.R. *et al.* (2009). Resolution of systemic hypertension after laparoscopic gastric bypass. *J Gastrointest Surg* 13(4): 793–797.
18. Ahmed, A.R., Rickards, G., Coniglio, D. *et al.* (2009). Laparoscopic Roux-en-Y Gastric Bypass and its early effect on blood pressure. *Obes Surg* 19(7): 845–849.
19. Bennett, J.C., Wang, H., Schirmer, B.D. *et al.* (2007). Quality of life and resolution of co-morbidities in super-obese patients remaining morbidly obese after Roux-en-Y gastric bypass. *Surg Obes Relat Dis* 3(3): 387–391.
20. Dall'Asta, C., Vedani, P., Manunta, P. *et al.* (2009). Effect of weight loss through laparoscopic gastric banding on blood pressure, plasma renin activity and aldosterone levels in morbid obesity. *Nutr Metab Cardiovasc Dis* 19(2): 110–114.

21. Brancatisano, A., Wahlroos, S., Brancatisano, R. (2008). Improvement in comorbid illness after placement of the Swedish adjustable gastric band. *Surg Obes Relat Dis* 4(3 Suppl): S39–S46.
22. Weiner, R., Blanco-Engert, R., Weiner, S. et al. (2003). Outcome after laparoscopic adjustable gastric banding — 8 years experience. *Obes Surg* 13(3): 427–434.
23. Mittermair, R.P., Weiss, H., Nehoda, H. et al. (2003). Laparoscopic Swedish adjustable gastric banding: 6-year follow-up and comparison to other laparoscopic bariatric procedures. *Obes Surg* 13(3): 412–417.
24. Dixon, J.B., O'Brien, P.E. (2002). Changes in comorbidities and improvements in quality of life after LAP-BAND placement. *Am J Surg* 184(6B): 51S–54S.
25. Pontiroli, A.E., Folli, F., Paganelli, M. et al. (2005). Laparoscopic gastric banding prevents type 2 diabetes and arterial hypertension and induces their remission in morbid obesity: a 4-year case-controlled study. *Diabetes Care* 28(11): 2703–2709.
26. Scopinaro, N., Marinari, G.M., Camerini, G.B. et al. (2005). Specific effects of biliopancreatic diversion on the major components of metabolic syndrome: a long-term follow-up study. *Diabetes Care* 28(10): 2406–2411.
27. Adami, G., Murelli, F., Carlini, F. et al. (2005). Long-term effect of biliopancreatic diversion on blood pressure in hypertensive obese patients. *Am J Hypertens* 18(6): 780–784.
28. Adami, G.F., Papadia, F., Carlini, F. et al. (2005). Effect of biliopancreatic diversion on hypertension in severely obese patients. *Hypertens Res* 28(2): 119–123.
29. Pontiroli, A.E., Laneri, M., Veronelli, A. et al. (2009). Biliary pancreatic diversion and laparoscopic adjustable gastric banding in morbid obesity: their long-term effects on metabolic syndrome and cardiovascular parameters. *Cardiovasc Diabetol* 8(1): 37.
30. Young, T., Palta, M., Dempsey, J. et al. (1993). The occurrence of sleep-disordered breathing among middle-aged adults. *N Engl J Med* 328(17): 1230–1235.
31. de Sousa, A.G., Cercato, C., Mancini, M.C. et al. (2008). Obesity and obstructive sleep apnoea–hypopnea syndrome. *Obes Rev* 9(4): 340–354.
32. Punjabi, N.M. (2008). The epidemiology of adult obstructive sleep apnoea. *Proc Am Thorac Soc* 5(2): 136–143.

33. Young, T., Skatrud, J., Peppard, P.E. (2004). Risk factors for obstructive sleep apnoea in adults. *JAMA* 291(16): 2013–2016.
34. Schwartz, A.R., Patil, S.P., Laffan, A.M. *et al.* (2008). Obesity and obstructive sleep apnoea: pathogenic mechanisms and therapeutic approaches. *Proc Am Thorac Soc* 5(2): 185–192.
35. Eckert, D.J., Malhotra, A. (2008). Pathophysiology of adult obstructive sleep apnea. *Proc Am Thorac Soc* 5(2): 144–153.
36. Rapoport, D.M., Sorkin, B., Garay, S.M. *et al.* (1982). Reversal of the "Pickwickian syndrome" by long-term use of nocturnal nasal–airway pressure. *N Engl J Med* 307(15): 931–933.
37. Riley, R.W., Powell, N.B., Guilleminault, C. *et al.* (1995). Obstructive sleep apnoea. Trends in therapy. *West J Med* 162(2): 143–148.
38. Schwartz, A.R., Gold, A.R., Schubert, N. *et al.* (1991). Effect of weight loss on upper airway collapsibility in obstructive sleep apnoea. *Am Rev Respir Dis* 144(3 Pt 1): 494–498.
39. Smith, P.L., Gold, A.R., Meyers, D.A. *et al.* (1985). Weight loss in mildly to moderately obese patients with obstructive sleep apnoea. *Ann Intern Med* 103(6 Pt 1): 850–855.
40. Varela, J.E., Hinojosa, M.W., Nguyen, N.T. (2007). Resolution of obstructive sleep apnoea after laparoscopic gastric bypass. *Obes Surg* 17(10): 1279–1282.
41. Rasheid, S., Banasiak, M., Gallagher, S.F. *et al.* (2003). Gastric bypass is an effective treatment for obstructive sleep apnoea in patients with clinically significant obesity. *Obes Surg* 13(1): 58–61.
42. Lankford, D.A., Proctor, C.D., Richard, R. (2005). Continuous positive airway pressure (CPAP) changes in bariatric surgery patients undergoing rapid weight loss. *Obes Surg* 215(3): 336–341.
43. Jensen, C., Tejirian, T., Lewis, C. *et al.* (2008). Postoperative CPAP and BiPAP use can be safely omitted after laparoscopic Roux-en-Y gastric bypass. *Surg Obes Relat Dis* 4(4): 512–514.
44. Dixon, J.B., Schachter, L.M., O'Brien, P.E. (2001). Sleep disturbance and obesity: changes following surgically induced weight loss. *Arch Intern Med* 161(1): 102–106.
45. Busetto, L., Angrisani, L., Basso, N. *et al.* (2008). Safety and efficacy of laparoscopic adjustable gastric banding in the elderly. *Obesity (Silver Spring)* 16(2): 334–338.

46. Rao, A., Tey, B.H., Ramalingam, G. *et al.* (2009). Obstructive sleep apnoea (OSA) patterns in bariatric surgical practice and response of OSA to weight loss after laparoscopic adjustable gastric banding (LAGB). *Ann Acad Med Singapore* 38(7): 587.
47. de Luis, D.A., Pacheco, D., Izaola, O. *et al.* (2005). Early clinical and surgical results of biliopancreatic diversion. *Obes Surg* 15(6): 799–802.
48. Simard, B., Turcotte, H., Marceau, P. *et al.* (2004). Asthma and sleep apnoea in patients with morbid obesity: outcome after bariatric surgery. *Obes Surg* 14(10): 1381–1388.
49. Manzato, E., Zambon, S., Zambon, A. *et al.* (1992). Lipoprotein sub-fraction levels and composition in obese subjects before and after gastroplasty. *Int J Obes Relat Metab Disord* 16(8): 573–578.
50. Zambon, A., Sartore, G., Passera, D. *et al.* (1999). Effects of hypocaloric dietary treatment enriched in oleic acid on LDL and HDL subclass distribution in mildly obese women. *J Intern Med* 246(2): 191–201.
51. Carmena, R., Duriez, P., Fruchart, J.C. (2004). Atherogenic lipoprotein particles in atherosclerosis. *Circulation* 109(23 Suppl 1): 1112–1117.
52. Kwiterovich, P.O. Jr (2002). Clinical relevance of the biochemical, metabolic, and genetic factors that influence low-density lipoprotein heterogeneity. *Am J Cardiol* 90(8A): 30i–47i.
53. Hunninghake, D.B., Stein, E.A., Dujovne, C.A. *et al.* (1993). The efficacy of intensive dietary therapy alone or combined with lovastatin in outpatients with hypercholesterolemia. *N Engl J Med* 328(17): 1213–1219.
54. Tang, J.L., Armitage, J.M., Lancaster, T. *et al.* (1998). Systematic review of dietary intervention trials to lower blood total cholesterol in free–living subjects. *BMJ* 316(7139): 1213–1220.
55. Maggard, M.A., Shugarman, L.R., Suttorp, M. *et al.* (2005). Meta-analysis: surgical treatment of obesity. *Ann Intern Med* 142(7): 547–559.
56. Zlabek, J.A., Grimm, M.S., Larson, C.J. *et al.* (2005). The effect of laparoscopic gastric bypass surgery on dyslipidemia in severely obese patients. *Surg Obes Relat Dis* 1(6): 537–542.
57. Nguyen, N.T., Varela, E., Sabio, A. *et al.* (2006). Resolution of hyperlipidemia after laparoscopic Roux-en-Y gastric bypass. *J Am Coll Surg* 203(1): 24–29.
58. Diniz, M.D., Passos, V.M., Barreto, S.M. *et al.* (2009). Different criteria for assessment of Roux-en-Y Gastric Bypass success: does only weight matter? *Obes Surg* 19(10): 1384–1392.

59. Zambon, S., Romanato, G., Sartore, G. et al. (2009). Bariatric surgery improves atherogenic LDL profile by triglyceride reduction. *Obes Surg* 19(2): 190–195.
60. Dixon, J.B., O'Brien, P.E. (2002). Health outcomes of severely obese type 2 diabetic subjects 1 year after laparoscopic adjustable gastric banding. *Diabetes Care* 25(2): 358–363.
61. O'Brien, P.E., Dixon, J.B., Brown, W. et al. (2002). The laparoscopic adjustable gastric band (Lap-Band): a prospective study of medium-term effects on weight, health and quality of life. *Obes Surg* 12(5): 652–660.
62. Bays, H.E. (2004). Current and investigational antiobesity agents and obesity therapeutic treatment targets. *Obes Res* 12(8): 1197–1211.
63. Garcia-Diaz, J., de, D., Lozano, O., Ramos, J.C. et al. (2003). Changes in lipid profile after biliopancreatic diversion. *Obes Surg* 13(5): 756–760.
64. Leibson, C.L., Williamson, D.F., Melton, L.J. III et al. (2001). Temporal trends in BMI among adults with diabetes. *Diabetes Care* 24(9): 1584–1589.
65. Turner, R.C., Cull, C.A., Frighi, V. et al. (1999). Glycemic control with diet, sulfonylurea, metformin, or insulin in patients with type 2 diabetes mellitus: progressive requirement for multiple therapies (UKPDS 49). UK Prospective Diabetes Study (UKPDS) Group. *JAMA* 281(21): 2005–2012.
66. Buchwald, H., Estok, R., Fahrbach, K. et al. (2009). Weight and type 2 diabetes after bariatric surgery: systematic review and meta-analysis. *Am J Med* 122(3): 248–256 e5.
67. Muscelli, E., Mingrone, G., Camastra, S. et al. (2005). Differential effect of weight loss on insulin resistance in surgically treated obese patients. *Am J Med* 118(1): 51–57.
68. Schernthaner, G., Morton, J.M. (2008). Bariatric surgery in patients with morbid obesity and type 2 diabetes. *Diabetes Care* 31(Suppl 2): S297–S302.
69. Silecchia, G., Casella, G., Rizzello, M. (2009). Surgical treatment of type 2 diabetes. *Acta Chir Belg* 109: 292–299.
70. Morinigo, R., Lacy, A.M., Casamitjana, R. et al. (2006). GLP-1 and changes in glucose tolerance following gastric bypass surgery in morbidly obese subjects. *Obes Surg* 16(12): 1594–1601.
71. Reinehr, T., Roth, C.L., Schernthaner, G.H. et al. (2007). Peptide YY and glucagon-like peptide-1 in morbidly obese patients before and after surgically induced weight loss. *Obes Surg* 17(12): 1571–1577.

72. Rosa, G., Mingrone, G., Manco, M. *et al.* (2007). Molecular mechanisms of diabetes reversibility after bariatric surgery. *Int J Obes (Lond)* 31(9): 1429–1436.
73. Bose, M., Olivan, B., Teixeira, J. *et al.* (2009). Do incretins play a role in the remission of type 2 diabetes after gastric bypass surgery: what are the evidence? *Obes Surg* 19(2): 217–229.
74. Schauer, P.R., Burguera, B., Ikramuddin, S. *et al.* (2003). Effect of laparoscopic Roux-en-Y gastric bypass on type 2 diabetes mellitus. *Ann Surg* 238(4): 467–84; discussion 84–85.
75. Pories, W.J., Albrecht, R.J. (2001). Etiology of type 2 diabetes mellitus: role of the foregut. *World J Surg* 25(4): 527–531.
76. Hickey, M.S., Pories, W.J., MacDonald, K.G. Jr *et al.* (1998). A new paradigm for type 2 diabetes mellitus: could it be a disease of the foregut? *Ann Surg* 227(5): 637–643; discussion 643–644.
77. Rubino, F., Gagner, M. (2002). Potential of surgery for curing type 2 diabetes mellitus. *Ann Surg* 236(5): 554–559.
78. Wittgrove, A.C., Clark, G.W. (2000). Laparoscopic gastric bypass, Roux-en-Y—500 patients: technique and results, with 3–60 month follow-up. *Obes Surg* 10(3): 233–239.
79. Pories, W.J., Swanson, M.S., MacDonald, K.G. *et al.* (1995). Who would have thought it? An operation proves to be the most effective therapy for adult-onset diabetes mellitus. *Ann Surg* 222(3): 339–350; discussion 350–352.
80. Diniz Mde, F., Diniz, M.T., Sanches, S.R. *et al.* (2004). Glycemic control in diabetic patients after bariatric surgery. *Obes Surg* 14(8): 1051–1055.
81. Rubino, F., Gagner, M., Gentileschi, P. *et al.* (2004). The early effect of the Roux-en-Y gastric bypass on hormones involved in body weight regulation and glucose metabolism. *Ann Surg* 240(2): 236–242.
82. Dixon, J.B., O'Brien, P.E., Playfair, J. *et al.* (2008). Adjustable gastric banding and conventional therapy for type 2 diabetes: a randomized controlled trial. *JAMA* 299(3): 316–323.
83. Singhal, R., Kitchen, M., Bridgwater, S. *et al.* (2008). Metabolic outcomes of obese diabetic patients following laparoscopic adjustable gastric banding. *Obes Surg* 18(11): 1400–1405.
84. Korenkov, M., Shah, S., Sauerland, S. *et al.* (2007). Impact of laparoscopic adjustable gastric banding on obesity co-morbidities in the medium- and long-term. *Obes Surg* 17(5): 679–683.

85. Pontiroli, A.E., Pizzocri, P., Librenti, M.C. et al. (2002). Laparoscopic adjustable gastric banding for the treatment of morbid (grade 3) obesity and its metabolic complications: a three-year study. *J Clin Endocrinol Metab* 87(8): 3555–3561.
86. Palomar, R., Fernandez-Fresnedo, G., Dominguez-Diez, A. et al. (2005). Effects of weight loss after biliopancreatic diversion on metabolism and cardiovascular profile. *Obes Surg* 15(6): 794–798.
87. Scopinaro, N., Adami, G.F., Marinari, G.M. et al. (1998). Biliopancreatic diversion. *World J Surg* 22(9): 936–946.
88. Fisher, B.L., Pennathur, A., Mutnick, J.L. et al. (1999). Obesity correlates with gastro-oesophageal reflux. *Dig Dis Sci* 44(11): 2290–2294.
89. Schauer, P.R., Ikramuddin, S., Gourash, W. et al. (2000). Outcomes after laparoscopic Roux-en-Y gastric bypass for morbid obesity. *Ann Surg* 232(4): 515–529.
90. Suter, M., Dorta, G., Giusti, V. et al. (2004). Gastro-esophageal reflux and esophageal motility disorders in morbidly obese patients. *Obes Surg* 14(7): 959–966.
91. Friedenberg, F.K., Xanthopoulos, M., Foster, G.D. et al. (2008). The association between gastro-oesophageal reflux disease and obesity. *Am J Gastroenterol* 103(8): 2111–2122.
92. Clements, R.H., Gonzalez, Q.H., Foster, A. et al. (2003). Gastrointestinal symptoms are more intense in morbidly obese patients and are improved with laparoscopic Roux-en-Y gastric bypass. *Obes Surg* 13(4): 610–614.
93. Foster, A., Laws, H.L., Gonzalez, Q.H. et al. (2003). Gastrointestinal symptomatic outcome after laparoscopic Roux-en-Y gastric bypass. *J Gastrointest Surg* 7(6): 750–753.
94. Jones, K.B., Jr, Allen, T.V., Manas, K.J. et al. (1991). Roux-en-Y Gastric Bypass: an effective anti-reflux procedure. *Obes Surg* 1(3): 295–298.
95. Perry, Y., Courcoulas, A.P., Fernando, H.C. et al. (2004). Laparoscopic Roux-en-Y gastric bypass for recalcitrant gastro-oesophageal reflux disease in morbidly obese patients. *JSLS* 8(1): 19–23.
96. Smith, S.C., Edwards, C.B., Goodman, G.N. (1997) Symptomatic and clinical improvement in morbidly obese patients with gastro-oesophageal reflux disease following Roux-en-Y gastric bypass. *Obes Surg* 7(6): 479–484.

97. Mejia-Rivas, M.A., Herrera-Lopez, A., Hernandez-Calleros, J. *et al.* (2008). Gastro-oesophageal reflux disease in morbid obesity: the effect of Roux-en-Y gastric bypass. *Obes Surg* 18(10): 1217–1224.
98. Bloomberg, R.D., Urbach, D.R. (2002). Laparoscopic Roux-en-Y gastric bypass for severe gastro-oesophageal reflux after vertical banded gastroplasty. *Obes Surg* 12(3): 408–411.
99. Cobey, F., Oelschlager, B. (2005). Complete regression of Barrett's esophagus after Roux-en-Y gastric bypass. *Obes Surg* 15(5): 710–712.
100. Csendes, A., Burgos, A.M., Smok, G. *et al.* (2006). Effect of gastric bypass on Barrett's esophagus and intestinal metaplasia of the cardia in patients with morbid obesity. *J Gastrointest Surg* 10(2): 259–264.
101. de Jong, J.R., van Ramshorst, B., Timmer, R. *et al.* (2004). The influence of laparoscopic adjustable gastric banding on gastro-oesophageal reflux. *Obes Surg* 14(3): 399–406.
102. Iovino, P., Angrisani, L., Tremolaterra, F. *et al.* (2002). Abnormal esophageal acid exposure is common in morbidly obese patients and improves after a successful Lap-band system implantation. *Surg Endosc* 16(11): 1631–1635.
103. Ovrebo, K.K., Hatlebakk, J.G., Viste, A. *et al.* (1998). Gastro-oesophageal reflux in morbidly obese patients treated with gastric banding or vertical banded gastroplasty. *Ann Surg* 228(1): 51–58.
104. Peternac, D., Hauser, R., Weber M. *et al.* (2001). The effects of laparoscopic adjustable gastric banding on the proximal pouch and the esophagus. *Obes Surg* 11(1): 76–86.
105. Suter, M., Dorta, G., Giusti, V. *et al.* (2005). Gastric banding interferes with esophageal motility and gastro-oesophageal reflux. *Arch Surg* 140(7): 639–643.
106. Weiss, H., Nehoda, H., Labeck, B. *et al.* (2000). Treatment of morbid obesity with laparoscopic adjustable gastric banding affects esophageal motility. *Am J Surg* 180(6): 479–482.
107. Suter, M., Giusti, V., Calmes, J.M. *et al.* (2008). Preoperative upper gastrointestinal testing can help predicting long-term outcome after gastric banding for morbid obesity. *Obes Surg* 18(5): 578–582.
108. McGoey, B.V., Deitel, M., Saplys, R.J. *et al.* (1990). Effect of weight loss on musculoskeletal pain in the morbidly obese. *J Bone Joint Surg Br* 72(2): 322–323.

109. Peltonen, M., Lindroos, A.K., Torgerson, J.S. (2003). Musculoskeletal pain in the obese: a comparison with a general population and long-term changes after conventional and surgical obesity treatment. *Pain* 104(3): 549–557.
110. Peluso, L., Vanek, V.W. (2007). Efficacy of gastric bypass in the treatment of obesity-related co-morbidities. *Nutr Clin Pract* 22(1): 22–28.
111. Mattar, S.G., Velcu L.M., Rabinovitz, M. *et al.* (2005). Surgically-induced weight loss significantly improves nonalcoholic fatty liver disease and the metabolic syndrome. *Ann Surg* 242(4): 610–617; discussion 618–620.
112. Dixon, J.B., Bhathal, P.S., Hughes, N.R. *et al.* (2004). Nonalcoholic fatty liver disease: improvement in liver histological analysis with weight loss. *Hepatology* 39(6): 1647–1654.
113. Sugerman, H.J., Felton, W.L. III, Sismanis, A. *et al.* (1999). Gastric surgery for pseudotumor cerebri associated with severe obesity. *Ann Surg* 229(5): 634–640; discussion 640–642.
114. Stein, I.F., Leventhal, N.L. (1935). Amenorrhea associated with bilateral polycystic ovaries. *Am J Obstet Gynecol* 29: 181–191.
115. Escobar-Morreale, H.F., Botella-Carretero, J.I., Alvarez-Blasco, F. *et al.* (2005). The polycystic ovary syndrome associated with morbid obesity may resolve after weight loss induced by bariatric surgery. *J Clin Endocrinol Metab* 90(12): 6364–6369.
116. Eid, G.M., Cottam, D.R., Velcu, L.M. *et al.* (2005). Effective treatment of polycystic ovarian syndrome with Roux-en-Y gastric bypass. *Surg Obes Relat Dis* 1(2): 77–80.
117. Karlsson, J., Sjostrom, L., Sullivan, M. (1998). Swedish obese subjects (SOS) — an intervention study of obesity. Two-year follow-up of health-related quality of life (HRQL) and eating behavior after gastric surgery for severe obesity. *Int J Obes Relat Metab Disord* 22(2): 113–126.
118. Dixon, J.B., Dixon, M.E., O'Brien, P.E. (2001). Quality of life after lap-band placement: influence of time, weight loss, and comorbidities. *Obes Res* 9(11): 713–721.
119. Kolotkin, R.L., Crosby, R.D., Gress, R.E. *et al.* (2009). Two-year changes in health-related quality of life in gastric bypass patients compared with severely obese controls. *Surg Obes Relat Dis* 5(2): 250–256.
120. Bond, D.S., Phelan, S., Wolfe, L.G. *et al.* (2009). Becoming physically active after bariatric surgery is associated with improved weight loss and health-related quality of life. *Obesity (Silver Spring)* 17(1): 78–83.

121. Dymek, M.P., le Grange, D., Neven, K. *et al.* (2001). Quality of life and psychosocial adjustment in patients after Roux-en-Y gastric bypass: a brief report. *Obes Surg* 11(1): 32–39.
122. Favretti, F., Cadière, G.B., Segato, G. *et al.* (1998). Bariatric analysis and reporting outcome system (BAROS) applied to laparoscopic gastric banding patients. *Obes Surg* 8(5): 500–504.
123. Adami, G.F., Ramberti, G., Weiss, A. *et al.* (2005). Quality of life in obese subjects following biliopancreatic diversion. *Behav Med* 31(2): 53–60.
124. Moneghini, D., Mittempergher, F., Terraroli, C. *et al.* (2004). Bariatric Analysis and Reporting Outcome System (BAROS) following biliopancreatic diversion. *Ann Ital Chir* 75(4): 417–420.

Chapter 13

Impact on Life Expectancy After Bariatric Surgery

Luca Busetto, Elisa Calo', Marco Mazza and Giuliano Enzi

Introduction

The use of bariatric surgery has increased exponentially in recent years. According to the data of the American Society of Bariatric Surgeons (ASBS), the total number of bariatric operations performed annually in the United States, stable at around 20,000 procedures per year throughout the 1990s, crossed the threshold of 100,000 annual procedures in the year 2003[1] and peaked to 121,055 in 2004.[2] At a lower scale, similar trends appeared to be present in most European countries and in Australia.[3] Two major driving forces may be hypothesized as the basis of the worldwide explosion of bariatric surgery. The first cause of this phenomenon is probably the fact that the prevalence of morbid obesity is increasing, at a pace that is even more accelerated than for obesity overall. According to the National Health and Nutrition Examination Survey (NHANES) 1999–2000, 3.1 per cent of adult American men and 6.3 per cent of adult American women suffer from morbid obesity.[4] From 1986 to 2000, the prevalence of obesity in general (BMI > 30 kg/m^2) approximately doubled in the United States, while that of morbid obesity (BMI > 40 kg/m^2) quadrupled and that of the so called 'super-obesity' (BMI > 50 kg/m^2) increased five-fold.[5]

The second force that may explain the wider clinical use of bariatric surgery is in our opinion the increasing acceptation of this type of therapy in the medical and surgical community. The reduction of the surgical risks, associated with newer technical skills, and the recognition of the clear clinical benefits produced by the sustained weight loss obtained by bariatric surgery on the global health of the morbidly obese patient are the basis of this change. In this chapter, we will briefly review the existing evidences about the effects of bariatric surgery on the metabolic and respiratory co-morbidities of morbid obesity. Newer data about the impact of bariatric surgery on health related quality of life and life expectancy will be also reported.

Impact of Morbid Obesity on Morbidity and Mortality

A large body of epidemiologic studies evidenced that overweight and obesity are associated with an increased risk of several metabolic disturbances, respiratory problems, cancers, cardiovascular diseases and death. However, more specific and precise data about the impact of severe obesity on health and longevity are far more scarce, giving the undersampling of morbidly obese people in the classic epidemiologic surveys. In the recruitment phase of the Swedish Obese Subjects (SOS) study, the first 1,006 morbidly obese patients included in a national obesity registry have been analysed with respect to morbidity and compared with on-going population studies of men and women.[6] The relative risks of diabetes associated with severe obesity in 50 year-old males and females were 4.3 and 4.7 respectively. Relative risks for hypertension were 2.1 and 4.5.[6] More recent epidemiologic surveys seem to confirm or even to enforce these figures. Of the 90,185 women recruited for the Women's Health Initiative Observational Study (WHIOS), the prevalence of diabetes at baseline was 18.0 per cent in the 3,234 women with BMI > 40 kg/m^2 and 2.3 per cent in the 36,217 normal weight women ($P < 0.001$).[7] Seemingly, the prevalence of hypertension was 58.6 per cent in the group with extreme obesity and 22.5 per cent in the group with normal body weight ($P < 0.001$).[7] At baseline, prevalence of coronary heart disease, previous myocardial infarction, congestive heart failure and cerebrovascular accidents were all significantly higher in the morbidly obese group.[7]

The much higher prevalence of metabolic and vascular disorders observed in morbidly obese patients translated in a clear excess mortality risk in longitudinal studies. In the WHIOS, with an average follow-up of seven years, the age-adjusted relative risk of death in white women with morbid obesity, as compared with normal weight white women, was 2.12 (95 per cent CI: 1.81–2.47), whereas the age-adjusted relative risk for coronary heart disease mortality was 3.13 (95 per cent CI: 1.90–5.15).[7] The association between BMI and the risk of death was recently examined also in 527,625 men and women from the United States aged 50–71, in the National Institutes of Health–American Association of Retired Persons (AARP) Diet and Health Study.[8] During a maximum follow-up of ten years, the multivariate relative risk of death in people with BMI > 40 kg/m^2 was 1.94 (95 per cent CI: 1.79–2.09) in women and 1.83 (95 per cent CI: 1.70–1.97) in men.[8] When the confounding effect of smoking on the relationship between BMI and mortality was taken into account, by analysing the risk of death specifically in people who never smoked, the effect of morbid obesity on mortality was even higher: multivariate relative risk of death in people with BMI > 40 kg/m^2 was 2.52 (95 per cent CI: 2.20–2.88) in women and 2.59 (95 per cent CI: 2.30–3.06) in men.[8] Therefore, we can conclude that morbid obesity was associated with at least a doubling of total mortality risk in both sexes. Excess relative risk may be even higher in younger patients, obviously at a lower absolute risk of death. The impact of severe obesity on morbidity and life expectancy is therefore clearly established. The major goal of bariatric surgery is the reduction of such disease and death burdens.

Effects of Bariatric Surgery on Metabolic Co-Morbidities

Type 2 diabetes

Most of the clinical studies showed a benefit of bariatric surgery on diabetes. In a recent systematic review and meta-analysis of the outcomes of bariatric surgery, Buchwald *et al.* pooled the results of 136 studies conducted with different types of bariatric procedures in a total dataset of 22,094 patients.[9] When defined as the ability to discontinue all diabetes-related medications and maintain the glucose levels within the normal range, strong evidence for improvement of type 2 diabetes was found across all the surgery types. Within studies reporting resolution of diabetes,

1,417 (mean 76.8 per cent; 95 per cent CI: 70.7–82.9 per cent) of 1,846 patients experienced complete resolution. Within studies reporting both resolution or improvement or only improvement of diabetes, 414 (mean 85.4 per cent; 95 per cent CI: 78.4–93.7 per cent) of 485 patients experienced resolution or improvement of diabetes.[9] The robustness of these estimations may be reduced by the acknowledgment that the large majority of the studies included in the review are observational, not randomized studies without appropriate control groups, and by the fact that in most of the studies the evaluation of outcomes is conducted shortly after surgery, typically less than two years later. However, the results of the few published long-term controlled trials seem to confirm this favourable picture.

The SOS study was launched in the early 1990s with the aim of prospectively evaluating total and cause-specific ten-year mortality in a large group of morbidly obese patients treated by several types of bariatric procedures. A well-matched group of highly comparable morbidly obese patients participating in a national obesity registry and not willing to undergo surgery was used as a control group.[6] Weight loss observed in the surgical arm of the SOS study was 23.4 per cent of baseline body weight two years after surgery and 16.3 per cent ten years after surgery. At the same time, the control group of morbidly obese patients treated by conventional medical treatment remained substantially weight stable (weight gain of 0.1 per cent at two years and 1.6 per cent at ten years).[10] In the first two years of the SOS study, 72 per cent of 342 diabetic surgically treated obese patients had a complete resolution of type 2 diabetes, while only 21 per cent of 248 diabetic obese controls did so. The odds ratio for being free from type 2 diabetes two years after surgery was 8.42 (95 per cent CI: 5.68–12.5) in the surgically treated as compared with the medically treated controls.[10] In the long-term, some of the benefits observed in the first years after surgery tend to vanish, maybe because of the slight tendency to weight regain observed in the surgical group as a whole and of the ageing of the study population. Anyway, the proportion of patients with type 2 diabetes at baseline still normoglycaemic without pharmacologic treatment ten years after surgery was higher in the surgically treated group (36 per cent) than in the control group (13 per cent). The probability of being free from diabetes ten years after surgery was still 3.45 (95 per cent CI: 1.64–7.28) times higher in the surgically treated group.[10]

The sustained weight loss observed in the surgical arm of the SOS study was not only associated with an improvement of the diabetic state, but also to the prevention of new cases of type 2 diabetes in those morbidly obese patients free from the disease at baseline. Indeed, the incidence of new cases of type 2 diabetes was 1 per cent in the surgically treated patients and 8 per cent in the control group at two years (OR 0.14; 95 per cent CI: 0.08–0.24), and it was 7 per cent and 24 per cent respectively at 10 years (OR 0.25; 95 per cent CI: 0.17–0.38).[10] The surgical induced weight loss seems thus to be able to prevent about 75 per cent of new type 2 diabetes cases over a ten year follow-up.

The results of the SOS study have been recently confirmed by a smaller prospective study evaluating the outcome of diabetes in 73 morbidly obese patients treated by laparoscopic adjustable gastric banding and in 43 eligible morbid obese patients who refused surgery for personal reasons.[11] From baseline to the end of the four-year follow-up, BMI decreased from 45 ± 0.89 to 37.7 ± 0.71 kg/m^2 in the gastric banding group and remained steady in the non surgical group. In patients without type 2 diabetes at baseline, the primary intervention study, 17.2 per cent of the subjects in the control group and none of the gastric banding patients (P = 0.0001) progressed to type 2 diabetes. In patients with type 2 diabetes at baseline, the secondary intervention study, type 2 diabetes remitted in 4.0 per cent of the patients in the control group and in 45 per cent of the surgically treated patients (P = 0.0052).[11]

In the SOS study, the degree of weight loss needed to obtain an effective prevention of type 2 diabetes is not so high. By pooling the surgical and the medical group all together, and analysing the two-year incidence of new cases of type 2 diabetes according to the level of weight loss in the entire study population, the SOS investigators showed that patients with no weight loss experienced a 7–9 per cent incidence of type 2 diabetes, patients with a weight loss of 7 per cent of the baseline body weight had a 3 per cent incidence, and patients with a 12 per cent weight loss did not experience any new cases.[12] In a study on the short term effects of weight loss on the cardiovascular risk factors in morbidly obese patients, we investigated the relationship between weight loss and the recovery from type 2 diabetes in 650 morbidly obese patients treated with laparoscopic adjustable gastric banding. The percentage of diabetic patients showing a

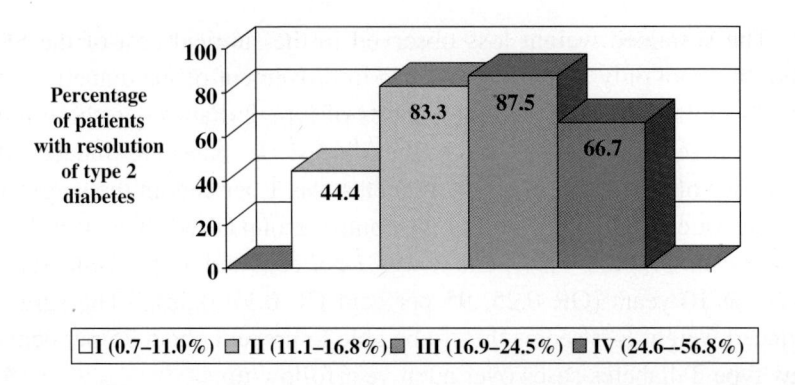

Figure 1. Percentage of morbid obese patients with type 2 diabetes at baseline showing normal glucose levels without pharmacologic 12–18 months after laparoscopic gastric banding according to quartiles of weight loss. The percentage of baseline body weight lost in each quartile is reported in the legend.[13]

normalization of glucose levels 12–18 months after surgery increased from 44.4 per cent in the lower quartile of weight loss (0.7–11.0 per cent of the baseline body weight) to 83.3 per cent in the 2nd quartile of weight loss (11.1–16.8 per cent of the baseline body weight), but no further improvements in the proportion of patients having a resolution of the diabetic state was observed with higher weight loss levels (Fig. 1).[13] According to these data, a 10–15 per cent weight loss seems to be sufficient to produce both recovery and prevention of type 2 diabetes in morbid obesity.

The factors influencing the degree of improvement in type 2 diabetes observed after bariatric surgery have been further recently analysed. An Australian study of type 2 diabetic subjects after laparoscopic adjustable gastric banding found, using strict criteria, a 64 per cent remission in type 2 diabetes one year after surgery, major improvements in blood glucose control in 26 per cent, and little change in 10 per cent.[14] Remission was predicted by greater weight loss and a shorter history of diabetes, with improvement in insulin sensitivity best predicted by extent of weight loss and improvement in β-cell function best predicted by a shorter duration of the disease.[15] This latter observation may be expected, given that progressive deterioration of β-cell function drives the progression from glucose intolerance to overt hyperglycaemia. If the bariatric procedure is performed before irreversible β-cell failure has occurred, then durable weight loss will be accompanied by a high likelihood of long-term remission.

In the large systematic review and meta-analysis of the outcomes of bariatric surgery produced by Buchwald et al., there was a difference in diabetes outcomes according to the type of operative procedure. With respect to diabetes resolution, there was a gradation of effect from 98.9 per cent (95 per cent CI, 96.8–100 per cent) for biliopancreatic diversion or duodenal switch to 83.7 per cent (95 per cent CI, 77.3–90.1 per cent) for gastric bypass and to 47.9 per cent (95 per cent CI, 29.1–66.7 per cent) for gastric banding.[9] These differences may be attributed to the corresponding differences in weight loss observed with the three procedures, but they may also be related to the existence in some type of operation of specific metabolic effects, independent from weight loss.

In particular, several studies showed that glycaemic control often occurs within days after gastric by-pass, long before significant weight loss was achieved,[16–18] suggesting that the control of diabetes may be a direct effect of the operation rather than a secondary outcome of body weight reduction. The key differential anatomical element between gastric by-pass and gastric banding is that in gastric by-pass the duodenum and part of the jejunum are excluded from the transit of food. Indeed, duodenal–jejunal exclusion without gastric restriction has been demonstrated to improve glucose tolerance in non obese diabetic rats, without inducing any change in body weight.[19] Because several peptides released in this part of the bowel are involved in glucose metabolism, changes in the so-called entero-insular axis might explain the superiority of gastric by-pass in diabetic control.[17,18] In particular, two hypotheses have been proposed to explain the effect of duodenal–jejunal bypass on type 2 diabetes.[20] The 'hindgut hypothesis' holds that diabetes control results from the expedited delivery of nutrients to the distal intestine, enhancing a physiologic signal that improves glucose metabolism. A potential candidate to be the mediator of this effect is glucagon-like peptide 1 (GLP-1), an incretin hormone secreted by L cells of the distal bowel in response to intestinal nutrients and a potent stimulator of insulin secretion and pancreatic β-cell proliferation. Indeed, the levels of GLP-1 were found to be elevated after gastric by-pass.[20] An alternative hypothesis is that the effect of selected bariatric procedures on glucose metabolism depends on the exclusion of the duodenum and proximal jejunum from the transit of nutrients, possibly preventing the secretion of some as yet unknown molecule promoting glucose intolerance ('foregut hypothesis').[21] Glucose-dependent insulinotropic polypeptide (GIP) levels are specifically increased in diabetic patients and are reduced very early after gastric by-pass.[18] GIP is synthesized and released in the duodenum and proximal jejunum in response to glucose or fat ingestion and stimulates insulin release and synthesis. Giving that the insulin-stimulating effect of GIP is characteristically attenuated in type 2 diabetes, possibly as a result of a decreased expression of the glucose-dependent insulinotropic polypeptide receptor (GIPR), it has been speculated that in susceptible individuals, chronic stimulation of the proximal gut with fat and carbohydrates may induce overproduction of an unknown factor that causes impairment of GIPR expression or GIP/GIPR interaction, leading to insufficient insulin secretion and glucose intolerance. Accordingly, the elevated GIP levels observed in diabetics may be a compensatory response to this phenomenon. The duodenal–jejunal exclusion typical of gastric by-pass might resolve this alteration, establishing normal GIP function and thus reducing circulating GIP levels.[18] Recent results from experimental animal surgery seems to support the 'foregut hypothesis' over the 'hindgut hypothesis' as an explanation for the very early improvement of type 2 diabetes after gastric by-pass.[21] However, the exact molecular mechanisms and the long-term sustainability of the entero-insular hormonal changes remain to be fully elucidated.

Other metabolic mechanisms may help to explain the superiority of biliopancreatic diversion or duodenal switch over pure restrictive procedures with respect to diabetes resolution. In these types of operations the malabsorption of fat produced by surgery is typically associated with a highly significant reduction of the plasma triglycerides levels both in the fasting and in the post-prandial states.[22] The reduced lipid overload of the entire body has been found to be associated with a reduced fat deposition in the non-adipose tissue organs, skeletal muscle in particular.[22] Intramyocellular fat deposition is associated with a reduced glucose uptake and utilization by the skeletal muscle, a clear metabolic marker of insulin-resistance. Indeed, in patients treated with bilio-pancreatic diversion the improvement of insulin sensitivity after surgery was more strictly associated with the reduction of the intramyocellular lipid content than to the fat mass loss.[22]

Hypertension

Short term studies consistently show a reduction of blood pressure levels and the need for anti-hypertensive medications after bariatric surgery.[9] Within studies reporting resolution of hypertension, 3,151 (mean 61.7 per cent; 95 per cent CI: 55.6–67.8 per cent) of 4,805 patients experienced complete resolution. Within studies reporting both resolution or improvement or only improvement of hypertension, 1,752 (mean 78.5 per cent; 95 per cent CI: 70.8–86.1 per cent) of 2,141 patients experienced resolution or improvement of hypertension.[9] The proportion of patients whose hypertension resolved seems to be strictly graded, at least in the short term, according to the weight loss produced by the operation, being 43.2 per cent (95 per cent CI: 30.4–55.9 per cent) for gastric banding, 67.5 per cent (95 per cent CI: 58.4–76.5 per cent) for gastric bypass, and 83.4 per cent (95 per cent CI: 73.2–93.6 per cent) for biliopancreatic diversion or duodenal switch.[9]

With respect to the control and the prevention of hypertension, the results of long-term studies are more confusing than for diabetes. In the four year prospective study of Pontiroli *et al.* evaluating the outcomes in morbidly obese patients treated by gastric banding and in morbidly obese patients who refused surgery, hypertension remitted in 20.5 per cent of the hypertensive patients in the surgical group and in 2.3 per cent of the patients in the control group (P = 0.0001).[11] New cases of hypertension occurred in 25.6 per cent of the patients with normal blood pressure levels at baseline in the control group and in 1.4 per cent of the patients with normal blood pressure levels at baseline in the surgical group (P = 0.0001).[11] In the first two years of the SOS study, 34 per cent of 1,204 hypertensive surgically treated obese patients had a complete recovery from hypertension, and the same happened in 21 per cent of 880 hypertensive controls. Therefore, the odds ratio for being free from hypertension two years after surgery was still significantly higher in the surgically treated than in the medically treated group (OR 1.72; 95 per cent CI: 1.40–2.12).[10] However, at the ten year evaluation, only 19 per cent of the surgically treated patients and 11 per cent of the control subjects still had normal blood pressure levels, with a relative risk of being free from hypertension that was only marginally higher in the surgical group (OR 1.68; 95 per cent CI: 1.09–2.58).[10] On the contrary, no benefits in the prevention of hypertension were observed for bariatric surgery in the SOS study. The incidence of new cases of hypertension was 24 per cent in the surgically treated patients and 29 per cent in the control group at two years (OR 0.78; 95 per cent CI: 0.60–1.01), and it was 41 per cent and 49 per cent respectively at ten years (OR 0.75; 95 per cent CI: 0.52–1.08).[10]

The differences between the two studies and the lack of a protective effect of surgery on new cases of hypertension observed in the SOS study may be related to the crucial role of body weight in the disease; in the SOS study, a significant regain of body weight was observed in the surgically treated group,[10] whereas in the study of Pontiroli *et al.* body weight remained substantially stable over the four years of follow-up.[11] Blood pressure levels are probably more dependent on the energy balance of the patient and the actual trend of his body weight (weight gain/weight stability/weight loss) than from the absolute level of body weight or BMI.[23] In a study on the effects of gastric banding on the cardiovascular risk factors in morbidly obese patients, we find a strict linear correlation between the degree of weight loss and the reduction of the blood pressure levels only in those patients actively losing weight, but not in patients who had reached body weight stabilization, or in weight regainers.[13] Maintenance of a stable body weight after surgery is therefore probably the most critical factor in the control of hypertension in the surgically treated morbidly obese patient.

Dyslipidemia

Hypercholesterolemia is not a specific feature of the morbidly obese patient. In the recruitment phase of the SOS study, total cholesterol levels was not increased in morbidly obese males and was in fact significantly lower in the morbidly obese compared with reference women.[6] By consequence, it is not surprising that in the intervention phase of the SOS study no significant differences were observed in the changes of cholesterol levels between the surgically treated and the weight stable medically treated groups.[10] The rates of recovery to normal cholesterol levels in patients with hypercholesterolemia at baseline were 22 per cent in the surgical group and 17 per cent in the control group two years after surgery (OR 1.22; 95 per cent CI: 0.98–1.51), and 21 per cent and

17 per cent respectively 10 years after surgery (OR 1.30; 95 per cent CI: 0.92–1.83).[10] The incidence of new cases of hypercholesterolemia was 27 per cent in the surgically treated patients and 24 per cent in the control group at two years (OR 1.27; 95 per cent CI: 0.95–1.69), and 30 per cent and 27 per cent respectively at ten years (OR 1.16; 95 per cent CI: 0.69–1.95).[10] In the total population analysed by Buchwald *et al.*, meta-analysis of the continuous measures demonstrated a significant decrease in total cholesterol level (mean change, 33.2 mg/dl; 95 per cent CI, 23.2–43.6 mg/dl) and low-density lipoprotein cholesterol level (mean change, 29.3 mg/dl; 95 per cent CI, 17.8–40.9 mg/dl).[9] However, most of the studies included in the meta-analysis did not have adequate control groups, and the lack of any difference in the changes of cholesterol levels between the two arms of the SOS study may suggest that any improvement observed after surgery may be related more to the changes in the quality of the diet than to weight loss *per se*. This consideration obviously does not apply to malabsorptive procedures. A pooled mean 99.7 per cent improvement of hypercholesterolemia was reported in three studies with biliopancreatic diversion or duodenal switch, with the majority of patients showing very low cholesterol levels after surgery.[24–26] In malabsorptive procedures the reduction of cholesterol levels was indeed the consequence of the disruption of the entero-hepatic cholesterol recycling caused by the operation and it was largely independent of weight loss.[26] The use of malabsorptive procedures with or without gastric restriction has been suggested for the treatment of severe hypercholesterolemia independently of the presence of obesity.[26]

The long-term results of the SOS study clearly demonstrated the efficacy of the weight loss induced by surgery in the treatment of the classic obesity-associated dyslipidemia: hypertriglyceridaemia with low HDL cholesterol levels. Recovery from hypertriglyceridaemia was observed in 62 per cent of the hypertriglyceridemic patients in the surgical group and in 22 per cent of the control group two years after surgery (OR 5.28; 95 per cent CI: 4.29–6.49), and in 46 per cent and 24 per cent respectively ten years after surgery (OR 2.57; 95 per cent CI: 1.85–3.57).[10] Recovery from low HDL cholesterol levels was observed in 76 per cent of the patients in the surgical group and 39 per cent in the control group two years after surgery (OR 5.28; 95 per cent CI: 3.85–7.23), and in

73 per cent and 53 per cent respectively ten years after surgery (OR 2.35; 95 per cent CI: 1.44–3.84).[10] The sustained weight loss induced by surgery not only normalized obesity-associated dyslipidemia in patients already dyslipidemic at baseline, but also prevented the occurrence of new cases. The ten-year incidence of new cases of hypertriglyceridaemia was 17 per cent in the surgically treated patients and 27 per cent in the control group (OR 0.61; 95 per cent CI: 0.39–0.95), while the new cases of low HDL cholesterol levels observed ten years after surgery were 3 per cent and 6 per cent respectively (OR 0.57; 95 per cent CI: 0.29–1.15).[10]

The long-term benefits of surgery on hypertriglyceridaemia observed in the SOS study were confirmed by the meta-analysis of a non-controlled short-term series. Within studies reporting improvement of hypertriglyceridaemia, 912 (mean 82.4 per cent; 95 per cent CI: 71.1–93.7 per cent) of 983 patients experienced an improvement, with a difference in outcome according to the type of operative procedure: 100.0 per cent (95 per cent CI, 98.1–100 per cent) for biliopancreatic diversion or duodenal switch, 91.2 per cent (95 per cent CI, 83.6–98.8 per cent) for gastric bypass, and 77.0 per cent (95 per cent CI, 54.1–99.9 per cent) for gastric banding.[9] On the contrary, the long-term benefits on HDL cholesterol levels observed in the SOS study were only partially confirmed in short-term studies. In the meta-analysis of Buchwald *et al.*, there was no significant increase in HDL cholesterol levels in the total population, while significant improvements were seen with gastric banding (mean change 4.63 mg/dl; 95 per cent CI, 1.54–7.72 mg/dl).[9] This discrepancy may be due to the particular relationship between weight loss and changes of HDL cholesterol levels. A meta-analysis of studies on blood lipids and lipoproteins designed to examine the effects of weight reduction by dieting demonstrated an increase of HDL cholesterol levels if patients were analysed at a stabilised, reduced weight, but a decrease of HDL cholesterol levels if patients were analysed when still actively losing weight.[27] We studied the short term effects of weight loss on the cardiovascular risk factors in morbidly obese patients, in order to investigate the effects of actual energy balance on the modifications of cardiovascular risk. Patients were divided into three groups according to the changes of body weight observed between the time after gastric banding in which the cardiovascular risk factors were determined, and the following clinical evaluation. We confirmed that HDL cholesterol levels significantly increased in patients with weight regain and in patients with stabilized body weight, whereas a small decrease in HDL cholesterol levels was observed in patients still actively losing weight (Fig. 2).[13] The null effect of bariatric surgery on HDL cholesterol levels reported by Buchwald et al.[9] may be therefore partly attributed to the fact that in most of the short-term studies included in the meta-analysis a significant proportion of patients was probably still in a phase of active body weight reduction.

Effects of Bariatric Surgery on Respiratory Disturbances

Pulmonary volumes and respiratory function

Evidence from several studies definitely proved that the respiratory complications of morbid obesity can be improved by bariatric surgery. Exertional dyspnoea is the most frequently reported symptom of morbid obesity and is typically of respiratory origin. In the recruitment phase of the SOS study, the relative risk of having dyspnoea in 50 year-old morbidly obese males and females were 4.3 and 4.7 respectively, in

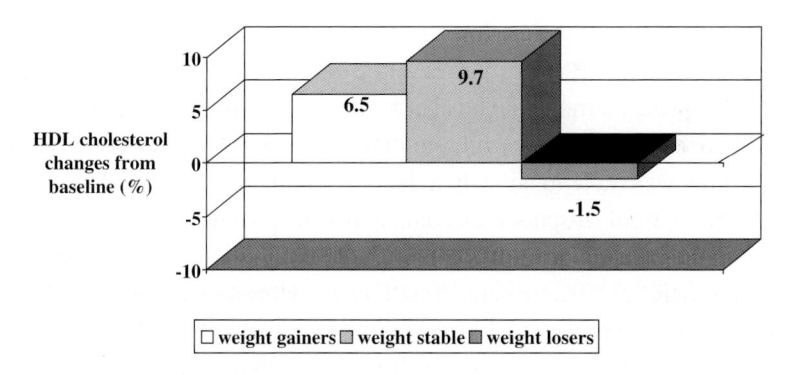

Figure 2. Modifications of HDL cholesterol levels in morbidly obese patients treated with laparoscopic gastric banding, according to actual energy balance 12–18 months after surgery. The percent changes from the baseline values were reported. Patients showing a ≥ 2.0 kg increase of body weight in the period immediately following the redetermination of blood lipids after surgery were classified as 'weight gainers', and patients with a ≥ 2.0 kg reduction of body weight as 'weight losers'. Patients with in between weight changes were classified as 'weight stable'.[13]

comparison with normal weight reference subjects.[6] In a subset analysis from the SOS study specifically devoted to the study of respiratory disturbances, 87 per cent of the first 1,260 morbidly obese patients enrolled in the intervention study complained at baseline with dyspnoea when climbing two flights of stairs and 24 per cent when performing simple activities of daily living such as washing or dressing. In these patients, a sustained surgically induced weight loss was able to drastically reduce the incidence of exertional dyspnoea, with only 19 per cent of patients still complaining with dyspnoea when climbing stairs and 3 per cent when washing or dressing.[28]

Morbidly obese patients are typically affected by a restrictive respiratory impairment, with the most characteristic pulmonary function abnormality being a reduction of the expiratory reserve volume (ERV).[29,30] Imaging studies conducted with the use of computed tomography demonstrated that the major determinant of ERV reduction was the amount of abdominal visceral adipose tissue, both in males and in females.[31] Small studies with determination of respiratory volumes before and after surgery demonstrated that the reduction of dyspnoea induced by bariatric surgery was related to increased vital capacity, FRV and ERV.[32,33]

It is also noteworthy that the respiratory complications of obesity, as well as the metabolic disorders, appeared to be positively affected, at least in the short term, by only a moderate level of body weight reduction. Dividing 1,087 morbidly obese patients according to quartiles of weight reduction, the SOS investigators were able to show that the larger reduction in the risk of continuing to suffer from dyspnoea as compared with patients with stable weight (+ 4.0 kg) was obtained in patients with a larger weight loss (− 41.5 kg) (RR 0.02; 95 per cent CI 0.01–0.03). However, a significant reduction of risk was also observed in the group of patients with only a moderate weight loss (RR 0.26; 95 per cent CI 0.18–0.33). In this group, mean weight loss was −7.9 kg, an apparently trivial level of weight loss in patients with severe obesity.[28] If pulmonary function impairment was more dependent on visceral fat accumulation than on the simple level of total fatness, it could be hypothesized that the improvements of respiratory complications observed with only a moderate body weight reduction could be ascribed to a selective reduction of visceral fat. Indeed, in a study with total body multi-slices NMR, we demonstrated a preferential mobilization of abdominal visceral fat with respect of total and regional subcutaneous fat in the first phase of weight loss in a small group of six pre-menopausal women with visceral obesity treated by laparoscopic gastric banding (Fig. 3).[34] In the first eight weeks after surgery, the relative reduction of visceral adipose tissue (19.6 ± 14.7 per cent) was significantly higher than the relative reduction of both total adipose tissue (11.5 ± 7.9 per cent) and gluteo-femoral subcutaneous adipose tissue (10.7 ± 8.1 per cent).[34] It is therefore possible that the improvements of pulmonary volumes observed after a modest weight loss should be a part of the better responsiveness of visceral than subcutaneous fat to caloric restriction. However, this hypothesis needs to be directly proven.

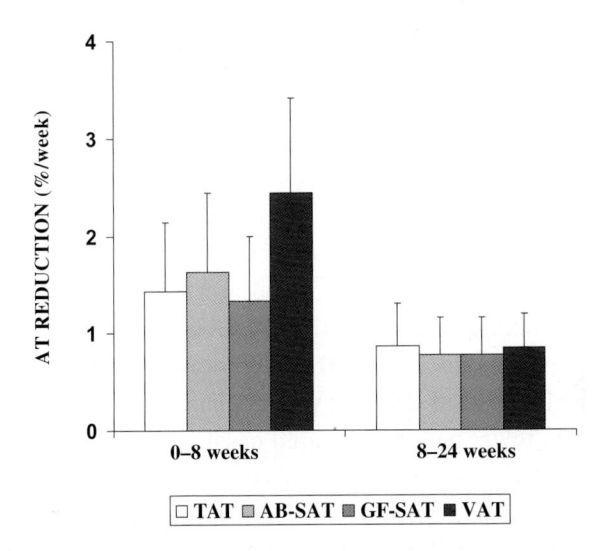

Figure 3. Relative reductions of total and regional adipose tissue (AT) volumes, expressed as percentage changes from baseline levels per week of observation, in the first eight weeks (weeks 0–8) and in the second 16 weeks (weeks 8–24) after surgery in six morbidly obese women with visceral obesity treated by laparoscopic gastric banding. TAT: total adipose tissue volume; AB-SAT: abdominal subcutaneous adipose tissue volume; GF-SAT: gluteo-femoral subcutaneous adipose tissue volume; VAT: abdominal visceral adipose tissue volume. Error bars represent standard deviations. Differences between total and regional adipose tissue volumes were tested by paired Student's t-test. Significant differences were found only in the 0–8 weeks period, between VAT and TAT (P < 0.05) and between VAT and GF-SAT (P < 0.05).[34]

Obstructive sleep apnoea syndrome

Obstructive sleep apnoea syndrome (OSAS) is particularly frequent in morbid obesity, with an estimated prevalence of 40 per cent.[35] In a subset analysis from the SOS, the prevalence of symptoms of OSAS, as evaluated by a specific questionnaire, was 23 per cent at baseline and it was significantly reduced to 8 per cent two years after surgery.[28] In a review and meta-analysis of the outcomes of bariatric surgery, when clinical diagnoses of sleep apnoea, sleep-disordered breathing, and pickwickian syndrome were combined as representative of obstructive sleep apnoea, OSAS was found to be resolved in 1,051 of 1,195 patients (mean 85.7 per cent; 95 per cent CI, 79.2–92.2 per cent).[9] However, these estimates may be flawed by the fact that in most studies the diagnosis of OSAS was made clinically, and not with a more objective instrumental registration of breathing disorders during sleeping.

Dixon *et al.* recently prospectively performed a polysomnographic overnight registration both before and at least one year after surgery in 25 morbidly obese patients with severe OSAS (apnoea–hypopnoea index [AHI] > 25 events/hour) treated by laparoscopic adjustable gastric banding. Subject baseline BMI was 52.7 ± 9.5 kg/m^2 and the second polysomnographic study was performed at a BMI of 37.2 ± 7.2 kg/m^2. The authors demonstrated a significant fall in AHI from 61.6 ± 31.9 to 13.4 ± 13.0 events/hour ($P < 0.001$), an improved sleep architecture with increased REM and stage III and IV sleep, and a reduced daytime sleepiness. Moreover, fewer patients required nasal continuous positive airways pressure (CPAP) after surgery than before (24 per cent versus 92 per cent; $P < 0.001$).[36] These new results substantially confirmed a previous meta-analysis of 4 studies, with a total population of 92 patients, in which the continuous objective variable of apnoeas or hypopnoea per hour was available, that demonstrated a reduction of 33.8 events/hour (95 per cent CI: 17.5–50.2 events/hour).[9]

We recently studied a small group of 18 middle-aged men with OSAS and severe visceral obesity (baseline BMI of 54.7 ± 9.5 kg/m^2) treated with the temporary insertion of an intragastric balloon in preparation for later laparoscopic adjustable gastric banding surgery, and we observed a high reduction of the number of apnoeic episodes during sleeping with a relatively modest level of weight loss and despite the fact the patients still remained affected by severe obesity after treatment.[37] A cardio-respiratory sleep study, which included assessment of air flow, thoracic and abdominal movements, snoring, pulse rate and oximetry, was performed at baseline and immediately after the removal of the balloon, six months apart, at a BMI of 48.6 ± 11.2 kg/m^2. The 14.5 ± 8.9 per cent reduction from baseline body weight produced by the intragastric balloon was associated in our study with a significant fall in AHI from 59.3 ± 18.1 to 14.0 ± 12.4 events/hour ($P < 0.01$). The reduction in the number of apnoeic episodes during sleep was accompanied by improvements of pulmonary function, standing and lying oxygen saturation, and the diurnal symptoms of OSAS. We also analysed the improvement in the severity of OSAS categorically, by evaluating how many patients were treated successfully by the intragastric balloon. We defined success as a reduction in AHI of at least 50 per cent with a reduction of the AHI to < 20 events/hour. According to these criteria, 10 of 17 patients (58.8 per cent) achieved success. The mean percentage weight loss after treatment with the intragastric balloon was higher in the responders than in the non responders (19.7 ± 7.6 versus 6.9 ± 3.3 per cent, respectively; $P < 0.001$). The lowest percentage weight loss that was associated with success was 8.8 per cent, and the highest percentage weight loss associated with failure was 12.2 per cent.[37] Therefore, in our study a moderate 10–15 per cent weight loss also appeared to be associated to a resolution of OSAS in patients with extreme levels of obesity.

The high prevalence of OSAS among obese patients has been attributed to a mass loading of the upper airway by adipose tissue.[38] In fact, obese patients with OSAS have been shown to have increased fat deposition adjacent to the upper airway[39,40] and reduced pharyngeal cross-sectional area[34] when compared to control subjects. We hypothesized that the higher than expected resolution of OSAS observed in our study may be related to changes of pharyngeal size in the first phase of weight loss, and therefore we measured the upper airways size by acoustic pharyngometry. The main finding of the study was that the pharyngeal cross-sectional area of the morbidly obese patient subjects, which was severely reduced at baseline as compared to a normal weight control group, increased after weight loss (Fig. 4).[37] The increase in the cross-sectional area of the pharynx was

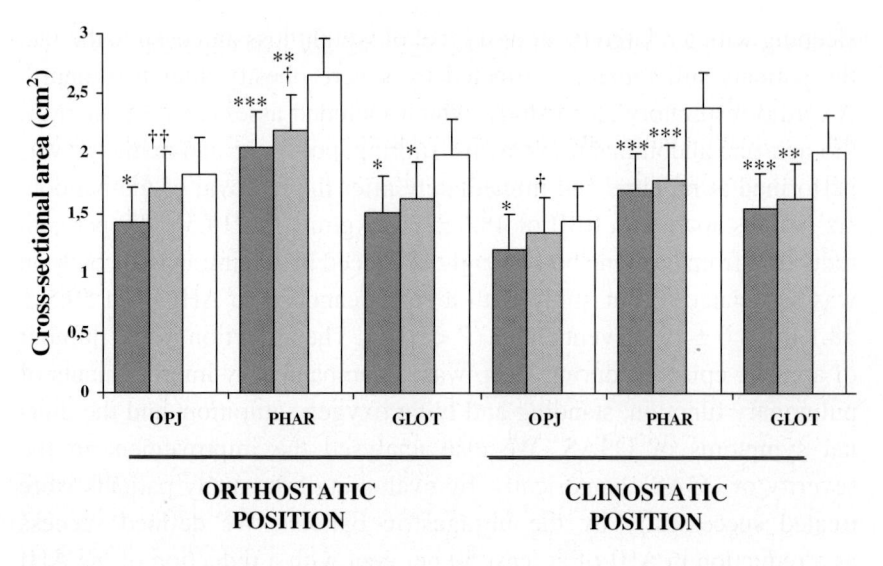

Figure 4. Cross-sectional pharyngeal areas determined by acoustic reflection in 17 morbidly obese patients in the upright and supine positions before intragastric balloon insertion (black bars) and after intragastric balloon removal (light grey bars). The pharyngometric measurements of 20 nonobese men were reported for comparison (white bars). OPJ = oropharyngeal junction cross-sectional area; PHAR = mean pharyngeal cross-sectional area; GLOT = glottis cross-sectional area. * = $P < 0.05$ (Mann–Whitney U test between obese patients and nonobese subjects); ** = $P < 0.01$ (Mann–Whitney U test between obese patients and nonobese subjects); *** = $P < 0.001$ (Mann–Whitney U test between obese patients and nonobese subjects). † = $P < 0.05$ (Wilcoxon rank sum test between obese patients before intragastric balloon insertion and after its removal); †† = $P < 0.01$ (Wilcoxon rank sum test between obese patients before intragastric balloon insertion and after its removal).[37]

significantly related to the level of weight loss (r 0.547; $P < 0.05$) and to the reduction of waist circumference ($r = 0.473$; $P < 0.05$), sagittal abdominal diameter ($r = 0.664$; $P < 0.01$), and neck circumference ($r = 0.506$; $P < 0.05$). However, the reduction of sagittal abdominal diameter, the best anthropometric index of visceral fat accumulation, was found to be the only variable that was significantly related to an increase in pharyngeal cross-sectional area in multivariate regression analysis.[37] We therefore suggest that the rapid improvements of pharyngeal patency may be another aspect of the better responsiveness of visceral than subcutaneous fat to caloric restriction observed in the first phase of body weight reduction.

Impact of Bariatric Surgery on Health Related Quality of Life

As previously shown, severe obesity is associated with a wide range of serious health complications. Consequently, it has been demonstrated that severe obesity produces profound impairments in health-related quality of life (HRQL). The harmful effects of obesity influence physical, psychological and social domains of HRQL and tend to be more severe at higher BMI levels.[41] Even after accounting for the pain and anxiety of surgery, the inconveniences of dietary restrictions, and possible complications including reoperation, quality of life improved for the majority of bariatric surgery patients.[9] The perception of wellbeing, social function, body self image, self-confidence, ability to interact with others, and time spent in recreational and physical activities have been also reported to increase after successful bariatric surgery.[9] It should be noted however that most of these assumptions are derived from the results of research studies reporting improvements in psychosocial areas after bariatric surgery, but suffering from important methodological limitations, principally represented by the small study samples and the short follow-up periods.[42]

Very recently, the SOS investigators reported on the ten-year trends in health-related quality of life after surgical and conventional treatment for severe obesity in the SOS intervention study.[43] HRQL was assessed before treatment and after six months, then after one, two, three, four, six, eight and ten years in a total of 655 of 851 surgically treated and 621 of 852 conventionally treated obese men and women who completed 10 years of the study, thus allowing for a long-term sequential analysis of the effects of bariatric surgery on quality of life. General health perceptions, mental well-being, mood disorders, health related dysfunctions in social life and the impact of obesity on psychosocial functioning were measured with the use of specific questionnaires. HRQL at baseline was generally poorer in the severely obese than in age-matched non-obese reference population. After surgery, changes in HRQL generally followed phases of weight loss, weight regain and weight stability. Poor HRQL before treatment was markedly improved after surgery and peak improvements during the ten-year observation period were noted after six months and one year, which corresponds with the maximal weight loss observed after the operation. Thereafter, a gradual regain of weight was observed, mainly up to six years, with about one-third of the initial weight reduction gradually regained. During this weight regain phase, a slow but steady decline in HRQL was noted. Finally, weight regain slowed down and body weight stabilized between six and ten years. Accordingly, quite stable HRQL ratings were observed in the surgical group between six and ten years. All the HRQL domains that were examined in the study were significantly improved in the surgical group after ten years. According to standard criteria for interpreting treatment-related changes of HRQL, ten-year improvements were in the small range for current health, social interaction, overall mood, depression and anxiety, whereas the improvement in psychosocial functioning was large.[43] The final comment of the authors concluded that bariatric surgery is a favourable option for the treatment of severe obesity, resulting in substantial long-term weight loss accompanied by improvements in health status and quality of life in a majority of patients. Nevertheless, the authors emphasized the difficulties that many surgical patients experienced to control and maintain weight loss over time and the possible negative impact that these difficulties and the associated weight regain may have on the physical and psychosocial well being of the patients. It is possible that these difficulties may be better coped with by the use of long-term behavioural support programmes in the postoperative management of patients.[43]

Impact of Bariatric Surgery on Life Expectancy

As summarized in the first part of this review, several longitudinal studies proved that the high prevalence of metabolic and vascular disorders observed in morbidly obese patients translates in a clear excess mortality risk. Morbid obesity was found to be associated with at least a doubling of total mortality risk in both sexes.[7,8] As reviewed above, a large body of clinical studies has proved that bariatric surgery may produce sustained and stable weight loss in morbidly obese patients and that this weight loss is accompanied by a long-term reduction in both the prevalence and the incidence of several obesity-related co-morbidities, type 2 diabetes in particular. However, reliable scientific evidence that these clinical benefits ultimately translate into a reduction of the excess mortality risk of morbid obesity is still scarce. To prove that bariatric surgery, notwithstanding the additional risks introduced by the operative procedures and the eventual post-operative complications, is able to cause a reduction in the excess mortality risk of the morbidly obese is clearly a key point in the development and acceptance of surgery as a first line therapeutic choice in severe obesity, but to comply with this task presents important technical and logistic problems. A randomized clinical trial prospectively comparing the mortality rate in morbidly obese patients treated by bariatric surgery and in comparable subjects treated by the best behavioural and pharmacologic methods should obviously provide the highest level of scientific evidence in this respect. However, conducting a randomized clinical trial of this sort may require a huge number of patients followed for a long time and may raise some ethical concern given the expected benefits of bariatric surgery on body weight, obesity-related co-morbidities and quality of life. To date, no such trials have been conducted and it seems highly improbable that this may happen in the future.

As previously described, the investigators of the SOS study tried to resolve this gap by planning and conducting a large prospective study in which the outcome of a large group of patients treated by several types of bariatric procedures was compared with the outcome of well-matched morbidly obese controls not choosing surgical treatment.[6] The primary aim of the study was to prospectively evaluate total and cause-specific ten-year mortality. The SOS study produced highly valuable data about the effect of surgery on co-morbidities and quality of life[10,23,28,43] and a very recent preliminary report from the SOS investigators declared a 24.6 per cent reduction of total ten-years mortality in the first 2,010 surgically-treated patients.[44] The scientific value of this observation is indisputable, but some concern about the applicability of the SOS results to current bariatric surgery has been raised.[45] The SOS study has a ten-year follow-up and additional years were needed for the enrolment of patients, so a significant proportion of the SOS patients were treated in the 1990s with procedures (vertical banded gastroplasty) and techniques (open surgery) that are now largely abandoned.

In a recent retrospective observational study, the five-year death rate of 1,118 morbidly obese patients surgically treated with Roux-en-Y gastric bypass (RYGB) at a single Canadian academic institution was compared with the death rate of 5,746 morbidly obese controls whose vital status was derived from the administrative records of the provincial health insurance database of Quebec.[46] In this study, the mortality rate in the bariatric surgery cohort, with the peri-operative mortality included in the calculation, was found to be 0.68 per cent, compared with a total mortality of 6.17 per cent in the control group. These figures translated into a highly significant 89 per cent reduction of the relative risk of death in the surgical group (relative risk 0.11; 95 per cent CI 0.04–0.27).[46] The results of retrospective observational studies may obviously be affected by selection biases and uncontrolled differences between the surgical and the control cohorts. In the Canadian study in particular, the baseline BMI of the subjects in the control cohort was not actually measured and all the control subjects were morbidly obese patients hospitalized for acute clinical problems. It could be argued that the five-year mortality rate of this control cohort of acutely sick morbidly obese patients (6.17 per cent) may be higher than the death rate of the general morbidly obese population, thus inflating the difference between the bariatric surgery group and the control group. Moreover, the peri-operative mortality rate in the Canadian study was very low, probably reflecting the top level of expertise of the surgical team. Much higher peri-operative mortality rates have been reported in morbidly obese patients treated by RYGB in the community,[47] raising some doubt about the applicability of the results to the current 'real-life' obesity surgery practice.

We recently tried to overcome the above methodological problems by comparing the mortality rate of 821 patients with BMI > 40 kg/m^2 consecutively treated by laparoscopic adjustable gastric banding at our institution with the mortality rate of 821 sex, age and measured BMI-matched morbidly obese patients observed at six Italian tertiary obesity care centres not using bariatric surgery.[48] Both our cohorts were therefore formed by morbidly obese patients seeking treatment at highly specialized institutions, but receiving a different type of therapy. Indeed, the seven-year mortality rate of our control cohort (4.38 per cent) was lower than the 6.17 per cent observed by Christou *et al.*[46] Nevertheless, we confirmed that bariatric surgery was associated with a significant reduction in total mortality. During a mean follow-up of 5.6 ± 1.9 years in the surgical group and 7.2 ± 1.2 years in the reference cohort, 8 and 36 deaths were recorded respectively, for a total mortality of 0.97 per cent in the surgical patients and 4.38 per cent in the controls. The difference in survival was statistically significant (P = 0.0004) at the log-rank test for comparison of Kaplan–Meier survival curves (Fig. 5), and the age, sex and BMI-adjusted relative risk of death in the surgical cohort, as compared with the reference cohort, was 0.36 (95 per cent CI: 0.16–0.79), with a statistically significant 60 per cent reduction in total mortality. It should be noted that patients in our surgical group had a zero operative mortality, a figure that is not unexpected for an operation, like laparoscopic banding, reported to have less operative risk than gastric by-pass[9] and that did not differ substantially from the low mortality rate (0.53 per cent) observed with laparoscopic gastric banding in an Italian study including centres with high as well low volumes of this operation.[49]

The results of our study seem to be confirmed by two other recent reports. Australian investigators compared the mortality rate in 1,468 morbid obese patients treated by laparoscopic gastric banding at the Monash University in Melbourne and in 5,960 patients with BMI > 35 kg/m² from the established population-based cohort of the Melbourne Cohort Collaborative Study, recruited between 1992 and 1994

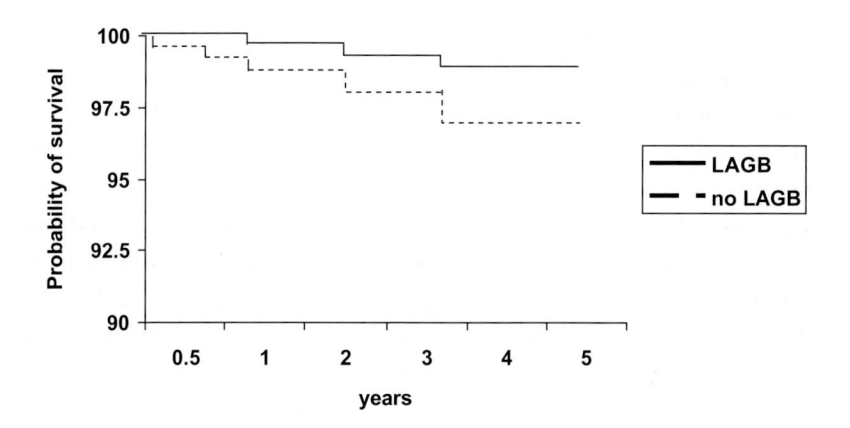

Figure 5. Kaplan–Meier estimates of survival in 821 obese patients with BMI > 40 kg/m² consecutively treated with laparoscopic adjustable gastric banding (LAGB) at the University of Padova and in 821 morbidly obese patients observed at six Italian tertiary obesity care centres not using bariatric surgery (no LAGB).[48]

to study the relationship between diet and cancer. They observed five deaths in 5,960 patient-years of follow-up in the surgical group, and 225 deaths in 25,280 patient-years of follow-up in the reference cohort. Cox regression analysis indicated that the surgical patients were 73 per cent less likely to die than the control subjects (age, sex and BMI-adjusted relative risk of death 0.27; 95 per cent CI: 0.09–0.81).[50] American investigators determined long-term mortality (18 years; mean 8.4 years) among 8,172 morbidly obese patients treated by gastric by-pass at a single surgical practice and in 8,172 population-based controls matched for age, gender and BMI. Total mortality was found to have reduced by 50 per cent in the surgical group (P < 0.0001).[51]

An additional important finding of our study was the absence of a clear dose-response relationship between the degree of weight loss and the observed reduction of mortality. In our surgical series, the mortality rate was significantly reduced in patients with a moderate weight reduction (10–20 per cent of baseline body weight) as compared with patients with no weight loss or weight gain (age, sex and BMI-adjusted relative risk of death 0.11; 95 per cent CI: 0.01–0.91), but a more pronounced weight loss (> 20 per cent of baseline body weight) seemed not to be associated with an additional reduction of mortality (age, sex and BMI-adjusted relative risk of death 0.27; 95 per cent CI: 0.06–1.29).[48] This observation is based on a very low number of events and should therefore be interpreted cautiously. However, it seems to be confirmed by epidemiologic studies investigating the relationship between intentional weight loss and total mortality in the general population. In women with obesity-related health problems, the reduction in the fully adjusted total mortality rate observed after intentional weight loss was similar in subjects with 0.5–9.0 or > 9.0 kg of weight loss.[52] In the overweight diabetic men enrolled in the American Cancer Society's Cancer Prevention Study I, the lowest mortality rate was found in patients experiencing a moderate 20–29 lb body weight reduction.[53] Finally, the observation that it may not be necessary to achieve massive levels of weight loss to obtain a reduction in total mortality of the morbidly obese patient fits very well with the previously presented observations demonstrating that significant improvements in metabolic and respiratory co-morbidities may be obtained with a moderate weight loss in severe obesity, as well as in obesity in general.

Conclusion

In conclusion, we summarized in this review the large body of scientific evidence definitively proving the sustained benefits of bariatric surgery on obesity-related metabolic and respiratory co-morbidities and on the health related quality of life. We finally presented more recent results suggesting that these benefits may actually translate into a reduction of total mortality in morbidly obese patients treated with bariatric surgery. In our opinion, providing that operative mortality was kept at the very low level now achievable by modern procedures, this evidence is sufficient to conclude that bariatric surgery really improves long-term survival in morbid obesity.

References

1. Steinbrook, R. (2004). Surgery for severe obesity. *N Engl J Med* 350: 1075–1079.
2. Zhao, Y., Encinosa, W. (2007). *Bariatric Surgery Utilization and Outcomes in 1998 and 2004*, Statistical Brief #23, Agency for Healthcare Research and Quality, Rockville, MD. www.hcup-us.ahrq.gov/reports/statbriefs/sb23.pdf. Accessed May 2, 2007.
3. Buchwald, H., Williams, S.E. (2004). Bariatric surgery worldwide. *Obes Surg* 14: 1157–1164.
4. Flegal, K.M., Carroll, M.D., Ogden, C.L. et al. (2002). Prevalence and trends in obesity among US adults, 1999–2000. *JAMA* 288: 1722–1723.
5. Sturm, R. (2003). Increases in clinically severe obesity in the United States, 1986–2000. *Arch Intern Med* 163: 2146–2148.
6. Sjöström, L., Larsson, B., Backmann, L. et al. (1992). Swedish obese subjects (SOS). Recruitment for an intervention study and a selected description of the obese state. *Int J Obes* 16: 465–479.
7. McTigue, K., Larson, J.C., Valoski, A. et al. (2006). Mortality and cardiac and vascular outcomes in extremely obese women. *JAMA* 296: 79–86.
8. Adams, K.F., Schatzkin, A., Harris, T.B. et al. (2006). Overweight, obesity, and mortality in a large prospective cohort of persons 50 to 71 years old. *N Engl J Med* 355: 763–778.
9. Buchwald, H., Avidor, Y., Braunwald, E. et al. (2004). Bariatric surgery. A systematic review and meta-analysis. *JAMA* 292: 1724–1737.

10. Sjöström, L., Lindroos, A.-K., Peltonen, M. *et al.* (2004). Lifestyle, diabetes and cardiovascular risk factors 10 years after bariatric surgery. *N Engl J Med* 351: 2683–2693.
11. Pontiroli, A.E., Folli, F., Paganelli, M. *et al.* (2005). Laparoscopic gastric banding prevents type 2 diabetes and arterial hypertension and induces their remission in morbid obesity. A 4-year case-controlled study. *Diabetes Care* 28: 2703–2709.
12. Sjöström, L. (2004). Surgical treatment of obesity: an overview and results from the SOS study. In: Bray G.A., Bouchard C. (eds.) *Handbook of Obesity: Clinical Application*, 2nd edition, pp. 359–389, Marcel Dekker Inc, New York.
13. Busetto, L., Sergi, G., Enzi, G. *et al.* (2004). Short term effects of weight loss on the cardiovascular risk factors in morbidly obese patients. *Obes Res* 12: 1256–1263.
14. Dixon, J.B., O'Brien, P. (2002). Health outcomes of severely obese type 2 diabetic subjects 1 year after laparoscopic adjustable gastric banding. *Diabetes Care* 25: 358–363.
15. Dixon, J.B., Dixon, A.F., O'Brien, P. (2003). Improvements in insulin sensitivity and beta-cell function (HOMA) with weight loss in the severely obese. *Diabet Med* 20: 127–134.
16. Pories, W.J., Swanson, M.S., MacDonald, K.G. *et al.* (1995). Who would have thought it? An operation proves to be the most effective therapy for adult-onset diabetes mellitus. *Ann Surg* 222: 339–352.
17. Pories, W.J., Albrecht, R.J. (2001). Etiology of type II diabetes mellitus: role of the foregut. *World J Surg* 25: 527–531.
18. Rubino, F., Gagner, M., Gentileschi, P. *et al.* (2004). The early effect of the Roux-en-Y gastric bypass on hormones involved in body weight regulations and glucose metabolism. *Ann Surg* 240: 236–242.
19. Rubino, F., Marescaux, J. (2004). Effect of duodenal-jejunal exclusion in a non-obese animal model of type 2 diabetes. *Ann Surg* 239: 1–11.
20. Le Roux, C.W., Aylwin, S.J.B., Batterham, R.L. *et al.* (2006). Gut hormone profiles following bariatric surgery favor an anorectic state, facilitate weight loss, and improve metabolic parameters. *Ann Surg* 243: 108–114.
21. Rubino, F., Forgione, A., Cummings, D.E. *et al.* (2006). The mechanism of diabetes control after gastrointestinal bypass surgery reveals a role of the proximal small intestine in the pathophysiology of type 2 diabetes. *Ann Surg* 244: 741–749.

22. Greco, A.V., Mingrone, G., Giancaterini, A. *et al.* (2002). Insulin resistance in morbid obesity. Reversal with intramyocellular fat depletion. *Diabetes* 51: 144–151.
23. Sjöström, C.D., Peltonen, M., Wedel, H. *et al.* (2000). Differentiated long-term effects of intentional weight loss on diabetes and hypertension. *Hypertension* 36: 20–25.
24. Hess, D.S., Hess, D.W. (1998). Biliopancreatic diversion with a duodenal switch. *Obes Surg* 8: 267–282.
25. Marceau, P., Hould, F.S., Simard, S. *et al.* (1998). Biliopancreatic diversion with duodenal switch. *World J Surg* 22: 947–954.
26. Scopinaro, N., Adami, G.F., Marinari, G.M. *et al.* (1998). Biliopancreatic diversion. *World J Surg* 22: 936–946.
27. Dattilo, A.M., Kris-Etherton, P.M. (1992). Effects of weight reduction on blood lipids and lipoproteins: a meta-analysis. *Am J Clin Nutr* 56: 320–328.
28. Karason, K., Lindroos, A.K., Stenlöf, K. *et al.* (2000). Relief of cardiorespiratory symptoms and increased physical activity after surgically induced weight loss. *Arch Intern Med* 160: 1797–1802.
29. Luce, J.M. (1980). Respiratory complications of obesity. *Chest* 78: 626–630.
30. Ray, C.S., Sue, D.Y., Vray, G. *et al.* (1983). Effects of obesity on respiratory function. *Am Rev Resp Dis* 128: 201–206.
31. Enzi, G., Vianello, A., Baggio, M.B. *et al.* (1990). Respiratory disturbances in visceral obesity. In: Oomura Y. *et al.* (eds). *Progress in Obesity Research*, pp. 335–339, John Libbey & Co, London.
32. Thomas, P.S, Owen, E.R., Hulands, G. *et al.* (1989). Respiratory function in the morbidly obese before and after weight loss. *Thorax* 44: 383–386.
33. Weiner, P., Waizman, J., Weiner, M. *et al.* (1998). Influence of excessive weight loss after gastroplasty for morbid obesity on respiratory muscle performance. *Thorax* 53: 39–42.
34. Busetto, L., Tregnaghi, A., Bussolotto, M. *et al.* (2000). Visceral fat loss evaluated by total body magnetic resonance in obese women operated with laparoscopic adjustable silicone gastric banding. *Int J Obes* 24: 60–69.
35. Rajala, R., Partinen, M., Sane, T. *et al.* (1991). Obstructive sleep apnoea syndrome in morbidly obese patients. *J Intern Med* 230: 125–129.
36. Dixon, J.B., Schachter, L.M., O'Brien, P.E. (2005). Polysomnography before and after weight loss in obese patients with severe sleep apnea. *Int J Obes* 29: 1–7.

37. Busetto, L., Enzi, G., Inelmen, E.M. *et al.* (2005). Obstructive sleep apnea syndrome in morbid obesity: effects of intragastric balloon. *Chest* 128: 618–623.
38. Shelton, K.E., Woodson, H., Gay, S. *et al.* (1993). Pharyngeal fat in obstructive sleep apnoea. *Am Rev Respir Dis* 148: 462–466.
39. Horner, R.L., Mohiaddin, R.H., Lowell, D.G. *et al.* (1989). Sites and sizes of fat deposits around the pharynx in obese patients with obstructive sleep apnoea and weight matched controls. *Eur Respir J* 2: 613–622.
40. Mortimore, I.L., Marshall, I., Wraith, P.K. *et al.* (1998). Neck and total body fat deposition in non-obese and obese patients with sleep apnea compared with that in control subjects. *Am J Respir Crit Care Med* 157: 280–283.
41. Kolotkin, R.L., Crosby, R.D., Williams, G.R. *et al.* (2001). The relationship between health-related quality of life and weight loss. *Obes Res* 9: 564–571.
42. Sarwer, D.B., Wadden, T.A., Fabricatore, A.N. (2005). Psychosocial and behavioral aspects of bariatric surgery. *Obes Res* 13: 639–648.
43. Karlsson, J., Taft, C., Ryden, A. *et al.* (2007). Ten-year trends in health-related quality of life after surgical and conventional treatment for severe obesity: the SOS intervention study. *Int J Obes* 31: 1–14.
44. Sjöström, K., Narbro, K., Sjöström, C.D. *et al.* (2007). Effects of bariatric surgery on mortality in Swedish obese subjects. *N Engl J Med* 357: 741–752.
45. Kral, J.G. (2006). Swedish obese subjects study — best available data to support antiobesity surgery? *SOARD* 2: 561–564.
46. Christou, N.V., Sampalis, J.S., Liberman, M. *et al.* (2004). Surgery decreases long-term mortality, morbidity, and health care use in morbidly obese patients. *Ann Surg* 240: 416–424.
47. Flum, D.R., Salem, L., Elrod, J.A. *et al.* (2005). Early mortality among medicare beneficiaries undergoing bariatric surgical procedures. *JAMA* 294: 1903–1908.
48. Busetto, L., Mirabelli, D., Petroni, M.L. *et al.* (2006). Comparative long-term mortality after laparoscopic adjustable gastric banding versus nonsurgical controls. *SOARD* 3: 496–502.
49. Angrisani, L., Furbetta, F., Doldi, S.B. *et al.* (2003). Lap Band adjustable gastric banding system: the Italian experience with 1863 patients operated on 6 years. *Surg Endosc* 17: 409–412.
50. Peeters, A., O'Brien, P., Laurie, C. *et al.* (2007). Substantial intentional weight loss and mortality in the severely obese. *Ann Surg* 246: 1028–1033.

51. Adams, T.D., Gress, R.E., Smith, S.C. *et al.* (2007). Long-term mortality after gastric bypass surgery. *N Engl J Med* 357: 753–761.
52. Williamson, D.F., Pamuk, E., Thun, M. *et al.* (1995). Prospective study of intentional weight loss and mortality in never-smoking overweight US white women aged 40–64 years. *Am J Epidemiol* 141: 1128–1141.
53. Williamson, D.F., Thompson, T.J., Thun, M. *et al.* (2000). Intentional weight loss and mortality among overweight individuals with diabetes. *Diabetes Care* 23: 1499–1504.

Index

abdominal 239, 247, 262, 273
    pain 236, 250, 262, 268, 272
abscess 239, 247, 262, 273
acute concentric 233, 234, 242
adhesion 261, 262, 264, 272
adiponectin 332, 339
adjustable gastric banding (AGB) 91, 92, 125, 149, 327, 330, 333–336, 338, 340, 342, 344, 345, 347
aldosterone 328, 330
alimentary
    behaviour 62, 72
    limb 161–163, 170, 184
anastomosis 245, 246, 248–254, 256, 257, 259, 262, 263, 266, 267, 269–272, 274
anastomotic
    leak 247, 249, 251
    obstruction 247, 252
    structure 245, 246, 248–254, 256, 257, 259, 262, 263, 266, 267, 269–272, 274
anatomy 224, 226, 245, 246, 248, 273
angiography 256

angiotensin 328
anterior slippage 235, 240
apnoea-hypopnea index (AHI) 331
associated disease 76

Ballobes Intragastric Balloon 63
balloon 224, 228, 230, 233, 234, 237, 241, 242, 244
    deflation 241, 242
band 223–242, 244, 262
    adjustment 224, 226, 230–232, 235, 241
    erosion 238, 239, 244
    removal 232, 238
    slippage 228, 235, 237, 240
band slip–hernia–pouch dilatation complex 234, 236, 240
Bariatric Analysis and Reporting Outcome System (BAROS) 347, 348
    BAROS MA II 317
bariatric surgery 223, 245, 247, 253, 261, 273, 285, 286, 291
barium 226–228, 230, 231, 233–237, 239, 248, 251, 253, 257, 258, 264–266

Barrett's oesophagus   343, 344
best practice care recovery model   306
beta cell   338
Bezoar   237, 261, 265
bilevel positive airway pressure (BIPAP)   51
biliopancreatic diversion (BPD)   327, 330, 334, 336–339, 343, 347, 348
biliopancreatic limb   245, 246, 253, 256, 258, 266, 267
BioEnterics Intragastric Balloon (BIB)   61, 64–86
   intolerance   83
   removal of   70, 74, 82, 84
bleeding   171, 175, 177, 247, 250
blood pressure (BP)   328–330
body mass index (BMI)   16, 17, 27, 46, 47, 51
bowel obstruction   244, 247, 249, 253, 256, 261, 262, 264, 265, 267, 269, 271, 272
Buchwald meta-analysis   337

cardiac output (CO)   26, 29–31
cholelithiasis   177
cholesterol   327, 330, 334–337
chronic concentric pouch dilatation   233
closed-loop obstruction   253
closing capacity (CC)   24, 25
clot   253, 255, 256
co-morbidity   2, 4, 5, 7, 9, 207, 213, 214, 327–329, 343, 346, 348
   metabolic   361

complications   125–130, 133, 136, 138, 140–142, 144, 146, 151, 152, 155, 160, 171, 179, 186, 202–205, 208–210, 215, 217, 223, 224, 226, 228, 230, 232, 238, 239, 241, 242, 244–247, 255–257, 262, 272, 273
   balloon   241
   band   238
   major   82, 84
   minor   82
computed tomography (CT)   223, 224, 226, 228, 229, 238, 240, 245, 247, 248, 251, 252, 255, 256, 259, 261–263, 265–274
congestive heart failure (CHF)   18, 20, 28
connecting tube   225, 227, 229, 242–244
continuous positive airway pressure (CPAP)   26, 51, 331–334

death   247, 252, 273
deficiencies   180
delayed gastric emptying   66, 69
depression   345
diabetes   157, 158, 173, 185, 187, 188
   type 2   336–343, 361–366, 378
'diet of thoughts'   300, 301, 308, 315, 321
discomfort   66
distribution volume (Vd)   31–36
duodenum   245, 253, 256, 270
dyslipidemia   334–336, 368–370
dysmotility   232
dysphagia   226, 233, 237, 264

eccentric pouch dilatation 233–236, 240
end tidal CO$_2$ (ETCO$_2$) 49
endobarrier 286
endoscopy 237, 239, 252, 255–257, 259, 264
Epworth sleepiness scale (ESS) 332, 333
evidenced based practice 320
exertional dyspnoea 371, 372
expiratory volume reserve (EVR) 24
extravasation 238, 250, 259

fibreoptic bronchoscope (FOB) 42, 45
fistula 247, 249, 250, 257–259, 261
fluid collection 228, 229, 240, 247, 252, 267, 273
fluoroscopic guidance 228, 230
food 224, 232, 234, 235, 237, 240, 245, 246, 258, 265
    intolerance 232, 234, 235, 240
forced expiratory volume in one second (FEV1) 24
forced vital capacity (FVC) 24
foregut 339
fractional inspired oxygen concentration (FiO$_2$) 33, 46, 48
free fatty acids (FFA) 31
fully stapled laparoscopic Roux-en-Y gastric bypass (FS-LRYGB) 164, 165
functional residual capacity (FRC) 24, 25

Garren-Edwards Gastric Bubble (GEGB) 62, 63
gastric
    dilation 69
    obstruction 82–84, 236, 237, 240
    perforation 83, 84, 238
    pouch 156, 157, 161–163, 165–168, 173, 174, 177, 181, 184, 224, 234, 245, 248–251, 254, 255, 258, 261, 262, 265, 269
    remnant 249, 252, 253, 259–261
gastrogastric fistula 247, 249, 257–259, 261
gastrografin 249, 251, 254, 255, 259, 260
gastrointestinal bleed 250
gastrojejunostomy 246–249, 251, 253–260, 262–265, 270
gastro-oesophageal reflux 230, 232–234
gastro-oesophageal reflux disease (GORD) 327, 329, 343, 344
ghrelin 157, 159, 332
glucagon-like peptide 1 (GLP-1) 157–159, 338, 339
glucose 330, 338–340, 342, 343
guidelines 4, 6

haematemesis 238, 239, 256, 272
haemorrhage 228, 238, 255–257
HbA1c 337, 342
HDL cholesterol 369–371

health related quality of life
  (HRQoL) 347, 360, 377, 383
heart rate (HR) 28, 41
Helicobacter pylori 257
hernia
  hiatal 232, 250, 265, 266
  internal 163, 164, 178, 179,
    267, 271, 272
  Petersen 267, 271
  port-site 273
herniation 223, 228, 230, 235–237,
  240, 242, 261, 267–272
  eccentric balloon 242
  gastric 228, 235–237, 240
  internal 261, 267–269, 271,
    272
high-density lipoprotein (HDL) 18,
  21, 334–337
hindgut 339
hypercholesterolemia 327, 335,
  368, 369
hypertension (IPT) 18, 21, 22,
  27–30, 49, 51, 327–330, 345, 360,
  367, 368
hypertriglyceridaemia 334, 335,
  369, 370

ideal body weight (IBW) 16, 33,
  35, 36, 47, 48, 50
imaging 223, 224, 226, 228, 242,
  251, 256, 261, 262, 264, 265, 268,
  272, 273, 275
indications 1, 5, 6, 8
infarction 223, 273
infection 223, 230, 239, 242, 244,
  250, 257

insulin 328, 337–340, 342, 346
  resistance 328, 338, 339, 346
  sensitivity 338, 339
intensive care unit (ICU) 49
interventional radiology 224
intragastric balloon 61–66, 68, 73,
  74, 76, 78, 79, 82, 85, 86
intraperitoneal leak 239
intravenous contrast 240, 248, 251,
  265, 268–270, 274
intussusception 261, 262, 272–274
investigation 244, 247, 255–257,
  259, 262, 264, 273
iron 181, 182

Jackson-Pratt drain 251, 255
jejunojejunal
  anastomosis 249, 252, 253,
    259, 262, 266, 267, 271, 272
  obstruction 253

laparoscopic 223–225, 229, 245,
  253, 262, 267, 273
  gastric banding 229
laparoscopic adjustable gastric
  banding (LAGB) 223, 224, 226,
  230, 232, 244
laparoscopy 91, 93, 126, 127, 129,
  134, 138, 144, 147
laparotomy 238, 252, 272, 273
LAP-BAND® 105, 108–110, 112,
  117, 120–122
L-cell 338
leak 171, 173–175, 226, 229, 238,
  239, 241, 242, 244, 247, 249–252,
  255, 259, 260, 273

lean body weight (LBW) 32, 33, 35
left ventricular end diastolic pressure (LVEDP) 27
left ventricular stroke work (LVSW) 49
leptin 332, 339, 340
life expectancy 359–361, 378
lipoprotein 334, 335, 337
long-term result 105, 110
low back pain 345
low-density lipoprotein (LDL) 334, 336, 337
lower oesophageal sphincter (LES) 343

marginal ulcer 176, 177, 256–258
mechanism of action 210
Medical Outcome Study Short Form-36 (MOS SF-36) 347
mental health evaluation/interview 311
metabolic syndrome 328, 330, 344
methylene blue 65, 68, 69
morbidity 164, 171
mortality 164, 171–174, 187, 188, 245, 247
multidisciplinary/interdisciplinary team 296, 300, 303
multiple treatment 71, 81, 82, 86
musculoskeletal 327, 344, 345
mushroom sign 263, 271

natural orifice transluminal endoscopic surgery (NOTES) 199, 214–217

negative self fulfilling prophecy 300
nitrous oxide (N_2O) 24, 36
non-alcoholic steatohepatitis (NASH) 345
non-invasive blood pressure (NIBP) 38
nuclear scintigraphy 224

obesity 1–7
    morbid 105, 110, 120, 285, 359–361, 364, 371, 374, 378, 383
obstruction 223, 226, 228, 230, 236–240, 244, 246, 247, 249, 251–256, 261–267, 269–272, 274
obstructive sleep apnoea (OSA) 18, 20, 22–24, 30, 41, 52, 327, 331–334
obstructive sleep apnoea syndrome (OSAS) 41
obstructive sleep hypopnoea (OSH) 18, 22, 23
oedema 228, 237, 252–254
oesophageal dilatation 232–234
oesophago–gastro–duodenoscopy 68–70
oesophagus 229, 232, 233, 235, 245, 249, 254, 262–265, 269, 271
oral contrast 248, 250, 252, 259, 261, 263, 266
orotracheal intubation (OTI) 40–44, 47

pain 232, 233, 236, 249, 250, 252, 257, 262, 264, 268, 272

partial pressure of carbon dioxide in arterial blood (PaCO$_2$)   23, 49
partial pressure of oxygen in arterial blood (PaO$_2$)   23, 25, 26, 43, 53
peptide YY (PYY)   157–159, 339
perforation   223, 228, 229, 238, 249, 257, 262, 271–273
peripheral nerve stimulator (PNS)   46
peritonitis   247, 250, 252, 268
physiology   156
pinch sign   268, 271
plasminogen activator inhibitor (PAI-I)   21, 22
pleural effusion   249, 250
political change agent   321
polycystic ovary syndrome (PCOS)   327, 346
polysomnography   332, 333
port   224–228, 230, 231, 239, 241–245, 273
   access   224, 228, 245
   complications   242, 244
   infection   239, 244
   injection   241, 243
POSE (Primary Obesity Surgery Endoluminal)   86, 286
positive end expiratory pressure (PEEP)   26, 48, 49
post surgical support   314
posterior slippage   240,
postoperative   226–228, 230, 237, 238, 247, 249, 251–253, 256, 258, 262, 264, 267, 272, 273

pouch   224–226, 228, 230, 232–236, 238, 240, 242, 245, 246, 248–251, 253–255, 257–266, 269–271, 273
   dilatation   230, 232–236, 240, 242, 262
predictive factor   75, 76
prejudice and discrimination   299
preoperative   232
   strategy   76
pressure end tidal CO$_2$ (PetCO$_2$)   49
prosthesis   230, 245
proton pump inhibitor   69, 82
pseudoachalasia   232
pseudotumor cerebri (PTC)   345, 346
psychological informed consent   312
psychological intolerance   85
pulmonary embolism   223, 230, 247, 250

quality of life (QoL)   327, 329, 346–348

radiological investigation   247, 257, 264
reflux   230, 232–234, 250, 252, 257, 259, 266
rennin   328
residual volume (RV)   24
respiratory rate (RR)   28
restrictive respiratory impairment   372
role of psychology   293, 295

Index

Roux limb 245, 246, 248, 249, 253–255, 257, 258, 260, 262–264, 266, 267, 269, 270, 273, 274
Roux-en-Y anastomosis 246, 274
Roux-en-Y gastric bypass (RYGB) 155–165, 171, 173, 174, 176, 178, 179, 181–188, 223, 232, 245, 247, 253, 261, 262, 266, 267, 272, 273, 327–329, 332, 333, 335, 337–341, 344–347

satiety 224, 232
saturation of arterial haemoglobin with oxygen (SaO_2) 23, 43, 48, 51
scintigraphy 224, 230, 242
sepsis 247, 252, 273
sequential treatment 76, 78, 85, 285, 290, 292
silicone band 224, 226, 230, 236, 238
single incision laparoscopic surgery (SILS) 199, 216, 217
sleep apnoea syndrome 374
sleeve gastrectomy 199–201, 204, 207, 213
slip 234, 236, 240
slippage 225, 228, 234–237, 240
small bowel 244, 245–247, 249, 251, 253, 261–272, 274
    obstruction 244, 247, 249, 253, 261, 262, 265, 267, 269, 271, 272
sphincter 232
standard of care 2, 8, 9

staple line 245, 247–249, 253, 256–261
    dehiscence 249, 253, 258–261
stapler 156, 162, 165, 166, 168–170, 176
stenosis 176, 233, 252
stoma 224–228, 232–235, 237, 242
stomach 224, 225, 227, 230, 233–236, 239, 240, 245, 253, 255, 256, 271
stomal
    adjustment 226, 228
    stenosis 233
    ulceration 247, 256, 258, 265
stricture 247, 261, 262, 264–266
stump 246, 248, 249
succinylcholine (SCH) 32, 35, 44, 47
sulphonylurea 337
super-obese patient 61, 68, 78–80, 85, 86
suprabursal 225
surgery 1–10
Swedish Obese Subjects study (SOS) 328, 335, 346
swirl sign 269, 271

Tc99-colloid 242
technique 94–97, 102, 199, 201, 214, 217
    operative 155, 164
total body weight (TBW) 35, 37
total lung capacity (TLC) 24, 25
'transfer of addiction' concept 312
transition point 262, 264

transmesenteric 267, 268, 271
transmesocolic 267, 271
triglyceride 330, 335–337

UK prospective diabetes study 337
ulcer 246, 256–258
ultrasonography 224
upper gastrointestinal series (UGI) 223, 224, 226, 228, 233, 234, 236–241, 245, 247–250, 252–262, 264, 266–269, 273

ventilation/perfusion ratio (V/Q) 24, 25
vertical banded gastroplasty (VBG) 344, 345
very low density lipoprotein (VLDL) 20

vitamin B12 160, 181
volvulus 236, 238, 240
vomiting 233, 234, 236, 240, 257, 262, 264, 268, 272

weight 223, 224, 226, 228, 230, 231, 233, 234, 239–241, 245, 246, 259, 267
   gain 239, 241
weight loss 2, 5–10, 202, 203, 206–208, 210, 212, 213, 223, 224, 226, 228, 231, 233, 234, 239, 240, 245–247
   excess 183, 184
   long-term 75
   preoperative 62, 79
work of breathing (WOB) 25
wound 230, 250
   infection 230, 250